COPING WITH BLAST-RELATED TRAUMATIC BRAIN INJURY IN RETURNING TROOPS

NATO Science for Peace and Security Series

This Series presents the results of scientific meetings supported under the NATO Programme: Science for Peace and Security (SPS).

The NATO SPS Programme supports meetings in the following Key Priority areas: (1) Defence Against Terrorism; (2) Countering other Threats to Security and (3) NATO, Partner and Mediterranean Dialogue Country Priorities. The types of meeting supported are generally "Advanced Study Institutes" and "Advanced Research Workshops". The NATO SPS Series collects together the results of these meetings. The meetings are co-organized by scientists from NATO countries and scientists from NATO's "Partner" or "Mediterranean Dialogue" countries. The observations and recommendations made at the meetings, as well as the contents of the volumes in the Series, reflect those of participants and contributors only; they should not necessarily be regarded as reflecting NATO views or policy.

Advanced Study Institutes (ASI) are high-level tutorial courses to convey the latest developments in a subject to an advanced-level audience.

Advanced Research Workshops (ARW) are expert meetings where an intense but informal exchange of views at the frontiers of a subject aims at identifying directions for future action.

Following a transformation of the programme in 2006 the Series has been re-named and re-organised. Recent volumes on topics not related to security, which result from meetings supported under the programme earlier, may be found in the NATO Science Series.

The Series is published by IOS Press, Amsterdam, and Springer Science and Business Media, Dordrecht, in conjunction with the NATO Emerging Security Challenges Division.

Sub-Series

A.	Chemistry and Biology	Springer Science and Business Media
B.	Physics and Biophysics	Springer Science and Business Media
C.	Environmental Security	Springer Science and Business Media
D.	Information and Communication Security	IOS Press
E.	Human and Societal Dynamics	IOS Press

http://www.nato.int/science
http://www.springer.com
http://www.iospress.nl

Sub-Series E: Human and Societal Dynamics – Vol. 86
ISSN 1874-6276 (print)
ISSN 1879-8268 (online)

Coping with Blast-Related Traumatic Brain Injury in Returning Troops

Wounds of War III

Edited by

Brenda K. Wiederhold, Ph.D., MBA, BCIA

Interactive Media Institute, San Diego, CA, USA
Virtual Reality Medical Institute, Brussels, Belgium

Amsterdam • Berlin • Tokyo • Washington, DC
Published in cooperation with NATO Emerging Security Challenges Division

Proceedings of the NATO Advanced Research Workshop on Wounds of War III: Coping with Blast-Related Traumatic Brain Injury in Returning Troops
Vienna, Austria
20-22 February 2011

ISBN 978-1-60750-796-3 (print)
ISBN 978-1-60750-797-0 (online)
Library of Congress Control Number: 2011933274

Publisher
IOS Press BV
Nieuwe Hemweg 6B
1013 BG Amsterdam
Netherlands
fax: +31 20 687 0019
e-mail: order@iospress.nl

Distributor in the USA and Canada
IOS Press, Inc.
4502 Rachael Manor Drive
Fairfax, VA 22032
USA
fax: +1 703 323 3668
e-mail: iosbooks@iospress.com

Foreword

"Wounds of War III: Coping with Blast-related Traumatic Brain Injury in Returning Troops"

On behalf of the Austrian Peacekeepers and the Austrian Ministry of Defense, I want to welcome each of you and extend a special welcome to our distinguished guests who we look forward to hearing from today.

Austria first engaged in peacekeeping operations in the Congo in 1960. In the last 50 years more than 90,000 Austrian soldiers have taken part in peacekeeping operations, amongst them also a large portion of reserve soldiers. In 1995 a veteran organisation of military and civilian peacekeepers was founded. As President of this association I have been involved with the problems of traumatic injuries quite recently. The Austrian Peacekeepers organize the Blue Helmet Forum Austria every year. In 2010 the topic of the Forum was "Stress Management and Peacesoldiering." On this occasion I had the pleasure to meet some of you. I must say I was extremely impressed by the high professional standard of the presentations and the lively discussions. I admit that as an ordinary soldier I sometimes felt that I had difficulties following the subject matter, but I realized the enormous importance of your expertise for the operational effectiveness of our troops and for the personal wellbeing of our soldiers.

By coincidence, the NATO sponsored Advanced Research Workshop held in Austria last year dealt also with Posttraumatic Stress Disorder. This time you will be discussing the effects of Traumatic Brain Injury and ongoing efforts to address the devastating impact of these injuries. Thanks to the sponsors of the workshop and to organizers Professor Brenda Wiederhold and Professor Walter Mauritz it has been possible to gather again a group of distinguished experts.

I believe these workshops are important because it is imperative that we continue to work together towards better and more effective strategies to both prevent and treat Traumatic Brain Injury. In the kind of asymmetric warfare we now have to face we must recognize the fact that Traumatic Brain Injuries will be a growing reality.

Dr. Norman Vincent Peale, an American minister and forefather of the power of positive thinking, once said, "When every physical and mental resource is focused, one's power to solve a problem multiplies tremendously." I could not agree more with Dr. Peale and I also believe that working collaboratively, we can share insights, accelerate discoveries, and more effectively prevent and treat Traumatic Brain Injuries. We have incredible resources here with us over the next three days, and I encourage each of you to recognize the potential outcomes of your interactions, lectures, and discussions. Your ideas, intelligence, commitment and devotion to solving these complex problems may directly save lives of our military service men and women and will help to offer hope for their families and friends.

I am sure we can discover the right answers and our efforts should be, and I believe will be, focused on finding them…together.

Today, blast injuries are the most common injury treated in the Iraq and Afghanistan theaters. In 2006, almost 22% of all injuries treated were Traumatic Brain

Injuries. At the time, that number was an estimate and many injuries from blasts were not categorized as Traumatic Brain Injuries but instead considered mere headaches, mood disorders or other "head and neck wounds." What is clear today is that these numbers were vastly underestimated. Why?

We know now there was a lack of ability to promptly and accurately diagnose such injuries. If someone is missing a limb, we know immediately it is serious and the treatment that must be followed is known. A brain injury is not as apparent. We have seen many cases in which a team of soldiers riding in a Humvee encounters a roadside bomb. These soldiers, after being slammed against the heavy armor of the vehicle, appear mostly unscathed and seemingly capable of returning to duty.

We know now that many of these soldiers who lack any outward sign may very well have suffered a Traumatic Brain Injury. It is likely that tens of thousands of our combat men and women are misdiagnosed, ignored, or dismissed completely.

We need, therefore, to pay more attention to education. Not long ago leaders in the field did not know of the effects of Traumatic Brain Injury and were wholly ill equipped to make such judgments. They did not know what to look for, how to detect Traumatic Brain Injury and most importantly, how to prevent and treat it. But times are changing and through education and vigilance, field commanders, doctors, and other staff can no longer ignore the effects of such injuries. These are injuries that MUST not go undiagnosed. We owe that to these brave men and women who put their lives on the line each and every day.

We must also address the fact that there is a stigma associated with brain injuries. Our military officials and policy writers cannot remain skeptical about the effects of Traumatic Brain Injury and how it endangers the members of our military families. We must insist that facts, on-going research, and the input of these injured personnel continue to show that Traumatic Brain Injury is real, dangerous, and a reality that must be understood and addressed.

The challenges are great. Properly diagnosing and treating these injuries in light of doubtful leadership may be the least of our worries. A recent study showed that even some military tests are failing to diagnose 40% of concussions. And we know that mild Traumatic Brain Injuries are harder to detect due to the damage and breakdown that can occur at the cellular levels, blocking important chemical processes.

We also know that even when there is a correct diagnosis, the documentation of the injuries might not even reach the soldier's permanent medical record. Often this is not the fault of the physicians in the field, but due to other circumstances. Regardless of how or why, it is clear that without that information on file, appropriate treatment will not be provided.

Today, it is estimated that 59% of all blast injuries involve Traumatic Brain Injuries. Reflect on that number…59% is nearly six out of ten. These figures are daunting but there is hope. More and more combat and medical personnel are recognizing that once a blast occurs, Traumatic Brain Injury is something that must be properly assessed and that it is something that requires immediate attention. While we still have far to go in regards to policies surrounding Traumatic Brain Injury, great strides have been made. The ability to immediately diagnose these injuries in the field and promptly evacuate the injured to proper treatment facilities has resulted in survival rates of almost 96%.

The good news is that those who have suffered from a mild Traumatic Brain Injury usually enjoy total recovery after a year. Again, the key is that we MUST not fail to diagnose. If we do fail, these injuries will likely become severe and will alter the lives of the wounded soldiers. Those injuries that are more severe can lead to depression and Posttraumatic Stress Disorder. Those injuries follow soldiers back from the field to their homes and families and have far reaching consequences as they are linked to future medical and socioeconomic realities.

The benefits from your work today will save and improve lives. I am convinced of that, and your work extends beyond the battlefield and finds application in other fields of battle, including sports. Only two weeks ago Austrians watched live on television the skiing race in Kitzbühel, the so called Streif downhill, where an Austrian downhill racer encountered a severe Traumatic Brain Injury after he did not land the famous Mausefalle jump and bumped his head heavily on the ground. While Traumatic Brain Injury is one of the signature wounds from the current conflicts in Iraq and Afghanistan, it is also a wound that affects thousands around the world in civilian life.

As many of you may know, I am a retired General with the Austrian Military and I have been commanding international operations in four different peacekeeping missions for more than 13 years. I have seen firsthand how Posttraumatic Stress and Traumatic Brain Injuries can affect our troops. When I was a young officer I do not remember anybody talking about Posttraumatic Stress or Traumatic Brain Injuries. We simply did not know. Now we know, but our challenges are still immense.

To speak with Dr. Peale, it is imperative that we remain focused on what we are about here – finding means, methods, protocols, ideas, and applications that will address the needs that face our brave war fighters who confront Traumatic Brain Injury.

Over the next three days you will work together to ensure these brave men and women have the best quality of life available to them. I wish you a productive meeting and a great stay in our beautiful city of Vienna.

Thank you,

General Günther Greindl (ret)
President, Austrian Peacekeepers

Preface

This Advanced Research Workshop (ARW), "Wounds of War III: Coping with Blast-related Traumatic Brain Injury in Returning Troops," was convened to discuss the topic of increased Traumatic Brain Injury (TBI) in service men and women around the world. Research has shown that those who have served in both combat missions and peacekeeping operations are at an increased risk for TBI. Research suggests that this may result from their "wounds of war." Some wounds may be more "invisible," such as suicide, depression, stress and chronic pain, while others are more visibly apparent, such as physical disabilities.

During this workshop, we discussed many aspects of military TBI and how to more effectively deal with this issue. Specifically, some of the questions addressed were:

1. Characterization of TBI: Which characteristics make up and help to classify TBI?
2. Diagnostic and Assessment Issues surrounding TBI: Which methods are used to diagnose and assess TBI?
3. Treatment of TBI: What are the latest treatment and therapy opportunities for soldiers after they have been diagnosed with TBI?
4. Quality of Life: How are the lives of TBI patients affected and in what ways can their quality of life be increased?

Through this workshop, we have come closer to understanding what programs are already in place in various countries for detection, assessment, prevention, and treatment. We have begun to learn from these existing plans and can start to formulate a more common set of best practices and guidelines which can be implemented throughout organizations in all our countries with the common goal to always seek to serve our service members more effectively.

This ARW has given participants an opportunity to foster essential international collaborative research on military TBI, a common and disabling consequence of war, terrorism, and natural disasters. As a result, it represents an important landmark in efforts to help soldiers and civilians of NATO and partner nations become more resilient in the face of international conflict.

This publication, which contains full papers focused on the key presentations during the workshop, acts as the permanent record of this event; a tangible documentation of the ideas that formed the basis of discussion and collaboration at the workshop. This text is organized to mirror the program from the event so as to provide an overview of the ideas of presenters and participants in the ARW.

Financial support for the workshop was provided by several sponsors. We would like to acknowledge the generous contributions of the NATO Science for Peace and Security Programme, the Croatian Ministry of Health and Social Welfare, the Austrian

Worker's Compensation Board, the United States Army Medical Research and Materiel Command, the Virtual Reality Medical Center, the Austrian Ministry of Defence (MOD), and the International Neurotrauma Research Organization.

The workshop was organized and this accompanying publication was compiled and edited jointly by the Interactive Media Institute, San Diego, California, USA and Virtual Reality Medical Institute, Brussels, Belgium. Professor Dr. Brenda K. Wiederhold and Professor Dr. Walter Mauritz, program co-organizers, conceived the overall design of the workshop and recruited co-chairs Professor Dr. Kresimir Cosic of the University of Zagreb in Zagreb, Croatia, Colonel Carl Castro of the United States Army Medical Research and Materiel Command, and Professor Dr. Mark D. Wiederhold of the Virtual Reality Medical Center. With the assistance of the co-chairs, Dr. Wiederhold and Dr. Mauritz selected and invited the majority of the speakers and participants, and conference coordinators Ms. Andreea Rimbu and Ms. Emily Butcher organized logistics including registration, travel, lodging and meals, assembling of workshop materials, and other arrangements for the ARW. Dr. Mauritz chose the beautiful Austrian location where the event took place and Ms. Franziska Riedler helped with registration and on-site direction for attendees. Ms. Iris Kai Lu was responsible for the artistic design of all event-related materials and Ms. Emily Butcher and Ms. Kate Bradley reviewed the conference program and full manuscripts, helping with editing and assembly of this and other associated texts.

Editorial

Brenda K. Wiederhold, Ph.D., MBA, BCIA
Interactive Media Institute &
Virtual Reality Medical Institute

Introduction

Thirty-five scientists and representatives from NATO and partner countries met in Vienna, Austria on 20-22 February 2011 for the three-day NATO Advanced Research Workshop titled *"Wounds of War III: Coping with Blast-related Traumatic Brain Injury in Returning Troops."* Formal scientific presentations were delivered by experts from ten different countries who were invited to take part in the workshop.

The workshop was divided into four scientific sessions:

1. Session I: Characterization of Traumatic Brain Injury
2. Session II: Diagnostic and Assessment Issues
3. Session III: Treatment
4. Session IV: Quality of Life

Papers and Presentations

Presenters were invited to submit a full paper for publication in this volume in order to enable those who could not attend the workshop to become educated on the issue of TBI in our troops. Their papers, which are in-depth descriptions of their presentations, are briefly described below.

The first session, "Setting the Stage: Characterization of Traumatic Brain Injury," discusses the characteristics of TBI. The opening paper "Developing a Valid Definition of Mild Traumatic Brain Injury (mTBI)/Concussion" by Colonel Dr. Carl A. Castro and Dr. Dallas Hack compares the definitions of Posttraumatic Stress Disorder (PTSD) and mTBI and discuss a strategic research plan for addressing the lack of definition. They look at five components (event, reaction, unique symptoms, impairment and time course) and discuss their importance in proper clinical diagnosis.

In the following paper, Professor Dr. Stanislaw Ilnicki presents "Mild Traumatic Brain Injury in Veterans of Polish Military Contingents, Psychiatrically Hospitalized with Combat Related Stress Disorders." In this study, they analyzed the treatment records of veterans of Polish Military Contingents (PMC) in order to evaluate the occurrence of mTBI in participants of military operations outside of Poland suffering from combat-related stress disorders. They used a Brief Traumatic Brain Injury Screen (BTBIS), analyzing such parameters as levels of injury, retrograde amnesia, and hospitalization in the Department of Psychiatry. Results of the analysis conducted highlight the importance of mTBI in PTSD diagnostics and therapy that has previously been underestimated in Poland.

The first session concludes with Professor Dr. Kemal Dizdarevic presenting the paper "War Head Injuries in Sieged Sarajevo." This study aimed to analyze head-penetrating injuries in sieged Sarajevo during the first part of the Bosnian War. Professor Dr. Dizdarevic also presents the prevailing operative strategies in the treatment of these patients. Their noninvasive early neurosurgical operative approaches in the forms of intracranial hematoma evacuation and reduced brain debridment without search for deep intracranial foreign bodies resulted in an acceptable treatment outcome during the Bosnian War.

Session two of the workshop, "Diagnostic and Assessment Issues," focuses on concerns related to diagnosis and assessment of TBI. Firstly, Dr. Wayne A. Gordon presents his paper "The Brain Injury Screening Questionnaire: An Approach to Screening for TBI that can be Applied to Soldiers." This study reviews an approach to screening for TBI – the Brain Injury Screening Questionnaire (BISQ) – and reviews the development, validity and research on the BISQ, as well as its potential diverse clinical applications.

Next, Dr. Robin Hurley presents the paper "Windows to the Brain: The Neuropsychiatry of Brain Injury and Common Co-morbidities." This study focuses on the occurrence of TBI in Afghanistan and Iraq, revealing that the vast majority of individuals who experience an mTBI attain recovery, but some have residual symptoms. These residual symptoms can affect the ability of Veterans to adjust to life after combat, and can lead to substance abuse, depression, PTSD and chronic pain.

Lastly, Dr. James L. Spira presents his paper "Predictors of Persistent Postconcussive Syndrome." In this paper, Dr. Spira discusses controversies and opinions surrounding the many facets of concussion and postconcussive syndrome, and states that there are record levels of postconcussive symptoms being reported. The studies presented in this paper suggest that more research is required before determining that screenings and treatments for concussion should discontinue.

In session three, "Treatment," presenters discuss different systems of treatment for TBI. Dr. Joshua Cantor presents the opening paper "Short-term Intensive Cognitive Rehabilitation in OIF/OEF Veterans Applying the STEP Model." This study suggests that executive dysfunction after TBI represents one of the most significant barriers to recovery, community reintegration and return to duty in military personnel. The presentation describes two theoretically and empirically-based intensive group cognitive rehabilitation interventions that combine attention, emotion regulation and problem solving training. Findings from these two intervention strategies are also presented.

Following Dr. Cantor's paper, Professor Dr. Micaiej Zbyszewski presents "Traumatic Stress and Injury of the Brain – the Dangerous Liaisons: Case Study." This presentation focuses on the case of a soldier evacuated from Iraq due to traumatic stress symptoms and somatic syndromes following exposure to a rocket explosion. The case presented shows that there might be co-morbidity of PTSD symptoms and mTBI, along with the disorder of some of the sensory receptors.

Next, Dr. Yusuf Izci presents the paper "Traumatic Brain Injury due to Landmine Explosions." This study analyzes 20 patients who sustained a head injury due to a landmine explosion in a Department of Neurosurgery between 2000-2010. The paper states that landmines occasionally cause TBI and that surgical intervention is seldom required. Survival is likely unless the patient is in a deep coma, in which case multidisciplinary approaches are required for treatment.

Following, Professor Dr. Nela Pivac presents the paper "Molecular Mechanisms in Traumatic Brain Injury," which focuses on the physical, cognitive, psychological, psychosocial and functional impairments imposed by TBI. Professor Dr. Pivac analyzes the various biological responses that occur in patients with TBI.

Next, Dr. Zeev Meiner presents the paper "Cognitive and Functional Outcomes of Terror Victims Who Suffered from Traumatic Brain Injury in Jerusalem." The purpose of this study was to record the effects of 17 cases of TBI generated from terrorist attacks in Jerusalem from September 2000-2004. As a control, 39 non-terror TBI patients who had been treated in the same department during the same period were evaluated. The results indicated that TBI terror victims had more severe injuries, but were still able to gain back most of their ADL functions, and their rehabilitation outcomes were similar to non-terror TBI patients.

Commander Dr. Jack Tsao then presents "U.S. Navy Program for Post-deployment Traumatic Brain Injury and Blast Exposure Screening." This paper discusses the use of surveys after deployment to ask questions about TBI events. Retrospective self-report surveys were used to evaluate blast exposure and related neurological symptoms associated with mTBI. These self-reports were given to U.S. Navy Sailors assigned to two weapons intelligence companies that were frequently exposed to vehicle-born and other types of improvised explosive devices as a part of their daily duties during a seven-month tour in Iraq.

Subsequently, Dr. Christoph Guger presents "Brain-computer Interface: Generic Control Interface for Social Interaction Applications." In this paper, Dr. Guger discusses the use of brain-computer interfaces (BCI) as a communication tool for those with disorders that inhibit their ability to interact with their environment. BCI can allow an individual to control a computer or specially prepared electronic device and stay in contact with friends through games and social networks. This paper presents a generic UDP, XML-based BCI command interface and its application to implement control interfaces enabling social interactions like spelling, virtual interaction in Second Life, operating Twitter and controlling a virtual smart home.

Next, William Elkins presents the paper "TBI Battlefield and Intensive Care Rapid and Selective Cerebral Hypothermia Using an Integrated Head-Neck Stabilization and Cooling Helmet System." This paper discusses the importance of ultra-early delivery of selective cerebral hypothermia by EMS personnel in the field in order to maximize the amount of neuroprotection. An integrated head-neck cooling and stabilization liner has been developed using NASA spin-off technology in order to address this issue. This program is designed to examine the effectiveness in improving the outcome of TBI-injured military personnel by creating moderate brain and mild body core hypothermia.

Professor Dr. Dragica Kozaric-Kovacic then presents "Biofeedback/neurofeedback Treatment of Psychiatric Disturbances Following Traumatic Brain Injury: Case Reports." The authors address the fact that psychiatric sequelae are increased for all types of TBI. Preliminary research on biofeedback/neurofeedback is encouraging for the treatment of different symptoms stemming from TBI such as anxiety, depression, cognitive difficulties (memory, concentration, attention), impulsiveness and sleep disorders.

Lastly, Colonel Dr. Eric Vermetten presents the paper "Longitudinal Effect of Blast Exposure in Dutch Soldiers: Preliminary Results." Recently, there has been an increase in interest in the prevalence of TBI due to exposure to blasts in combat. Exposure to blast/IED incidents in Iraq and Afghanistan is so frequent that TBI has been called the "signature injury" of these conflicts. Despite the increased academic interest, there are still important gaps in knowledge about the epidemiology, diagnosis, pathogenesis, and the relationship with co-morbid problems such as PTSD and depression. The purpose of this study is to design and implement a protocol for the assessment, differential diagnosis and long-term follow-up of soldiers that are exposed to IED blasts.

In session four, "Quality of Life," speakers present their research on the quality of life outcomes of TBI patients. The first paper, presented by Professor Dr. Rael Lange, is titled "12-Month Outcome from Mild Traumatic Brain Injury in Military Service Members." This study examined the 12-month outcome following polytrauma and mTBI in service members injured and medically evacuated during Operations Iraqi Freedom and Enduring Freedom. The research follows the recovery process of service members at the Walter Reed Army Medical Center, but there is still very limited longitudinal data on outcome from mTBI in service members injured in and evacuated from combat.

Following, Dr. Nikolaus Steinhoff presents "Loneliness and Emptiness after TBI: Mechanism, Access and Solutions to This Underestimated Condition and to All Underlying Problems after Traumatic Brain Injury." The paper discusses the issue of TBI patients overcoming the sudden change of emotions and acceptance of new situations with memories in the body corresponding to the time before the incident. This study concludes that caregivers and case managers are often not skilled enough to deal with emptiness, reorientation, the mourning process and the issue of responsibilities when TBI patients have a duty to national or international interests.

Working Group Sessions

In addition to the presentations, the workshop provided ample opportunities for informal discussions and brainstorming. As part of the meeting, four specialized working groups convened on the third day to allow participants to further examine the research presented during the sessions. Working group leaders presented summaries of their discussions to the conference on the final day and time was provided for open discussion.

The first work group, focusing on Characterization of TBI, was moderated by Dr. Wayne Gordon and Professor Dr. Nela Pivac. Conclusions reached by the group pointed to the need to assess the long-term trajectory of recovery, as well as injury-related factors, in order to adequately address characterization needs for TBI. Additionally, TBI needs to be better understood as a disease, rather than an injury.

The second work group, led by Dr. Robin Hurley and Professor Dr. Kemal Dizdarević, focused on Diagnostic and Assessment Issues. Recommendations included the need to create a standardized package of clinical examinations for TBI, a patient tracking database, and an efficient way to share best practices, perhaps in the form of a phone application. Through these actions and collecting categorized blast-related information, collecting comprehensive information on the clinical/natural trajectory of the impact of TBI (recording clinical changes over time), and using predeployment clinical information to assess changes in performance as a result of TBI, the findings could be translated to address not only military and academia needs, but also effects on civilian populations, such as the field of sports.

Dr. Joshua Cantor acted as the moderator for the third work group, which addressed Treatment of TBI. The group concluded that due to the heterogeneity of TBI and frequent occurrence of co-morbidities, individualization and specialization of treatment is very important. Additional recommendations included the importance of delivering psychoeduation on TBI and its consequences to practitioners, patients, and their families, removing symptomatic soldiers from operations for 7-10 days, delivering cognitive remediation to soldiers whose symptoms do not resolve, delivering psychotherapy to soldiers with psychiatric disorders secondary to TBI, and maximizing social support of those afflicted by TBI.

Lastly, the fourth work group, led by Dr. Lou French, addressed Quality of Life for TBI sufferers. The group pointed to the benefits or utilizing the Quality of Life after Brain Injury (QOLIBRI), the first TBI disease-specific patient reported outcome tool for clinical trials and individual use. Furthermore, Quality of Life issues in need of further attention and development include the ways in which civilian and military populations are affected differently (also, how the context of wartime differs from times of peace), the differing severity of TBI cases, multiple mechanisms of injury, cultural issues, the problem of disability and resilience.

The sessions encouraged informal debate and discussion in the hopes of creating new ideas and solutions for the problem of TBI in returning troops. In this way, the groups helped to provide a general overview of areas in need of improvement in the field of TBI and directions for future growth.

Summary

The fundamental aim of the ARW was to critically assess the existing knowledge on TBI and identify directions for future actions. Experts who presented their findings indicated that those who have served in both combat missions and peacekeeping operations are at an increased risk for TBI.

Final conclusions reached by participants at the conference indicate that: 1) TBI research must begin to look 5-10 years ahead instead of 3-6 months ahead in regards to training, assessment, diagnosis, and treatment; 2) Countries must work together to pool research on both prevention and treatment strategies for dealing with at-risk active duty and Veteran populations; 3) Additional workshops are required for a more detailed discussion of each "wound of war." Recommended specialized workshop topics were chronic pain, physical disability, substance abuse, and impact on military families and relationships.

Co-Chairs

Professor Brenda K. Wiederhold, PhD, MBA, BCIA
Interactive Media Institute
9565 Waples Street, Suite 200
San Diego, CA 92121
Tel: +1 858 642 0267, Fax: +1 858 642 0285
Virtual Reality Medical Institute
64 Rue de l'Eglise, Bte 3
1150 Brussels, Belgium
Tel: +32 2 770 93 33, Fax: +32 2 762 93 33
E-mail: office@vrphobia.eu

Professor Walter Mauritz, MD, PhD
Trauma Center "Lorenz Boehler"
International Neurotrauma Research Organization
E-mail: walter.mauritz@igeh.org

Professor Kresimir Cosic, PhD
University of Zagreb
Faculty of Electrical Engineering & Computing
Head of the Delegation to the NATO Parliamentary Assembly
E-mail: kcosic@sabor.sabor.hr

Colonel Carl Castro, PhD
United States Army Medical Research and Materiel Command
Tel: +1 301 619 7301
E-mail: Carl.Castro@amedd.army.mil

Professor Mark D. Wiederhold, MD, PhD, FACP
Virtual Reality Medical Center
E-mail: frontoffice@vrphobia.com

Main Lectures/Presentations Given

Session I: Setting the Stage: Characterization of Traumatic Brain Injury

"Defining Mild Traumatic Brain Injury"
Colonel Dr. Carl A. Castro

"Mild Traumatic Brain Injury in Veterans of Polish Military Contingents Psychiatrically Hospitalized with Combat Related Stress Disorders"
Professor Dr. Stanislaw Ilnicki

"War Head Injuries in Sieged Sarajevo"
Professor Dr. Kemal Dizdarević

Session II: Diagnostic and Assessment Issues

"The Brain Injury Screening Questionnaire: An Approach to Screening for TBI that Can be Applied to Soldiers"
Dr. Wayne Gordon

"Neurobiology of Traumatic Brain Injury"
Dr. Robin Hurley

"Predictors of Persistent Postconcussive Syndrome"
Dr. James L. Spira

Session III: Treatment

"Short-Term Intensive Cognitive Rehabilitation in OIF/OEF Veterans Applying the STEP Model"
Dr. Joshua Cantor

"Traumatic Stress and Injury of the Brain – the Dangerous Liaisons: Case Study"
Professor Dr. Maciej Zbyszewski

"Head Injuries Due to Landmines"
Dr. Yusuf Izci

"Molecular Mechanisms in Traumatic Brain Injury"
Professor Dr. Nela Pivac

"Cognitive and Functional Outcomes of Terror Victims Who Suffered from Traumatic Brain Injury in Jerusalem"
Dr. Zeev Meiner

"U.S. Navy Program for Post-deployment Traumatic Brain Injury and Blast Exposure Screening"
Commander Dr. Jack Tsao

"Brain-computer Interface: Generic Control Interface for Social Interaction Applications"
Dr. Christoph Guger

NATO RTG 193 – A Brief Update
Colonel Dr. Eric Vermetten

"Traumatic Brain Injury Battlefield and Intensive Care Rapid and Selective Cerebral Hypothermia Using an Integrated Head-Neck Stabilization and Cooling Helmet System"
Bill Elkins

"Biofeedback/neurofeedback Treatment of Psychiatric Disturbances Following Traumatic Brain Injury: Case Reports"
Professor Dr. Dragica Kozarić-Kovačić

"Using the MACE in Theatre with Follow Up after 3-6 months"
Colonel Dr. Eric Vermetten

Session IV: Quality of Life

"12-Month Outcome from Mild Traumatic Brain Injury in Military Service Members"
Professor Dr. Rael Lange

"Loneliness and Emptiness after Traumatic Brain Injury: Mechanism, Access and Solutions to This Underestimated and to all Problems after Traumatic Brain Injury Underlying Phenomenon"
Dr. Nikolaus Steinhoff

"Psychological Disinhibition in Posttraumatic Stress Disorder With and Without Prior Concussion"
Professor Dr. Mark D. Wiederhold

"Early Management of Patients with Traumatic Brain Injury in Austria"
Professor Dr. Walter Mauritz

Sponsors

Workshop organizers Interactive Media Institute and Virtual Reality Medical Institute would like to thank the sponsors of this Advanced Research Workshop listed below. Without their support, this event could not have taken place.

North Atlantic Treaty Organization (NATO)

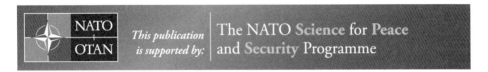

Austrian Ministry of Defence (MOD)

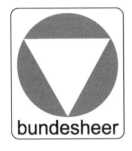

Social Welfare Croatia

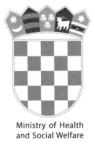

Virtual Reality Medical Center

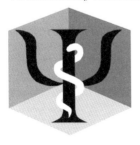

International Neurotrauma Research Organization

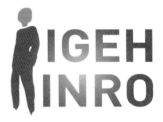

U.S. Army Medical Research and Materiel Command

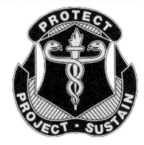

Austrian Worker's Compensation Board

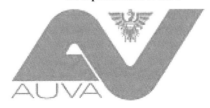

Contents

Section I: Characterization of Traumatic Brain Injury

Section II: Diagnostic and Assessment Issues

Section III: Treatment

Section IV: Quality of Life

Section I

Characterization of Traumatic Brain Injury

Coping with Blast-Related Traumatic Brain Injury in Returning Troops
B.K. Wiederhold (Ed.)
IOS Press, 2011
© 2011 The authors and IOS Press. All rights reserved.
doi: 10.3233/978-1-60750-797-0-3

The Importance of Developing a Valid Definition of Mild Traumatic Brain Injury/Concussion

Carl Andrew CASTRO [a,1], Brenda K. WIEDERHOLD [b,c]

aU.S. Army Medical Research and Materiel Command, Ft. Detrick, Maryland, U.S.A.
bVirtual Reality Medical Center, San Diego, CA, U.S.A.
cVirtual Reality Medical Institute, Brussels, Belgium

Abstract. A valid definition of a symptom-based injury requires five components – an event, a reaction, unique symptoms, impairment, and a time course. In the case of mild traumatic brain injury (mTBI) or concussion, existing clinical definitions lack one or several of these components, thus hindering proper clinical diagnosis and research into the mechanisms, cause and treatment of mTBI/concussion. Recommendations for addressing this lack of definition validation are discussed.

Keywords. Traumatic Brain Injury, concussion, service members, veterans, PTSD, blast, post-concussive syndrome

There is a widely-held perspective that mild traumatic brain injury (mild TBI or mTBI) is part of a medical continuum with moderate and severe TBI. This perspective guides interventions, despite strong evidence that the two conditions are distinct clinically and epidemiologically. It is due to this common conflation that use of the term "concussion" instead of "mild traumatic brain injury" is presently encouraged.

Concussion/mild TBI is an important combat injury. In some patients, concussion can lead to persistent/chronic post-concussive symptoms (PCS), including headache, sleep disturbance, irritability, dizziness, imbalance, fatigue, inattention, and problems with concentration and memory. Multiple concussions may have cumulative effects. There is an increased risk of dementia from concussions involving loss of consciousness (LOC) or highly repetitive blows to the head (e.g., boxing). Immediate intervention is important to facilitate healing; however, clinical recovery from concussion is usually rapid (hours to days).

The case definition of mild TBI—a blow or jolt to the head resulting in brief alteration in consciousness, loss of consciousness (lasting less than 30 minutes, or post-traumatic amnesia)—may be useful at the time of acute injury. Yet the case definition lacks three essential criteria for use months after injury: symptoms, time course, and impairment. A valid definition of a symptom-based injury requires five components— an event, a reaction, unique symptoms, impairment, and a time course. In the case of mild TBI/concussion, existing clinical definitions lack one or several of these components, thus hindering proper clinical diagnosis and research into the

---

[1] Corresponding Author: COL Carl A. Castro. Medical Research and Materiel Command, Ft. Detrick, Maryland, U.S.A. Telephone: 001-301-619-7304; E-mail: carl.castro@us.army.mil.

mechanisms, cause and treatment. The definition of mild TBI does not include symptoms nor an impairment. Thus, a service member who has had a mild TBI doesn't necessarily ever have any symptoms or impairments that need to be treated. A service member only receives a diagnosis for post-concussive syndrome, not for a mild TBI.

Complicating matters, there is an overlap of post-concussion syndrome and posttraumatic stress disorder (PTSD) symptoms. But while the symptomotology of PTSD has been well validated for over a decade, the symptoms for post-concussion syndrome have not. Emerging findings indicate that the definition needs significant revision in terms of the reaction, symptoms, and possibly the time course. Hoge and Castro reported in 2008 [1] that PTSD symptoms accounted for nearly all mild TBI symptoms. These findings were replicated and extended by Schneiderman et al. [2], who found that PTSD was almost three times more strongly associated with PCS than with mild TBI (loss of consciousness). A small independent effect remained for LOC. Marx et al. [3] subsequently reported that only PTSD associated with objective post-deployment neurocognitive deficits (history of LOC had no effect). The evidence in these studies has been minimized in favor of a consensus that mild TBI is on par symptomatically with more serious types of TBI.

Post-deployment screening is based on the assumption that a causal connection has been established between concussion/mild TBI and persistent post-concussive symptoms. To identify those who sustained a concussion/mild TBI during deployment, the post-deployment screening form asks service members and veterans to recall whether they were "dazed" or "confused" at the time of an injury or blast "experience." Positive responses to this single unvalidated question have accounted for two-thirds of all reported cases of concussion/mild TBI. The remaining cases are clinically similar to sports concussions, involving brief LOC (usually lasting seconds to a few minutes) or post-traumatic amnesia.

A 2008 U.K. study [5] further substantiated the need to re-examine generalizations about the effects of "TBI." Fear et al. reported that post-concussional syndrome was associated with blast exposure, but also with other non-specific markers of deployment ("depleted uranium" and "aiding wounded"). Pietrzak, et. al. [6] replicated these findings, concluding that PTSD "mediated" the association of mild TBI with poor general health and functional impairment. LOC had a small independent association with work impairment. Lippa et al. [7] found no difference between blast and non-blast mild TBI/concussion groups in terms of symptom severity or symptom profile and no difference between blast and non-blast mild TBI/concussion groups in terms of distance from blast or number of blast injuries. Similar findings were again replicated by Luethcke et al. (2010) who found no difference between blast and non-blast mild TBI/concussion in terms of concussive symptoms, psychological symptoms or neurocognitive function [8]. A longitudinal study by Polusny the following year concluded that after adjusting for PTSD symptoms, concussion/mild TBI was not associated with post-deployment symptoms or outcomes [9]. Clearly, a separate, validated definition of mild TBI is needed for a comprehensive understanding of its likely effects, or lack thereof.

Table 1. Definitions of mTBI, Post-Concussion Syndrome and PTSD.

Disorder/ Syndrome	Characteristics	Component	Characteristics	Disorder/ Syndrome
mTBI (PDHA/PDHRA 10-20%)	1. History of Head Trauma: –Impact –Blast/Non-Impact	**Event**	1. Life Threatening/Traumatic Experience	
	2. Manifestation: -Dazed/confused lasting up to 24 h -Loss of consciousness (lasting up to 30 min) -Amnesia (up to 1 day) -Normal structural imaging	**Reaction**	2. Manifestation: -Feelings of Lack of Control, Horror, Helplessness	
Post-Concussion Syndrome (3-5%)	3a. **Impaired Cognition** (Attention/Memory)	**Symptoms**	3a. **Intrusive Recollection** (1 or more) Recurrent and intrusive recollections of event; recurrent distressing dreams of event; acting or feeling as if the event is reoccurring; intense psychological distress at exposure to event cues; physiologic reactivity upon exposure to event cues	**PTSD**
	3b. Other Symptoms (3 or more) **Fatigue, sleep disturbance,** headache, dizziness, **irritability, affective disturbance,** personality change, **apathy** Other symptoms: light headedness, blurred vision/tired eyes, ringing in the ears, bad taste in the mouth		3b. Avoidant/Numbing (3 or more) Efforts to avoid thoughts, feelings, or conversations associated with trauma; efforts to avoid activities, places or people associated with trauma; inability to recall an important aspect of the trauma; **markedly diminished interest or participation in significant activities; restricted range of affect;** sense of foreshortened future	
			3c. Hyper-arousal (2 or more) **Difficulty falling asleep; irritability; difficulty concentrating;** hyper-vigilance; exaggerated startle response	
	4. Symptoms that begin or worsen after injury; interference with **social and occupational functioning**	**Impair-ment**	4. Clinically significant distress or impairment in **social, occupational,** or other important areas of functioning	
	5. Symptoms lasting ≥3 months	**Time Course**	5. Acute: symptoms lasting <3 months Chronic: symptoms lasting ≥ 3 months Specify with or without delay onset: > 6 months after stressor	

The goal of post-deployment screening is to identify and treat service members and veterans with persistent post-concussive physical, neurocognitive, and behavioral symptoms. But without symptoms or a time course in the definition, clinicians' attribution of such non-specific symptoms to concussion/mild TBI is subjective. The screening process has led to reports that 40% of service members who have had concussions experience one or more persistent symptoms—much higher than the 3-5% rate expected on the basis of studies in civilians. Service members and veterans with suspected post-concussive symptoms are referred to specialty TBI or polytrauma clinics designed for moderate and severe TBI—contrary to evidence-based best practices centered in primary care that were established after the first Gulf War for the treatment of postwar symptoms. Cognitive or multidisciplinary rehabilitation designed for moderate and severe TBI has not been effective for mild TBI, and the treatment of symptoms such as headaches, irritability, or sleep problems does not vary according to the presence or absence of a history of mild TBI. Health initiatives that assume that mild TBI approximates moderate and severe TBI are thus likely to be causing unintended consequences.

Post-deployment screening is administered within a structure of care encompassing communication, treatment, and disability initiatives—influenced by definitional issues—all of which are likely to promote negative expectations for recovery. Multiple studies have shown that expectations exert a powerful effect on the persistence of symptoms after concussion. Further, the consequences of misattributing symptoms include the side effects of medications and inappropriate treatment, including a failure to address underlying conditions (e.g., depression, PTSD, or substance abuse), the use of unproven rehabilitation procedures, and the prescribing of medications for nonapproved indications (such as an atypical antipsychotic for sleep) [4]. Unproductive and time-consuming tests, including neurocognitive assessments, may reinforce patients' negative perceptions of illness.

The care of veterans who have any war-related injury or health concern is of the highest priority. Management of mild TBI or deployment-related cognitive effects focuses largely on alleviation of symptoms, yet the most compelling efficacy data highlight the importance of education to normalize symptoms and provide expectation of rapid recovery. Devoting increasingly more personnel and time to the illusory demands of mild TBI could hinder service members' and veterans' recovery. Thus, a different public health approach is recommended. This approach should include validated risk-communication approaches, education strategies, and evaluation procedures. The current approach, which lacks definition yet guides policy on mTBI, risks unintended negative impacts on those returning from service.

References

[1]   Hoge, C.W., McGurk, D., Thomas, J.L., Cox, A.L., Engel, C.C., & Castro, C.A. (2008). Mild traumatic brain injury in U.S. soldiers returning from Iraq. *The New England Journal of Medicine 355*(5), 453–463.
[2]   Schneiderman, A.I., Braver, E.R., & Kang, H.K. (2008). Understanding sequelae of injury mechanisms and mild traumatic brain injury incurred during the conflicts in Iraq and Afghanistan: Persistent post-concussive symptoms and posttraumatic stress disorder. *American Journal of Epidemiology 167*, 1446–1452.

[3]   Marx, B.P., Doron-Lamarca, S., Proctor, S.P., & Vasterling, J.J. (2009). The influence of pre-deployment neurocognitive functioning on post-deployment PTSD symptom outcomes among Iraq-deployed Army soldiers. *Journal of the International Neuropsychological Society 15*, 840–852.

[4]   Hoge, C.W., Goldberg, H.M., & Castro, C.A. (2009). Care of war veterans with mild traumatic brain injury—Flawed perspectives. *New England Journal of Medicine 360*(16), 1588–1591.

[5]   Fear, N.T., Jones, E., Groom, M., Greenberg, N., Hull, L., Hodgetts, T.J., & Wessely, S. (2008). Symptoms of post concussional syndrome are non-specifically related to mild traumatic brain injury in U.K. armed forces personnel on return from deployment in Iraq: An analysis of self-reported data. *Psychological Medicine 39*, 1379–1387.

[6]   Piertrzak, R.H., Johnson, D.C., Goldstein, M.B., Malley, J.C., & Southwick, S.M. (2009). Posttraumatic stress disorder mediates the relationship between mild traumatic brain injury and health and psychosocial functioning in veterans of Operations Enduring Freedom and Iraqi Freedom. *Journal of Nervous and Mental Disease 197*(10), 748–753.

[7]   Lippa, S.M., Pastorek, N.J., Benge, J.F., & Thornton, G.M. (2010). Postconcussive symptoms after blast and nonblast-related mild traumatic brain imjuries in Afghanistan and Iraq war veterans. *Journal of the International Neuropsychological Society 16*, 856–866.

[8]   Luethcke, C.A., Bryan, C.J., Morrow, C.E., & Isler, W.C. (2011). Comparison of concussive symptoms, cognitive performance, and psychological symptoms between acute blast versus nonblast-induced mild traumatic brain injury. *Journal of the International Neuropsychological Society 17*(1), 36–45.

[9]   Polusny, M.A., Kehle, S.M., Nelson, N.W., Erbes, C.R., Arbisi, P.A., & Thuras, P. (2011). Longitudinal effects of mild traumatic brain injury and posttraumatic stress disorder comorbidity on postdeployment outcomes in National Guard soldiers deployed to Iraq. *Archives of General Psychiatry 68*(1), 79–89.

Coping with Blast-Related Traumatic Brain Injury in Returning Troops
B.K. Wiederhold (Ed.)
IOS Press, 2011
© 2011 The authors and IOS Press. All rights reserved.
doi: 10.3233/978-1-60750-797-0-8

Mild Traumatic Brain Injury in Veterans of Polish Military Contingents, Psychiatrically Hospitalized with Combat Related Stress Disorders

Stanisław ILNICKI[a,1], Andrzej K. RADZIKOWSKI[a] and
Dorota WOJTŁOWSKA-WIECHETEK[a]
[a]*Department of Psychiatry and Combat Stress of the
Military Medical Institute, Warsaw*

Abstract. In order to evaluate the occurrence of Mild Traumatic Brain Injury (mTBI) in participants of military operations outside of Poland suffering from combat-related stress disorders, treatment records of veterans of Polish Military Contingents (PMC) hospitalized in the Department of Psychiatry and Combat Stress (DP&CS) of the Military Institute of Medicine in Warsaw were reviewed. During the period of 2006-2010, a total of 144 PMC veterans were hospitalized. Firstly, we excluded from this group: those with confirmed examination and observation of evident brain damage; those whose mental condition made it impossible to obtain a credible anamnesis; those who were serving at posts without direct contact with combat operations during deployment, and those who had received a head injury prior to the deployment or after deployment. Basing on the above-presented criteria, 18 patients have been eliminated from further examinations. Medical records of the remaining 126 were analyzed by means of Brief Traumatic Brain Injury Screen (BTBIS). The analysis conducted showed that 53 (42.1%) out of 126 patients evaluated had, at the deployment, one or more injuries caused by an external force directly related to combat operations. Patients with a positive result of BTBIS (mTBI) made up 20 out of 53 (37.7%) injured veterans.

It was stated that mTBI veterans – compared to non-TBI veterans – were diagnosed with Posttraumatic Stress Disorder (PTSD) more often (60% vs 34.9%), with prevailing symptoms of increased arousal (30% vs. 4.7%), disorder was persistent, rehospitalization was necessary, (30.0% vs 4.7%) and usage of selective serotonin reuptake inhibitor (SSRI) (75% vs 56%) mood stabilizers was required (40.0% vs 27.4%).

Keywords. Mild Traumatic Brain Injury, Brief Traumatic Brain Injury Screen, Posttraumatic Stress Disorder, Polish Military Contingents, Iraq, Afghanistan

1. Introduction

In total, 48,180 Polish soldiers participated in international military operations of various types in the period of 2003-2010. The highest number of Polish military contingents (PMC) was deployed to Iraq (15,100 soldiers) and to Afghanistan (12,800 soldiers). Forty-six soldiers have been killed within these missions. Three hundred ninety-

---

[1] Corresponding Author: Stanislaw Ilnicki, Department Psychiatry and Combat Stress, Military Medical Institute, Szaserow Street 128, 04-141 Warszawa, Poland; E-mail: silnicki@wim.mil.pl.

six soldiers were evacuated back to Poland due to medical indications including 141 wounded in combat, 204 due to injuries and diseases experienced beyond the battlefield and 51 with diagnosed Combat and Operation Stress Reaction.

Conversion of these figures into loss per 1,000 participants of the deployments shows that NATO's operations in Afghanistan generate higher mission losses than in Iraq (killed – 1.9 vs. 1.5, wounded in combat – 7.7 vs. 2.8, non-combat casualties and diseases – 9.1 vs. 5.8). Comparing to this number, the ratio of evacuation due to psychiatric indications (0.6 vs. 2.9) is surprisingly low. However, analysis of that phenomenon is beyond the scope of this paper.

The Department of Psychiatry and Combat Stress (DP&CS) of the Military Institute of Medicine is one of five military wards in Poland specialized in the treatment of combat-stress related disorders. Approximately 80% of all veterans suffering from these disorders are being treated in our clinic. Therefore, the data on hospitalized veterans can be considered to be representative of the total population of hospitalized PMC veterans.

During the time when our clinic was established in 2006, treatment was provided to 144 veterans. Twenty-five of them (17.4%) were sent directly from the war operation theatre, 81 (56.2%) were admitted due to their health worsening after return from deployment, 30 (20.8%) were admitted on request of military medical commissions and eight (5.6%) due to other reasons (e.g. on request of the court or military prosecutor office).

The dominating group among those hospitalized in our clinic for the first time consisted of veterans of PMC Iraq, 102 soldiers (70.6%), and PMC Afghanistan, 31 soldiers (21.4%), while the remaining 11 soldiers (8.0%) had served within other missions.

In terms of the structure of our patients the most numerous group were non-commissioned officers, 93 patients (64.6%), while the number of private contractors was 27 patients (18.7%) and the number of both junior officers, 12 patients (8.3%), and senior officers, nine patients (6.2%), was much smaller [1].

2. Materials and Methods

In order to evaluate the occurrence of Mild Traumatic Brain Injury (mTBI) in participants of military operations outside of Poland suffering from combat-related stress disorders, treatment records of PMC veterans hospitalized in the DP&CS of the Military Medical Institute in Warsaw were reviewed.

During the period of 2006-2010, a total of 144 PMC veterans were hospitalized. Firstly, the following patients were excluded from this group: those with confirmed examination and observation of evident brain damage; those whose mental condition made it impossible to obtain a credible anamnesis; those who were serving at posts without direct contact with combat operations during deployment, and those who had received a head injury prior to the deployment or after deployment (having returned to Poland). Basing on the above-presented criteria, 18 patients have been eliminated from further examinations. Medical records of the remaining 126 were analyzed by means of the Brief Traumatic Brain Injury Screen (BTBIS) (Figure 1) [2].

3 Question DVBIC TBI Screening Tool

1. **Did you have any injury(ies) during your deployment from any of the following?**
    (check all that apply):

    A. ☐ Fragment
    B. ☐ Bullet
    C. ☐ Vehicular (any type of vehicle, including airplane)
    D. ☐ Fall
    E. ☐ Blast (Improvised Explosive Device, RPG, Land mine, Grenade, etc.)
    F. ☐ Other specify: _____

2. **Did any injury received while you were deployed result in any of the following?**
    (check all that apply):

    A. ☐ Being dazed, confused or "seeing stars"
    B. ☐ Not remembering the injury
    C. ☐ Losing consciousness (knocked out) for less than a minute
    D. ☐ Losing consciousness for 1-20 minutes
    E. ☐ Losing consciousness for longer than 20 minutes

    > **NOTE:** Endorsement of A-E meets criteria for positive TBI Screen

    F. ☐ Having any symptoms of concussion afterward
        (such as headache, dizziness, irritability, etc.)
    G. ☐ Head Injury

    > **NOTE:** Confirm F and G through clinical interview

    H. ☐ None of the above

3. **Are you currently experiencing any of the following problems that you think might be related to**
    a possible head injury or concussion?
    (check all that apply):

    A. ☐ Headaches   E. ☐ Ringing in the ears
    B. ☐ Dizziness   F. ☐ Irritability
    C. ☐ Memory problems   G. ☐ Sleep problems
    D. ☐ Balance problems   H. ☐ Other specify:_____

Schwab, K. A., Baker, G., Ivins, B., Sluss-Tiller, M., Lux, W., & Warden, D. (2006). The Brief Traumatic Brain Injury Screen (BTBIS):
Investigating the validity of a self-report instrument for detecting traumatic brain injury (TBI) in troops returning from deployment in
Afghanistan and Iraq. Neurology, 66(5)(Supp. 2), A235.

Figure 1. The Brief Traumatic Brain Injury Screen (BTBIS) [1]

We analyzed BTBIS in order to obtain answers to the following questions:

1. Has the patient being evaluated experienced one or more injuries due to causes specified in item 1 (A-F) of the BTPIS Questionnaire?

2. Did the injury experienced during deployment result in loss of consciousness that met the criteria specified in item 2 (A-H) of the above-mentioned questionnaire?

3.Did the symptoms specified the item 3 (A-H) of the BTBIS questionnaire occur in patients for whom affirmative answers to questions 1 and 2 were obtained during their stay in the clinic?

3. Results

The analysis conducted shown that 53 (42.1%) out of 126 patients evaluated had, at the time of deployment, one or more injuries caused by an external force directly related to combat operations. Patients with positive result of BTBIS (mTBI) made up 20 out of 53 (37.7%) injured veterans.

Among patients who met the criteria for mTBI, 12 subjects (60%) sustained an injury without a blast injury and eight (40%) sustained an injury with blast injury. Eleven (55%) suffered a head injury. Taking into account the severity of the injury, 13 (65%) cases were classified as "mild" and seven (35%) as "moderate or severe" according to Helmick criteria [3].

3.1. Neurological Condition of the Evaluated Patients

In a neurological examination 16 out of 20 subjects (80%) patients did not exhibit characteristics of damage to the central and peripheral nervous system and four out of 20 (20%) did have characteristic of damage of the peripheral nervous system.

In neuroimaging studies only two out of 20 (10%) showed in their MRI "small, scattered vascular outbreaks in the frontal lobes."

The EEG was abnormal in one out of 20 (5%). Suspicion of organic brain damage in psychological tests was confirmed in three out of 20 subjects (15%) (Table 1).

Table 1. Results of examination of somatic condition of patients with mTBI. diagnosis (n=20).

Type of deviation from the standard	mTBI	
	n	%
Symptoms of the peripheral nervous system damage	4	20.0
Abnormal EEG record	1	5.0
Small, scattered vascular changes in MRI	2	10.0
Suspicion of an organic brain damage resulting from psychological tests	3	15.0

3.2. Psychiatric Diagnoses of the Evaluated Patients

There were 49 (38.9%) patients with a diagnosis of PTSD in the analyzed group, 28 (22.2%) patients with adjustment disorders and 49 (38.9%) with neurotic disorders and personality disorders. PTSD was diagnosed more often in the mTBI group compared to the non-mTBI (60% vs. 34.9%) (Table 2).

Table 2. Distribution of psychiatric diagnoses in the mTBI and non-mTBI group.

Main diagnosis	mTBI		non-mTBI		Total	
	n	%	n	%	N	%
PTSD (F43.1)	12	**60.0**	37	34.9	49	38.9
Adjustment disorders (F43.2)	4	20.0	24	22.6	28	22.2
Other (F41, F42, F45, F60)	4	20.0	45	42.5	49	38.9
Total	20	100.0	106	100.0	126	100.0

3.3. The Course of mTBI

Compared to non-mTBI, mTBI veterans were significantly and repeatedly (>2) hospitalized more often (30% vs 4.7%). It can be considered an evidence of persistence of occurring posttraumatic disorders (Table 3).

Table 3. Number of hospitalisations of patients with mTBI and non-mTBI.

Number of hospitalisations	mTBI		non-mTBI		Total	
	n	%	n	%	N	%
1	11	55.0	76	71.7	87	69.1
2	3	15.0	25	23.6	28	22.2
>2	6	**30.0**	11	4.7	11	8.7
Total	20	100.0	106	100.0	126	100.0

3.4. Pharmacotherapy of mTBI Patients vs. non-mTBI Patients

Medical treatment was similar among all veterans. Treatment applied consisted of: antidepressants for 12 out of 20 patients (60%), mood stabilizers for five out of 20 patients (25%), anxiolytics and sedative for 14 out of 20 patients (70%). No medical treatment was applied in four out of 20 patients (20%) (Table 4).

Table 4. Groups of medicines applied for patients with mTBI and non-mTBI.

Main diagnosis	mTBI n=20		non-mTBI n=106		Total n=126	
	n	%	n	%	n	%
SSRI, SNRI	15	**75.0**	60	56.6	75	59.5
Mood stabilizers	8	**40.0**	29	27.4	37	29.4
Non-benzodiazepine anxiolytic medicines	10	50.0	63	59.4	73	57.9
No medicines	5	25.0	26	24.5	31	24.6

Due to simultaneous application of a few medicines the sum of percentage points exceeds 100.

3.5. Clinical Picture of PTSD with mTBI and non-mTBI

Using the scale 1-3 as a basis of the rank of the intensity of symptoms belonging to the PTSD clinical picture, that is "B" – persisted re-experiencing, "C" – persistent avoidance and "D" – increased arousal, it was stated that patients with PTSD plus mTBI, compared to non-mTBI patients, had more dominant symptoms from cluster "D", e.g., impulsivity, irritability, aggressive behavior etc. (30% vs 4.7%) (Table 5).

Table 5. Dominating groups of symptoms in patients with PTSD + mTBI and PTSD + non-mTBI .

Main diagnosis	PTSD+ mTBI n=12		PTSD + non-mTBI n=37		Total n=49	
	pkt	%	pkt	%	pkt	%
B. Persistent re-experiencing	40	55.0	159	71.7	199	67.7
C. Persistent avoidance	11	15.0	52	23.6	63	21.4
D. Increased arousal	21	**30.0**	11	4.7	32	10.9

3.6. Clinical Pictures of Veterans with mTBI Diagnosis

We provide descriptions for three cases to illustrate the clinical pictures, the course of disorders and the results of therapy of veterans who, on the basis of the analysis of their medical records, were classified as mTBI, according to BTBIS criteria.

3.6.1. Case 1

Platoon Leader J.R., 33-years old, a rifleman and veteran of PMC Iraq. In April 2004, while on sentry duty, was knocked down by a bus in a terrorist attack. He experienced a crushing trauma of the abdomen and pelvis. The patient reported: *The bus was driving right on me. I was trying to jump to the side but it was driving fast and I was too tired. I felt a blow and heard strange noises. Probably all my bones that could be broken were broken. Somebody gave me morphine but the first ampoule flew out with blood. Only the second dose helped, so I could begin to think logically. I woke up from a coma after three weeks in the U.S. base in Ramstein, Germany. I could hardly find out where I was and I was already being taken to the operating table.* He underwent many surgeries. J.R. was admitted to the Clinic of Psychiatry and Combat Stress four times during 2006-2009. He was diagnosed with a chronically depressed mood, quick temper, moodiness and conflicts with family. The patient was abusing alcohol periodically. No CNS damage was detected by means of neuroimaging examination and psychological tests. J.R. participated in psychotherapeutic sessions and was administered medication including sertraline 100 mg/die and carbamazepine 400 mg/die. Currently, he is a disability pensioner with a certificate of 100% damage to his health. He divorced his wife and then remarried. J. R. went to college. He is an activist in the Association of Wounded and Injured Veterans.

3.6.2. Case 2

Senior Private P.S., 28-years old, a sapper and veteran of PMC Iraq. In June 2004, during mortar shelling of the base, an explosion of UXO picked up by the sappers. Pulled out from under a burning vehicle, he experienced an acoustic injury and burns covering 85% of his body. He reported: *Having been brought back to Poland I was laying unconscious for the first month. I had burns of the first, second and third degree. I do not want to revisit this subject. My fingers were going numb once I left the hospital. My eardrum was ripped and I did not have one ear at all. In the first moment I did not know what happened. When I was asking doctors what had happened to me they were giving me something and I was falling asleep again.* P.S. stayed in the Clinic of Psychiatry and Combat Stress twice in 2006 and 2007. He complained of fear, hypersensitivity to stimuli, nightmarish dreams and irritability. The patient was avoiding conversations and situations recalling events from the deployment. No features of CNS damage were detected by means of neuroimaging examination and psychological tests. He participated in group therapy sessions. P.S. was treated with valproic acid 1500 mg/die, perazine 300 mg/die and lorazepam 2 mg/die. Reduction of the suffering and an improvement in functioning has been achieved. In 2007 the patient retired as a disability pensioner with a certificate on 85% personal injury. He was decorated by the President of the Republic of Poland with the Medal for War Heroism. Having left the armed forces, he was hired by his home military unit as a training equipment warehouseman. Once attaining the health category "fit for military service with limitations," he was allowed to return to active military service and qualified for a training course for non-commissioned officers.

3.6.3. Case 3

Senior Warrant Officer, 45-year old veteran PMC in former Yugoslavia (1995), Syria (1999/2000) and Iraq (2005). In the sixth week of his duty in Iraq, due to a mortar projectile explosion, he suffered an acoustic injury that resulted in hearing loss and ASD symptoms. Because of these symptoms, he was evacuated to Poland. After a short stay in the military hospital in Wroclaw he was transferred to our clinic. During his first stay, symptoms of PTSD, lowered mood and somatic ailments were observed. He took part in individual and group psychotherapy and was treated with mianserin 60 mg/die and carbamazepine 400 mg/die. He was discharged from the hospital, having made a remarkable recovery. He continued with his duty in a previous unit as an audiovisual maintenance technician. He was admitted to the hospital once again because of increasing irritability, suspiciousness, aggressive behavior toward his wife and two suicide attempts. Slight, unspecified changes in a central nervous system were revealed in MRI, EEG and neuropsychological tests. After being discharged from the clinic with the diagnosis of "organic personality disorder," the patient was discharged from the army, divorced and settled in with his mother in another town. Thanks to the help of the Veterans' Association he got a job as a civilian in a military unit in his new place of residence. After few months he quit and went abroad with his new partner. He came back after few months and made an effort to be admitted to the army again. As the army medical advisory board stated the he does not fulfill needed health conditions, he actively fought a change in this decision.

4. Discussion

There are numerous publications on organically conditioned mental and behavioral disorders in soldiers in Polish literature. They refer to disorders caused by mechanic injuries of the central nervous system, vibrations, an influence of electromagnetic fields, toxic substances and, something which might be considered as something of an oddity, perinatal microinjuries [4, 5, 6]. Traditional names for these disorders like "encephalopathy," "characteropathy," and "cerebrasthenia" are slowly being replaced with modern terminology defined in ICD-10 and DSM-IV. A diagnosis of "mild Traumatic Brain Injury" has not become a part of Polish military medical language, however, the essence of this term is taken into account in the diagnostic process, both in therapy and military-medical expertise.

The retrospective analysis of medical documentation of veterans hospitalized with combat-stress related mental disorders, despite methodology objections resulting from the non-uniform nature of the compared data and small number of subjects in the researched group, indicate a need for more systematic research including mTBI symptoms in current clinical analysis [7, 8, 9]. It is especially important for acoustic trauma injuries with psychiatric consequences that have not been noticed by Polish military researchers [10].

In connection with the subject of this conference, it is hard not to recall the discussion that took place in 1916 in München within so-called Kriegstagung der Gesellschaft deutsche Nervenärzte. In a voting at this meeting, a thesis on an organic background of "traumatic neurosis," presented by Professor Hermann Oppenheim (1858-1919), was rejected by the majority of votes (91 to 3). The result of this vote not only forced Prof. Oppenheim to step down from the position of the President of the Association but also contributed to his premature death [11]. Taking up this issue again nearly 100 years later shows that, given scientific progress, no important medical question can be resolved once and for all, especially by a vote. Today's truth may turn out to be false tomorrow.

5. Conclusions

1. Among 126 PMC veterans psychiatrically hospitalized due to mental disorders connected to combat stress, 53 (42.1%) were directly injured in battle.
2. Retrospective analysis of the medical records of injured patients made by means of BTBIS showed that 20 (37.7%) patients met diagnostic criteria for mTBI.
3. Patients with mTBI compared to non-mTBI patients suffered from PTSD more often (60.0% vs 34.9%), with a particular intensity of hyperarousal symptoms (20% vs 4.7%); their ailments were persistent and resulted in rehospitalization (30% vs 4.7%).
4. The need for a systematic screening of injured veterans with regard to mTBI was confirmed to improve diagnostics, therapy and military-medical expertise of stress injuries.

References

[1] S. Ilnicki, A. Radzikowski, S. Szymanska, M. Zbyszewski, R. Tworus, P. Ilnicki, A. Laskowska: Spra
    wozdanie z działalności Kliniki Psychiatrii i Stresu Bojowego Wojskowego Instytutu Medycznego
    w Warszawie w latach 2006-2010. Lekarz Wojskowy **89** (2011), in print.
[2] K.A. Schwab, B. Ivins, G. Cramer, W. Johnson, Wayne; M. Sluss-Tiller, K. Kiley, W. Lux, D. Warden,
    Screening for Traumatic Brain Injury in Troops Returning From Deployment in Afghanistan and Iraq:
    Initial Investigation of the Usefulness of a Short Screening Tool for Traumatic Brain Injury. Journal of
    Head Trauma Rehabilitation **22** (2007), 377-389.
[3] K. Helmick. Cognitive rehabilitation for military personnel with mild traumatic brain injury and chronic
    post-concussional dis order: Results of April 2009 consensus conference. *NeuroRehabilitation* **26** (2010),
    239-255.
[4] J. Terelak, *Człowiek i stres*, Oficyna Wydawnicza Branta, Bydgoszcz-Warszawa, 2008.
[5] A. Florkowski, W. Gruszczyński (Ed.), *Zdrowie psychiczne żołnierzy*, Wojskowa Akademia Medyczna,
    Łódź, 2000.
[6] W. Gruszczyński, M. Lepak. Problemy adaptacyjne do służby wojskowej uwarunkowane obciążającym
    wywiadem okołoporodowym i wczesnodziecięcym. *Lekarz Wojskowy* **82** (2006) 189-198.
[7] *VA/DoD Clinical Practice Guideline for Management of Concussion/Mild Traumatic Brain Injury*. De
    partment of Veterans Affairs & Department of Defense, Washington D.C., 2009.
[8] C.W. Hoge, D. McGurk, J.L. Thomas, A.L. Cox, C.C. Engel, C.A. Castro. Mild traumatic brain injury in
    U.S. soldiers returning from Iraq. *The New England Journal of Medic*ine **358** (2008), 453-463
[9] C.W. Hoge, H.M. Goldberg, C.A. Castro. Care of war veterans with mild traumatic brain injury – flawed
    perspectives, *The New England Journal of Medicine* **360** (2009), 1588.
[10] K. Korzeniewski, Health hazards in Iraq. *Lekarz Wojskowy* **81** (2007), 176-180.
[11] E. Jones, S. Wessely, *Shell shock to PTSD: military psychiatry from 1900 to the Gulf War*. Maudsley
    Monograph No. 47, Psychology Press, New York 2005

Coping with Blast-Related Traumatic Brain Injury in Returning Troops
B.K. Wiederhold (Ed.)
IOS Press, 2011
doi: 10.3233/978-1-60750-797-0-17

War Head Injuries in Sieged Sarajevo

Kemal DIZDAREVIC[a,1], Alhafidz HAMDAN[b],
Josip JURISIC[a] and Kemal CUSTOVIC[a]
[a] *Department of Neurosurgery, Clinical Centre University of Sarajevo,*
Bosnia-Herzegovina
[b] *Institute of Neuroscience, Newcastle University, Newcastle upon Tyne,*
United Kingdom

Abstract. Objective: We aimed to analyze the penetrating war head injuries in sieged Sarajevo during the first part of Bosnian war and to present our operative strategies in treatment of patients. **Method and patients:** We conducted a retrospective study of injured patients in sieged Sarajevo during the first two years of the Bosnian war (April 1992-July 1994) using a review of the hospital data. Our typical surgical strategy was craniectomy with reduced debridement of the brain injury without search and removal of the deep intracranial foreign fragments. In 34% of cases, operation was performed based only on clinical examination due to lack of electricity in the sieged city. **Results:** A total of 1,728 neurosurgical injured patients were admitted to our department from the region of central Sarajevo (361,179 inhabitants) with an almost equal divide of civilians and military personnel. Eighty-four percent of patients were admitted within 3 hours of injury and operated without any delay. Diagnosis was largely dependent on clinical examination (35% of cases) and plain radiography (47%). Computed tomography scan was only used 18% of the time due to lack of availability. The majority of neurosurgical injuries were head injuries (80%). Spine injuries comprised only 6% patients and peripheral nerve injuries 14%. Over 80% of head-injured patients had a penetrating injury. The patients with head injuries were operated on in 70% of the cases. Mortality of patients that were operated on with head injuries was 13.3%. The number of severely brain-injured patients with Glasgow Coma Scale (GCS) 3 and GCS 4 who died were 143 (35%) and 122 (30%) respectively, giving a total of 265. The GCS 4 patients were operated on only in the case that compressive intracranial haematomas had been detected. A total mortality of the patients with head injury was 30%. Over 60% of injured patients who died were under 50 years old. The most common cause of death were excessive penetrating brain injury (85%) caused by high velocity missiles. Metal grenade fragments were the cause of injury in 73% of cases. Good outcome without any focal neurological deficit was found in 42.6% of all patients with head injuries. **Conclusion:** Our noninvasive early neurosurgical operative approach in the form of intracranial haematomas evacuation and reduced brain debridment without search for deep intracranial foreign bodies resulted in an acceptable treatment outcome during the Bosnian war.

Keywords. seiged, war surgery, craniectomy, neurosurgical debridement, head injury, penetrating injury, noninvasive approach, Sarajevo

---

[1] Corresponding Author: Kemal Dizdarevic, Associate Professor of Neurosurgery, Department of Neurosurgery, Clinical Centre University of Sarajevo, Bolnika 25, 71000 Sarajevo, Bosnia-Herzegovina; E-mail: kemaldiz@bih.net.ba.

Introduction

American military neurosurgeons, Matson, and later Hayes, based on their experiences in World War II and Korea, emphasized the importance of extensive brain debridement strategy in the management of patients with penetrating head injuries during war conditions [1]. This approach is known as a traditional one and it includes thorough wound debridement, removal of all in-driven bone fragments, meticulous dural closure to prevent cerebrospinal fluid (CSF) leakage and postoperative infection, and scalp closure without tension [1,2]. Many American neurosurgeons in Vietnam were trained by Hayes and followed his abovementioned neurosurgical strategy in times of war. Carey et al., who reported extensive experience from the Vietnam War, utilized this traditional thorough debridement with meticulous watertight dural closure [3, 4]. The approach was later followed by Aarabi during the Iran-Iraq war (1980-1988) who also presented his experience based on the concept of thorough brain debridement [5,6,7].

Levi, Feinsod and Brandvold introduced minimal brain debridement in the 1980s. Their surgical strategy, derived from experiences from the Israel-Lebanon war, included two important factors: a) minimal manipulation of brain tissue without searching for in-driven fragments and b) the consideration that dural closure was not important [8]. Taha and later Amirjamshidi favored no brain debridement at all in selected cases [9, 10]. Taha reported the series of patients with minor wounds (mean scalp entrance site of 0.7 cm) and average Glasgow Coma Scale (GCS) of 14. Amirjamshidi's patients had scalp wounds less than 2-3 cm and GCS ≥ 8.

After comparing traditional and minimal brain debridement strategies, Carey stated that minimal brain debridement strategy without attention to dural closure was up to 20 to 30 times more likely to require an additional operative debridement than the traditional debridement strategy [2]. The former resulted in 10 to 15 times higher incidence of life-threatening CSF leakage. Also, Carey presented that minimal operative strategy was connected with a fivefold increase in postoperative meningitis and two to three times greater risk of fatal meningitis [2]. He stressed that populations in underdeveloped countries wounded during the war must be particularly protected from these postdebridement complications because of lack of antibiotics, computed tomography (CT) scans and neurosurgical care. However, from this analysis, we did not learn much about the most important factor on which our decision regarding treatment strategy should be relied i.e. postoperative total mortality rate for all categories of head-injured patients. In the context of war head injuries based only on both postoperative mortality and complication rates, we can choose proper neurosurgical strategy and balance between different treatment modalities and their benefits.

Today, elective neurosurgery tends to be minimalistic and less invasive. With regard to the current neurosurgical thinking, minimal brain debridement without removal of all intracerebral bones or dural repair seems timely and wanted strategy. But in reality, during the war, we should be flexible and capable of adopting ourselves to different surgical maneuvers depending on the war circumstances and not to be so strict in following any defined strategy [11].

Our experiences from seiged Sarajevo showed that neurosurgical war practices could be influenced by different and unpredictable situations. We were negatively influenced by many limiting factors including lack of CT scans and exposure of the hospital to direct military attack of the enemy. On the other hand, we had some positive influences on our work from local the war environment, such as small distances between frontline and definitive places of treatment, neurosurgical operations performed only by trained and experienced neurosurgeons in a department with a university background, possibility for medical operative staff to leave the hospital after the shift to spend some time with family, etc. [12].

Objective

We aimed to analyze penetrating head injuries in sieged Sarajevo during the first part of Bosnian war and to present our operative strategies in patient treatment with short-term outcome.

Method and Patients

Patients with head injuries who were wounded in the region of sieged central Sarajevo during the first two years of Bosnia & Herzegovina (BH) war were enrolled in this clinical study [12]. Review of hospital data covering only the patients from proper Sarajevo were used. The war in BH started in April 6, 1992 and ended in December 1995 with the Dayton peace agreement signed in the USA which was officially confirmed in Paris, France two months later. The study included the period of time from April 6, 1992 to July 1, 1994 and collected data were analyzed retrospectively. During this period the population of central Sarajevo was continuously shelled and sniped by Serb militants (supported by Serbian Army) located on the nearby hills surrounding the city.

In central Sarajevo (the capital of BH under the control of the Bosnian Army), the number of injured patients was 56,720. According to a census conducted in BH in 1991, central Sarajevo had 361,179 inhabitants. In total, during the two-year time period, 22,241 injured patients were hospitalized in three major Hospitals (18,641 patients at the Clinical Center University of Sarajevo and 3,600 patients at the General Hospital and War Hospital). Patients with minor injuries (34,741 patients) were not hospitalized but only received medical services in these Hospitals.

Our study was based on mortality rate and short-term outcome. We did not conduct long-term follow-ups for the majority of our patients due to many reasons. The two main reasons are: a vast number of patients left Sarajevo after the signing of the Dayton Peace Accord hence they were out of our reach and also, after the war, many patients were sent to medical centers outside BH.

The dominant operative strategy applied in our management of penetrating head-injured patients was a combination of traditional and minimal brain debridement strategy [11, 12]. It included: a) broad craniectomy, b) minimal manipulation of brain tissue without searching for in-driven fragments, c) irrigation of missile trajectory with saline and removal of superficial fragments, d) urgent removal of all compressive intracranial haematomas, e) dural watertight closure with autografts (fascia lata, pericranium), e) debridement of entrance and exit wounds with scalp closure without tension, f) early definitive surgery (up to 6 hours after injury), and g) no operation of patients with GCS of 3 and GCS of 4 who did not harbor any intracranial haematomas.

Results

A total of 1,728 (Table 1) neurosurgical injured patients were admitted to our Department of Neurosurgery, Clinical Centre University of Sarajevo, from the region of central Sarajevo (361,179 inhabitants) with an almost equal divide of civilians and military personnel (Table 2). Neurosurgical patients comprised 7.8% of all war-injured patients admitted to the hospitals in central Sarajevo during this period (1,728/22,241). Majority of patients (84%) were admitted within three hours of injury (Table 3). Diagnosis was largely dependant on clinical examination and plain radiography. In 34% of cases operation was performed based only on clinical examination due to lack of electricity in the sieged city (Table 4). CT was only used 18% of the time due to lack of availability.

Table 1. Number of admitted patients according the type of neurosurgical injury.

Total neurosurgical hospital admission	1,728 (100%)
Head injury	1,385 (80.15%)
Spine injury	101 (5.84 %)
Peripheral nerves	242 (14 %)

Table 2. Civilians/soldiers ratio of neurosurgical patients.

Civilians	860 (49.76%)
Soldiers	822 (47.56%)
Unknown	46 (2.66 %)

Table 3. Time spent from the moment of injury to the Hospital admission.

Up to 3 hours	83.98%
3 - 6 h	3.97%
6 – 12 h	2.96%
12 – 24 h	2.75%
24 h	3.90%
Unknown	2.42%

Table 4. Percentage of diagnostic procedure used by neurosurgeons during the siege.

Clinical examination only	34.72%
Plane radiography	47.37%
Computed tomography	17.90 %

Patients with head injuries included 80% of all neurosurgical admittance in this series (1,385) or 6.2% of all war-injured patients admitted to the hospitals. The spine cases comprised only 6% and peripheral nerves 14% of patients (Table 1). Over 80% of head-injured patients had a penetrating injury (1,130/1,385) (Table 5). Mortality of penetrating head injury was 35.4% (401/1,130). Intracranial metal fragments were found in 835 patients or 60.3% of all head-injured patients. Brain prolapse was a frequent clinical manifestation of penetrating head injury and it was noted in 38.5% of cases. A total of 967 patients (69.8%) with head injuries were operated on. Patients that underwent operation mainly underwent broad craniectomy (88.2%). Mortality of patients that were operated on with a head injury was 13.3% (Table 6). During the first two months of the war, we performed 64 extensive brain operations (6.6%) with traditional debridement including removal of all in-driven fragments. Mortality rate for these patients was 23%.

Table 5. Type of injury.

Penetrating injury	81.58%
Nonpenetrating injury	13.57%
Closed	4.83%
Total head injury	100%
Associated injuries (other systems together with nervous system)	45.96%

Table 6. Number and mortality of operated patients.

Number of patients with head injury	1,385
Operated patients with head injury	967 (70.46%)
Mortality of operated patients with head injury	129 (13.34%)

The number of severely brain-injured patients with GCS 3/4 who died was 265 (143 and 122 respectively). These GCS 3/4 patients were operated on only in the case that the compressive intracranial haematomas had been detected. A total mortality of patients with a head injury was 30%. Over 60% of patients who died were under 50 years old (Figure 1). Patients in the age group 21–40 comprised 47.5% of all victims. Children and young adults (≤ 20) consisted of 22.3% injured individuals. Regarding sex distribution, it was noted that 31% of all victims were female (Table 7). Most of the injured patients were Bosniaks (Table 8). The most common cause of death was excessive penetrating brain injury (85%) caused by shell shrapnels from a short distance (Table 9). Another frequent cause of excessive injury was sniper missile. The metal grenade fragment (shell shrapnels) was the cause of injury in 73%, blast in 5% and sniper missile in 22% of cases (Figure 2). Good outcome with mild focal neurological deficit or without any deficit was found in 42.6% of all patients with a head injury (Figure 3).

Frequency of infective complication was 2.1%. The group of patients who were admitted to the hospital 6 hours after the injury had infection in 8.1% of cases, those patients admitted before 6 hours had infection rate of 1.5%. (1,307) (Table 10). Head-penetrating injuries were associated with other organ system injuries in 44% of patients. Majority of associated injuries were in extremities (13.5%), thorax (8.4%) and abdomen (6.7%). From the July 1, 1994 to the end of the war, 567 new patients with penetrating head injuries were noted. These patients were not included in our study.

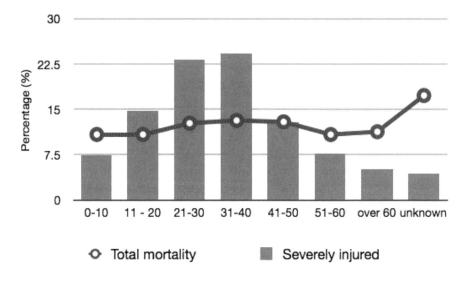

Figure 1. Age and mortality of severely brain injured patients

Table 7. Sex distribution of neurosurgical patients.

Male	69% (1193)
Female	31% (535)

Table 8. Ethnic and religious distribution of injured patients.

Bosniaks (Islam)	1384 (80.11%)
Serbs (Orthodox Church)	125 (7.23%)
Croats (Catholic Church)	95 (5.49%)
Others	124 (7.17%)

Table 9. Causes of neurosurgical death.

Excessive brain injury	84.52% (366)
Intracranial haematomas	5.54% (24)
Brainstem ischaemia	2.54 % (11)
Infection	1.61% (7)
Injury in others systems	1.15% (5)
High cervical lesion	4.38% (19)
Unknown	0.23 % (1)

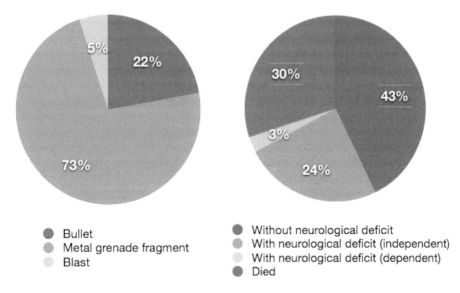

Figure 2. Causes of neurosurgical injury

- Bullet
- Metal grenade fragment
- Blast

Figure 3. Outcome of operative and conservative treatment of head injuries

- Without neurological deficit
- With neurological deficit (independent)
- With neurological deficit (dependent)
- Died

Table 10. Time of hospital admission as a factor of infection rate.

Up to 6 hours	1.45 %
More than 6 hours	8.1 %

Discussion

Patients with penetrating head injuries and GCS≤8 received cardiopulmonary resuscitation, endotracheal tube placement and venous access with fluid administration without any delay to reach haemodynamic stabilization. All patients received intravenous antibiotics and anticonvulsant therapy (phenobarbital). Surgery was indicated for all patients with CGS≥5 as soon as possible. Patients with CGS 3/4, intracranial haematomas and presence of brainstem reflexes were operated on as well. A large craniectomy with exposure of the entrance wound and all dural lacerations were accomplished. Also, the exit wound was approached in a similar way.

At the beginning of the war we started to use extensive brain surgery (performed in 6% of cases) (Table 11). It utilized a broad resection of all necrotic tissue, removal of foreign bodies (metal and bone fragments, and missiles) including the search for those deeply located, haematoma evacuation, vigorous cleaning of missile tract, dural repair with fascia or pericranium using watertight suture and appropriate repair of bone and soft tissue. The operative results of this small series of patients were disappointing. This was the reason for our decision to change operative strategy focusing on minimal manipulation of neuronal tissue without searching for deeply located in-driven fragments. Dural closure stayed meticulous and watertight preventing postoperative CSF leakage.

Table 11. Type of operation.

Decompressive procedure only	11.78%
Craniectomy with extensive debridement of the brain injury and removal of all intracranial foreign fragments	6.61%
Craniectomy with reduced debridement of the brain injury without search and removal of the deep intracranial foreign fragments	81.59%

The proximity of hospitals to the scene of a majority of injuries meant that there was a very short time period between the moment of injury and definitive neurosurgical treatment. The reason for this was the fact that the aggressor shelled the population on the street and in the apartments. Also, the frontline was not outside the city but in the city proper. Severe lack of resources including electricity and running water, which were cut off by the aggressor, had an influence on general neurosurgical management and restricted operative indications.

The main cause of penetrating head injuries in our series was shrapnel and sniper bullets. Shell shrapnel is considered a low-velocity missile but it behaves like high velocity ones if the distance between shell explosion and the victim is less than 100 meters. In accordance with the findings of some other authors, we noted the important characteristics of penetrating head injuries having an absolute influence on outcome including: multilobular lesion, missile trajectory through basal ganglia and supratentorial ventricles (lateral and third) and posterior fossa involvement with brainstem damage. In fact, there are three main factors which are connected with severity of the lesions. These include a) brain stem/diencephalic damage, b) malignant citotoxic diffuse edema accompanied by refractory intracranial hypertension and c) lacerations of magisterial intracranial arteries/large sinuses with profuse haemorrhage and serious secondary ischaemia. The most important isolated clinical sign which is directly associated with mortality is bilateral dilated fixed pupil. Almost 100% of patients from our series died if this sign was found in the head-injured patients with GCS 3. In general, our patients who had a low GCS (GCS of 3-6) and a wound tract that crossed the midline had a bad prognosis.

Based on Narayan's scale [13] for predicting outcome in severe head injuries, we introduced our simple scoring system, which was easily understandable for general surgeons, and other medical doctors who participated in sorting casualties together with neurosurgeons [11, 12, 14, 15]. This score was the foundation for our neurosurgical triage principles. Patients were classified into four groups as follows:

- Group A (trivial closed head injuries, there is no need for neurosurgeons involvement in any form)
- Group B (there is a need for neurosurgical short observations, scalp wound with or without loss of consciousness; cranial fracture)
- Group C was divided in three subgroups: C1 = urgent surgery: open penetrating head injury and/or compressive intracranial haematoma with declining consciousness and focal neurological deficits; C2 = patients who need reanimation before surgery, C3 = patients who can wait for surgery; closed impressive fracture)
- Group D (patients who did not receive operative treatment, brain death patients and GCS of 3 and 4 without compressive haematoma).

We were forced to observe some patients for 24 hours due to lack of CT availability. Urgent surgery was required in 36% of head-injured patients. In group D, 17.1% of patients were triaged. These cases were not operated on but their scalp wounds were sutured outside the operating room. All patients from group D died.

Martins et al. showed that patients with penetrating gunshot head injuries and GCS score ranging from 3-5 have a mortality rate reaching 98.5%. The total mortality rate of all patients from the Martins' series who sustained penetrating head injuries with GCS score ranging from 3-15 was 65% [16]. The total mortality rate in our series including 20 patients with GCS 3/4 was 30%. This mortality rate applies not only to penetrating head-injured patients but also to all head-injured patients admitted to our department.

Current management protocol for patients with penetrating head injuries does not include performing skull X-rays as a diagnostic procedure. In these cases, CT scan is the procedure of choice. CT of the brain can easily identify a compressive haematoma and show the extension of brain injury as well as retained intracranial bone fragments. We were forced to perform the majority of our surgery based only on clinical examination and skull X-ray. This means that planning of our operations was insufficient in detail but this did not show any significant impact on our surgical performance. Contrary to elective neurosurgical operations, major characteristics of penetrating head injury is obvious and there is no need for anticipating all possible problems, which can be met during surgery. Performing X-rays and clinical examinations before surgery were shown to be sufficient to justify subsequent operative procedures. One problem concerning neuroimaging (CT scans) was encountered in the deeply comatose patients (mainly from group D). The intracranial haematomas in some of them were not diagnosed so they did not receive appropriate surgery.

As we mentioned before, 6.6% of our patients underwent extensive brain operation (traditional debridement) and mortality rate for them was 23%. This is a 10% higher mortality rate compared with our total mortality postoperative rate (13%) which was mainly derived from less invasive operations. Obviously, vigorous manipulation of neuronal tissue and extensive debridement of severe injured brain characterized by malignant citotoxic edema, intracerebral bleeding and serious secondary ischaemia can additionally disturb brain volume regulation and consequently chance for recovery.

We did not find any difference in immediate infective rate between these two groups. Also, we found that metal fragments were less connected with deep brain infections and abscesses. Our operative series clearly shows that there is a difference of infective rates between patients operated within 6 hours post-injury compared with other operated patients. Carey determined that 45% of soldiers operated upon within 4 hours of acquiring the wound had bacterially contaminated bone fragments within their brains [4]. We routinely administrated antibiotics pre- and postoperatively. In the first few months of the war, third generation of cephalosporines were used but afterward, we used a combination of penicilline and gentamycine. All neurosurgical patients in the hospital received antibiotics and 34% of them had antibiotics during transportation from the scene to our department.

The finding of intracerebral metal fragments in vast number of head-injured or in almost all penetrating head-injured patients in which we performed skull X-ray or CT scans shows that head wounds in our series were mainly caused by shell shrapnels. Frequent general postoperative complication of patients with penetrating head injury was pneumonia [17]. We had the same problem with patients that underwent operations.

CSF leakage was the most important complication associated with surgical treatment. The presence of CSF fistula could be complicated by meningitis, sepsis and death [18, 19]. We did not have serious problems with CSF fistula. The treatment for CSF leakage was made by lumbar drainage and/or direct surgical repair. Infections of wounds also involved brain abscess, subdural empyema and cranial osteomyelitis.

The high mortality rates were a result of not only the primary brain lesion but also of the secondary brain injury generated due to intracranial/extracranial reasons and particularly due to the brainstem damage caused by extensive brain shift and herniation. We also noted that brainstem distortion during missile impact was a recognized mechanism leading to death.

Conclusion

Our less invasive neurosurgical operative strategy in the form of obligatory intracranial compressive haematomas evacuation, broad craniectomy, reduced brain debridement without search for deep intracranial in-driven fragments and meticulous dural closure resulted in acceptable short-term outcome in terms of mortality and surgical complications during the Bosnian war.

References

[1]   Matson DD.The menagement of acute craniocranial injuries due to missiles.In: Coates JB,ed. Surgery in World War II, Neurosurgery, Volume I. Washington,DC: Office of the Surgeon General, Department of the Army, 1958:123-82.
[2]   Carey ME. The treatment of wartime brain wounds: Traditional versus minimal debridement. Surg Neurol 2003;60:112-9.
[3]   Carey ME,Young HF,Rish BL,Mathis JL.Follow up study of 103 American soldiers who sustaned a brain wound in Vietnam. J.Neurosurg 1974;41:542-9.
[4]   Carey ME,Young HF,Mathis JL. The neurosurgical treatment of craniocerebral missile wounds in Vietnam.Surg Gynec Obstet 1972;135:386-90.
[5]   Aarabi B: Surgical outcome in 435 patients who sustained missile head wounds during the Iran-Iraq War. Neurosurgery 1990; 27: 692- 695
[6]   Aarabi B. Comparative study of bacteriological contamination between primary and secondary exploration of missile head wounds.Neurosurgery 1987;20:610-5.
[7]   Aarabi B.Causes of infections in penetrating head wounds in the Iran-Iraq war.Neurosurgery 1989;923-6.
[8]   Brandvold B,Levi L,Feinsod M,George E. Penetrating craniocerebral injuries in the Israel involvement in the Lebanese conflict,1982-1985. J Neurosurg 1990;72:15-21.
[9]   Taha JM, Saba MI, Brown TA: Missile injuries to the brain treated by simple wound closure: results of a protocol during the Lebanese conflict. Neurosurgery 1991; 29: 380-383
[10] Amirjamshidi A, Abbassioun K, Rahmat H: Minimal debridement or simple wound closure as the only surgical treatment in war victims with low-velocity penetrating head injuries. Indications and menagement protocol based upon more than 8 years follow-up of 99 cases from Iran-Iraq conflict.Surg Neurol 2003;60:105-11.
[11] Dizdarević K, Apok V and Custovic K : Clinical study of neurosurgical casualties in sieged Sarajevo: Date from Bosnian war. British Journal of Neurosurgery 2009; Proceedings of the 153rd Meeting of the British Neurological Surgeons, p 124
[12] Konjhodzic F: Neurosurgical injuries in the defensive war in Bosnia and Herzegovina. Monographic book, Oko, Sarajevo 1994
[13] Narayan RK: Emergency room management of the head injury. Philadelphia: WB Saunders, 1989
[14] Sisic F, Konjhodzic F Duric O: Principles of surgical war doctrine. Sarajevo: Avicena 1993
[15] Husum H et al. : War Surgery, field manual. Third Word Network, Penang 1995

[16] Martins RS, Siqueira MG, Santos MTS, et al. Prognostic factors and treatment of penetrating gunshot wounds to the head. Surg Neurol 2003;60:98-104.

[17] Hammon WM.Analysis of 2187 consecutive penetrating wounds of the brain from Vietnam. J Neurosurg 1971;34:127-31.

[18] Meirowsky AM, Caveness WF, Dillon JD, et al. Cerebrospinal fluid fistulas complicating missile wounds of the brain. J Neurosurg 1981;54:44-8.

[19] Rish BL, Dillon JD, Weiss GH. Mortality following penetrating craniocerebral injuries. An analysis of the deaths in the Vietnam Head Injury Registry population. J Neurosurg 1983; 59:775-80

Section II

Diagnostic and Assessment Issues

Coping with Blast-Related Traumatic Brain Injury in Returning Troops
B.K. Wiederhold (Ed.)
IOS Press, 2011

doi: 10.3233/978-1-60750-797-0-31

The Brain Injury Screening Questionnaire: A Methodology to be Applied to Soldiers

Wayne A. GORDON[1, a]

[a]*Mount Sinai School of Medicine, New York, NY*

Abstract. Traumatic Brain Injury (TBI) is extremely prevalent in the soldiers returning from Iraq and Afghanistan. Although some soldiers in the United States are currently being screened for TBI both before and after they are deployed, there are many factors that limit the validity of these screenings. For example, many soldiers are reluctant to "step up" because they are concerned that a positive screen will delay their return home. Additionally, many of the symptoms of mild TBI may not emerge until the soldiers have returned home and picked up the fabric of their former life. This paper will review an approach to screening for TBI, the Brain Injury Screening Questionnaire (BISQ). Additionally, the development, validity and research on the BISQ, as well as its potential diverse clinical applications, will be reviewed.

Keywords. Traumatic Brain Injury, screening, mild Traumatic Brain Injury

Introduction

Traumatic Brain Injury (TBI) has been described as "the signature injury" of the war in Iraq and Afghanistan [1,2]. The rate of TBI in both Operation Enduring Freedom (OEF) and Operation Iraqi Freedom (OIF) is believed to be higher than in any previous war [2]. It is estimated by the Defense and Veterans Brain Injury Center (DVBIC) at Walter Reed that of all OEF and OIF veterans returning from their overseas deployments, 30% had experienced a TBI [3]. Of those patients transferred back to the U.S. for treatment, 56% had moderate to severe TBI while 44% struggled with mild TBI [3]. Due to the fact that mild TBI in particular is difficult to diagnose because of its symptoms overlap with other combat-related trauma such as Posttraumatic Stress Disorder, it is believed that current estimates of the prevalence of TBI in veterans could be grossly underestimated. Thus, the brain injuries that are described in the media of

---

[1] Corresponding Author: Wayne A. Gordon, Ph.D., ABPP/Cn Jack Nash Professor, Department of Rehabilitation Medicine Mount Sinai School of Medicine, One Gustave Levy Place, Box 1240, New York, NY 10029; E-mail: wayne.gordon@mountsinai.org.

The preparation of this manuscript is supported by Grant#1R 49CE 001171-01 from The Centers for Disease Control and Prevention (CDC).

soldiers returning home with multiple grievous injuries represent only those who have been counted or identified as having a TBI.

Unidentified TBI occurs in soldiers and/or civilians whenever the injured person is not recognized or identified as having sustained a brain injury. The person may be experiencing physical, cognitive, behavioral and/or emotional symptoms that are secondary to their injury, yet they remain unidentified. Unidentified TBI is a common phenomenon, one that needs attention from medical, educational and military systems — the last because TBI is "the signature injury" [4] of the wars in Iraq and Afghanistan. The prevalence of unidentified TBI is difficult to determine both in civilian and in military populations because it is difficult to count those who are not systematically reported and therefore remain unknown. The best civilian estimates of known TBI are based on data published by the Centers for Disease Control and Prevention (CDC). Estimates that there are 5.3 million cases or 2% of the U.S. population has sustained a TBI [5]. CDC acknowledges that these numbers underestimate the true prevalence of TBI, since only those seen in Emergency Rooms and those who die are counted. Those who receive care outside of hospitals (e.g., in medical offices) or who do not receive medical attention at all (e.g., people injured in assaults, domestic violence, sports, falls and the like) are not counted. Research suggests that for every person hospitalized with a brain injury, three to five others are injured but do not receive any care [6,7]. Among people who have sustained a brain injury, do we have any idea how many continue to experience symptoms attributable to mild TBI but fail to causally link the symptoms to the injury? In a recent population-based survey in New Haven, Connecticut, Jonathan Silver and colleagues [8] found that 8.5% of the 5,034 people surveyed reported a brain injury with continuing challenges. An unpublished study at the Mount Sinai School of Medicine in New York City found a similar level of unidentified TBI – about 7% of a sample of people identifying themselves as non-disabled met criteria for TBI and also reported numerous symptoms associated with known TBI. In another study conducted at Mount Sinai [9] it was found that 9% of a sample of high school students was identified as having sustained a TBI. If we consider such data in the context of the current U.S. population, they suggest that unidentified TBI may affect as many as 20-25 million Americans. Clearly, more studies are needed to refine these estimates and get a better handle on the extent of the problem among civilians. Mild TBI is the most common form of undiagnosed brain injury [10]. Although it has been suggested [11,12,13,14] that the effects of mild TBI are "mild to non-existent" [15] (p. 586), a substantial body of evidence contradicts this claim [16,17,18].

As would be expected, the number of unidentified TBIs in the military is also difficult to determine. We have learned in the past few years, thanks to media coverage, to expect large numbers of soldiers to have a known TBI. In reality, the prevalence of "probable" TBI is estimated at 19.5%, which translates to possibly 320,000 of those returning from Iraq and Afghanistan [19]. However, these numbers are probably underestimates because post-deployment screening is implemented too close in time to the soldier's returning home. Thus, many post-TBI challenges do not emerge until the soldier has returned home and picked up the fabric of his/her pre-deployment life.

The large number of estimated injuries in both civilian and military venues should raise concern, as the consequences of TBI, whether known or unidentified, are typically life changing. TBI is strongly associated with multiple, often overwhelming, challenges that can undermine a person's efforts to live a productive life, leading to "social failure." For example, among prisoners, estimates of the prevalence of TBI range from 42% to 87%. [11,12,13,30,31,32] For most, the brain injury preceded the start of criminal activity. TBI is also common in inpatient psychiatric and substance abuse populations, and, similarly, the injury often precedes onset of psychiatric symptoms [14,15] or substance abuse. TBI is associated with high levels of co-occurring depression, anxiety and Posttraumatic Stress Disorder, or PTSD.[19,25] (While some symptoms of TBI and PTSD are similar, such as fatigue and difficulty sleeping, other symptoms are unique to each disorder — heightened startle response and night sweats are unique to PTSD, for example). Although the overlap between the estimated 320,000 returning soldiers with known TBI and the 300,000 returning with depression and/or PTSD is relatively small (7%), this figure includes only those with identified TBI. In Silver's study, individuals reporting TBI attempted suicide four times more often than those with no brain injury, they were more likely to be receiving public assistance or disability benefits, and they experienced poorer overall emotional and physical health [8]. Additionally, those who are substance abusers often have a history of early TBI [26,27]. Simpson and Tate [28] found suicide 21 times more likely in those with combined TBI, substance abuse and major depression. At the extreme, Lewis and colleagues [29] found that all of the inmates they interviewed on death row had experienced one or more TBIs. Finally, children with TBI are at increased risk for social failure as they mature into adulthood. TBI in children is associated with poor academic performance [33] as well as problem behaviors [34]. Glang and colleagues [35] estimate that 130,000 U.S. children need special education classes because of TBI, but that, in fact, only 11% of children with TBI are currently enrolled. These children truly remain "hidden" to their schools or are misidentified as having other types of emotional or learning disorders [36]. TBI is strongly associated with multiple, often overwhelming, challenges that can undermine the person's efforts to live a healthy, productive life. Combined, these challenges often result in the person with TBI experiencing "social failure."

TBI is a heavy burden for the individual who is injured, but the costs to society, estimated at $60 billion annually – 15% of the total cost of all types of injuries in the United States – are also astronomical [37]. As these estimates do not include the costs associated with unidentified TBI, the real figures are likely to be even higher. Screening of at-risk populations to detect hidden TBI is needed in order to facilitate referral of those with unidentified TBI for appropriate services. The only instrument of which we are aware designed to screen for TBI in both military and civilian populations that integrates information related to concussion history with current symptoms is the *Brain Injury Screening Questionnaire* (BISQ) [38]. The BISQ was developed by the Research and Training Center on Community Integration of Individuals with Traumatic Brain Injury at Mount Sinai School of Medicine to conduct brain injury screening in a variety of populations. The BISQ incorporates elements of symptom checklists developed by Lehmkuhl [39] at The Institute for Rehabilitation and Research and the Medical College of Virginia, [40] as well as the structure of the HELPS card developed by Picard, Scarisbrick and Paluck [41].

Part I of the BISQ allows users to determine whether American Congress of Rehabilitation Medicine (ACRM) minimal criteria are met for brain injury, including a blow to the head, a loss of consciousness (LOC) or a period of being dazed and confused (DAC) [42]. In Part II, the BISQ documents functional impairments (symptoms) that are present and how frequently they occur. Finally, in Part III, factors other than brain injury (e.g., psychiatric disorders, medication use, substance abuse) that might account for the impairments are documented. The BISQ can be used as a self-report measure or can be completed by a proxy.

The BISQ is inexpensive and easy-to-use. It takes 5-20 minutes to complete depending on whether or not the person has a history of TBI. Thus, if the person does not report any events in Part I, the person does not go on to Part II and the BISQ has been completed for this person. Thus, when a person screens negative because of the absence of events the BISQ takes about five mintues to complete. The BISQ can easily be administered by social service agencies, in schools and among at-risk populations such as military personnel, athletes, prison inmates, victims of domestic violence and individuals seeking mental health or substance abuse services. Indeed, it has already been used in several of these settings. Ultimately, it is a tool that has the potential to improve access to care.

The BISQ was developed based on a core set of symptoms from the TIRR Symptom Checklist [39]. Initial studies [43, 44] focused on the identification of hidden TBI using these symptoms and information about history of blows to the head and alterations in mental status. A subsequent study examined the sensitivity and specificity of these symptoms [45]. Based on this research, the current form of the BISQ was developed, incorporating additional symptoms and information on events that might result in a TBI. Subsequent investigations used the BISQ to screen "at risk" groups of people not previously identified as having a brain injury.

In the first of the studies, using the earlier version of the BISQ, Gordon et al. [43] found that 7% of a group of individuals who did not identify as having a TBI screened positive for brain injury using BISQ items – they had experienced a blow to the head, loss of consciousness and had large numbers of continuing problems associated with known TBI. In a study using the same items, Jaffe and colleagues [44] identified extensive hidden brain injury in a group of individuals with HIV.

Gordon and colleagues [45] compared self-reported symptoms (cognitive, physical, behavioral/affective) across six groups: 135 individuals with mild TBI, 275 with moderate/severe TBI, 287 with no disability, 104 with spinal cord injury, 197 who were HIV positive and 107 who had undergone a liver transplantation. The participants with TBI and SCI were at least one-year post injury. The TBI groups reported significantly more symptoms than the others. Symptom reports in the TBI groups were not related to demographic variables, time since injury or depression. Logistic regression was used to assess each of the 67 symptoms. It was determined for each symptom whether it was significantly more likely to occur in the TBI groups than the non-TBI groups. Six covariates (age, sex, ethnicity, education, income and depression) were controlled for. Criteria for sensitivity and specificity were then applied to symptoms that occurred significantly more often in individuals with TBI. Sensitivity was defined as the true positive rate and was based on the percentage of individuals in the TBI groups who reported a given symptom. Specificity was defined as the true negative rate and was based on the percentage of individuals in *each* respective non-TBI group who did *not* report the symptom. The criteria adopted for a symptom to be deemed "sensitive and specific" were as follows: sensitivity = 33% or more of the relevant TBI group report the symptom; specificity = 10% or less of the non-disabled group report the symptom (i.e., 90% specificity) and 25% or less in the SCI, HIV and liver transplant groups report the symptom (i.e., 75% specificity). Five of the 67 symptoms were found to be sensitive and specific to TBI in general and 25 symptoms were sensitive and specific to mild TBI (23 were cognitive, one physical and one behavioral/affective).

Logistic regression models predicting the dichotomous variables – Mild TBI vs. no disability and moderate/severe TBI vs. no disability – were then applied to the symptoms found to be sensitive/specific. These logistic regressions were repeated in models predicting mild and moderate/severe TBI vs. a combined group of other disabilities. Odd ratios were calculated indicating that a report of one of the five symptoms sensitive to TBI significantly increased the likelihood of having a mild TBI (3.28 vs. non-disabled and 2.38 vs. disabled) or moderate/severe TBI (2.39 vs. non-disabled and 1.17 vs. disabled). Reporting one of the 25 symptoms sensitive and specific to mild TBI increased the likelihood of belonging to the mild TBI group by 1.45 compared to non-disabled individuals and by 1.26 compared to persons with disabilities. Increased symptom report increased the likelihood of TBI. Adding depression as a covariate or demographic covariates made little difference in the predictive power of the models.

Based on this study, the current version of the BISQ was developed, including 57 of the 67 TIRR items and adding other symptoms from the symptom checklists developed at the Medical College of Virginia, [40] as well as items based on the collective clinical experience of our research team. In addition, the response options were changed to increase the measure's sensitivity.

The BISQ was used to screen individuals in drug abuse treatment programs in New York State; about 50% of those screened were found to have had probable brain injuries [26]. Those who screened positive were more likely to have had multiple admissions to substance abuse treatment programs and had more mental health diagnoses, suggesting that they were more difficult to treat and more likely to be treatment failures.

The BISQ has been used with the homeless population in New York City by Common Ground, a non-profit organization whose mission is to combat homelessness by providing access and referrals to medical services, housing and employment. BISQs were administered to homeless persons by trained Common Ground field personnel. At the time of writing, 14 of 48 individuals screened (29%) were found to have a moderate or high probability of having TBI-related impairments.

Cantor and colleagues [9] examined the utility of the BISQ in screening for brain injury in children over 12 and to determine whether children and parents reported differently on the BISQ. They recruited 137 children ages 12-19 in two New York City public schools. Fourteen (10%) of the children provided information on the BISQ that suggested that they were "at risk" for having sustained a brain injury. "At risk" status was determined by the presence of two factors. They or their parent (or both) reported an alteration in mental status (LOC or DAC), and five or more symptoms sensitive and specific to TBI [45]. BISQ reports indicated that most of the participants had experienced blows to the head and about half had experienced an alteration in mental status. Parents and children did not report significantly different numbers of symptoms, head injuries or alterations in mental status. These findings suggest that there may be significant numbers of children with undetected brain injury in schools.

In a second study, Cantor and colleagues [9] continued to examine the BISQ's utility with schoolchildren. An ethnically diverse convenience sample of 174 children ages 12–19 recruited in three urban public schools participated in the study, none of whom had previously been identified by the school system as having a brain injury. BISQs were completed by the parent and child for 74% of the sample, by the child alone for 21% of the sample and by the parent alone for 5% of the sample. Forty-eight percent of the sample completed a neuropsychological test battery. BISQ findings indicated that 9% of the participants had a "high probability" of having sustained a brain injury. A significantly greater number of cognitive, behavioral and physical symptoms (as well as behavioral problems) were reported by the children in the "high probability" group than in the "low probability" group. Eighty percent of the "high probability" children tested demonstrated neuropsychological evidence of cognitive impairment.

Overall, these findings support the utility of the BISQ as part of a screening process to identify adults and children who may have experienced a brain injury. There are currently no validated screening tools for TBI. The BISQ is the only such screening instrument. When applied to diverse groups who are "at risk" for TBI, the BISQ can identify those in need of further diagnostic evaluation and potentially prevent secondary conditions that can result in social failure. The BISQ currently is available as either a paper form or on the Internet from Dr. Gordon for a nominal fee. The paper form needs to be returned to Dr. Gordon for scoring. A report is generated from the web-based form as soon as it is submitted. Obviously, the BISQ has many applications when employed in military settings. For example, it can provide a comprehensive report of concussion history prior to deployment and when re-administered post-deployment, can document incidents that are deployment-related. In addition, the symptom report can be used to develop a treatment plan. Finally, it should be made available to returning soldiers, as these individuals may gain awareness of their difficulties once they return home and have difficulty functioning outside of the structure provided by military. In other words, some symptoms may not become apparent until the soldier attempts to pick-up the fabric of his/her previous life and finds that tasks that were easily completed prior to their service are now a source of daily challenge.

References

[1]   M. McCrea, N. Pliskin, J. Barth, D. Cox, J. Fink, L. French, T. Hammeke, D. Hess, A. Hopewell, D. Orme, M. Powell, R. Ruff, B. Schrock, L. Terryberry-Spohr, R. Vanderploeg, R. Yoash-Gantz. Official position of the military TBI task force on the role of neuropsychology and rehabilitation psychology in the evaluation, management, and research of military veterans with traumatic brain injury. *Clinical Neuropsychology* **22(1)** (2008), 10-26.
[2]   D. Warden. Military TBI during the Iraq and Afghanistan wars. *Journal of Head Trauma Rehabilitation* **21(5)** (2006), 398-402.
[3]   D. Warden, L.M. Ryan, K.M. Helmick, K. Schwab, L.M. French, W. Lu, et al. War neurotrauma: The Defense and Veterans Brain Injury Center (DVBIC) experience at Walter Reed Army Medical Center (WRAMC). *Journal of Neurotrauma* **22(10)** (2005), 1178.
[4]   S. Okie. Reconstructing lives: A tale of two soldiers. *New England Journal of Medicine* **355** (2006), 2609–2615.
[5]   J.A. Langlois, W. Rutland-Brown, K.E. Thomas. *Traumatic brain injury in the United States: Emergency department visits, hospitalizations and deaths.* Centers for Disease Control and Prevention, National Center for Injury Prevention and Control, Atlanta, GA, 2004.
[6]   J.F. Kraus and D.L. McArthur. Epidemiologic aspects of brain injury. *Neurologic Clinics* **14** (1996), 435-450.
[7]   D.M. Bernstein. Recovery from mild head injury. *Brain Injury* **13** (1999), 151-172.
[8]   J.M. Silver, R. Kramer, S. Greenwald, M. Weissman. The association between head injuries and psychiatric disorders: Findings from the New Haven NIMH epidemiologic catchment area study. *Brain Injury* **15** (2001), 935–945.
[9]   J.B. Cantor, W.A. Gordon., T.A. Ashman. Screening for brain injury in schoolchildren [abstract]. *Journal of Head Trauma Rehabilitation* **21(5)** (2006), 424.

[10] *National Center for Injury Prevention and Control Report to Congress on mild traumatic brain injury in the United States: Steps to prevent a serious public health problem.* Centers for Disease Control and Prevention, Atlanta, GA 2003.

[11] L.M. Binder. A review of mild head trauma. Part II: Clinical implications. *J Clin Exp Neuropsychol* (1997), 432-457.

[12] L.M. Binder, M.L. Rohling, J. Larrabee. A review of mild head trauma. Part I: Meta-analytic review of neuropsychological studies. *J Clin Exp Neuropsychol.* **19** (1997), 421-431.

[13] S.S. Dikmen, B.L. Ross, J.E. Machamer, N.R. Temkin. One year psychosocial outcome in head injury. *J Int Neuropsychol Soc.* **1** (1995), 67-77.

[14] G.L. Iverson, M.R. Lovell, S. Smith, M.D. Franzen. Prevalence of abnormal CT-scans following mild head injury. *Brain Injury* **14** (2000), 1057-1061.

[15] P.R. Lees-Haley, P. Green, M.L. Rohling, D.D. Fox, L.M. Allen, 3rd. The lesion(s) in traumatic brain injury: Implications for clinical neuropsychology. *Arch Clin Neuropsychol.* **18** (2003), 585-594.

[16] M.D. Lezak, D.B. Howieson, D.W. Loring. *Neuropsychological Assessment.* Fourth ed. Oxford University Press, 2004.

[17] E.D. Bigler. Neurobiology and neuropathology underlie the neuropsychological deficits associated with traumatic brain injury. *Arch Clin Neuropsychol.* **18** (2003), 595-621.

[18] A. Sterr, K. Herron, C. Hayward, D. Montaldi. Are mild head injuries as mild as we think? neurobehavioral concomitants of chronic post-concussion syndrome. *BMC Neurol.* **6(7)** (2006).

[19] T. Tanielian, L.H. Jaycox. *Invisible Wounds of War: Psychological and Cognitive Injuries, Their Consequences and Services to Assist Recovery.* RAND Corporation, MG-720-CCF, Santa Monica, CA, 2008.

[20] K. Brewer-Smyth, A.W. Burgess, J. Shults. Physical and sexual abuse, salivary cortisol and neurologic correlates of violent criminal behavior in female prison inmates. *Biological Psychiatry* **55** (2004), 21–31.

[21] M. Sarapata, D. Herrmann, T. Johnson, R. Aycock. The role of head injury in cognitive functioning, emotional adjustment and criminal behaviour. *Brain Injury* **12** (1998), 821–842.

[22] B. Slaughter, J.R. Fann, D. Ehde. Traumatic brain injury in a county jail population: Prevalence, neuropsychological functioning and psychiatric disorders. *Brain Injury* **17** (2003), 731–741.

[23] J.S. Burg, L.M. McGuire, R.G. Burright, P.J. Donovick. Prevalence of a head injury in an outpatient psychiatric population. *Journal of Clinical Psychology in Medical Settings* **3** (1996), 243–251.

[24] L.M. McGuire, R.G. Burright, R. Williams. Prevalence of traumatic brain injury in psychiatric and non-psychiatric patients. *Brain Injury* **12** (1998), 207–214.

[25] M. Hibbard, S. Uysal, K. Kepler, J. Bogdany, J. M. Silver. Axis I psychopathology in individuals with TBI. *Journal of Head Trauma Rehabilitation* **13(4)** (1998), 24–39.

[26] A. Sacks, C. Fenske,., W.A. Gordon, M.R. Hibbard, K. Perez, S. Brandau, J. Cantor, T. Ashman, L. Spielman. Co-morbidity of substance abuse and traumatic brain injury. *Journal of Dual Diagnosis* **5** (2009), 404-417.

[27] R. Walker, M. Hiller, M. Staton, C.G. Leukefeld. Head injury among drug abusers: An indicator of co-occurring problems. *J Psychoactive Drugs* **35** (2003), 343-353.

[28] G. Simpson, R. Tate. Clinical features of suicide attempts after traumatic brain injury. *J Nerv Ment Dis* **193** (2005), 680-685.

[29] D.O. Lewis, J.H. Pincus, M. Feldman, L. Jackson, B. Bard. Psychiatric, neurological, and psychoeducational characteristics of 15 death row inmates in the United States. *Am J Psychiatry* **143** (1986), 838-845.

[30] K. Brewer-Smyth, A.W. Burgess, J. Shults. Physical and sexual abuse, salivary cortisol, and neurologic correlates of violent criminal behavior in female prison inmates. *Biol Psychiatry* **55** (2004), 21-31.

[31] M. Sarapata, D. Herrmann, T. Johnson, R. Aycock. The role of head injury in cognitive functioning, emotional adjustment and criminal behaviour. *Brain Injury* **12** (1998), 821-842.

[32] B. Slaughter, J.R. Fann, D. Ehde. Traumatic brain injury in a county jail population: Prevalence, neuropsychological functioning and psychiatric disorders. *Brain Injury* **17** (2003), 731-741.

[33] L. Ewing-Cobbs, M.A. Barnes, J.M. Fletcher. Early brain injury in children: Development and reorganization of cognitive function. *Dev Neuropsychol* **24** (2003), 669-704.

[34] H.G. Taylor. Research on outcomes of pediatric traumatic brain injury: Current advances and future directions. *Dev Neuropsychol* **25** (2004), 199-225.

[35] A. Glang, J. Tyler, S. Pearson, B. Todis, M. Morvant. Improving educational services for students with TBI through statewide consulting teams. *NeuroRehabilitation* **19** (2004), 219-231.

[36] M.R. Hibbard, T. Martin, J. Cantor, A. Moran. Students with acquired brain injury: Identification, accommodations and transitions in schools. In: J. Farmer, J. Donders, S. Warchausky, eds. *Neurodevelopmental Disabilities.* First ed. Guilford, New York (2006), 209-233.

[37] E. Finkelstein, P. Corso, T. Miller, & associates. *The Incidence and Economic Burden of Injuries in the United States.* Oxford University Press, New York, NY 2006.

[38] *Brain Injury Screening Questionnaire.* Research and Training Center on Community Integration, Mount Sinai School of Medicine, New York, NY, 1998.

[39] D. Lehmkuhl. *The TIRR Symptom Checklist.* The Institute for Rehabilitation Research, Houston, Texas, 1998.

[40] Rehabilitation and Neuropsychological Service, Department of Physical Medicine and Rehabilitation, Medical College of Virginia. *TBI Symptom Checklist.* Rehabilitation and Neuropsychological Service, Richmond, VA, (undated).

[41] M. Picard, D. Scarisbrick, R. Paluck. *HELPS.* New York: Comprehensive Regional TBI Rehabilitation Center (1991).

[42] Mild Traumatic Brain Injury Committee of the Head Injury Interdisciplinary Special Interest Group of the American Congress of Rehabilitation Medicine. Definition of mild brain injury. *J Head Trauma Rehabil* **8** (1993), 86-87.

[43] W.A. Gordon, M. Brown, M. Sliwinski, et al. The enigma of "hidden" traumatic brain injury. *J Head Trauma Rehabil* **13** (1998), 39-56.

[44] M.P. Jaffe, J. O'Neill, D. Vandergoot, W.A. Gordon, B. Small. The unveiling of traumatic brain injury in an HIV/AIDS population. *Brain Injury* **14** (2000), 35-44.

[45] W.A. Gordon, L. Haddad, M. Brown, M.R. Hibbard, M. Sliwinski. The sensitivity and specificity of self-reported symptoms in individuals with traumatic brain injury. *Brain Injury* **14** (2000), 21-33.

[46] J.B. Cantor, W.A. Gordon., & T.A. Ashman. Screening for brain injury in schoolchildren [abstract]. *Journal of Head Trauma Rehabilitation* **21** (2006), 424.

Coping with Blast-Related Traumatic Brain Injury in Returning Troops   39
B.K. Wiederhold (Ed.)
IOS Press, 2011
© 2011 The authors and IOS Press. All rights reserved.
doi: 10.3233/978-1-60750-797-0-39

Deployment-Related Brain Injuries: Neurobiology and Clinical Management

Katherine H. TABER[a,1] and Robin A. HURLEY[b]

[a] *VISN 6 Mental Illness Research, Education and Clinical Center, W.G. Hefner VAMC Salisbury NC, Virginia College of Osteopathic Medicine Blacksburg VA*
[b] *VISN 6 Mental Illness Research, Education and Clinical Center, W.G. Hefner VAMC Salisbury NC, Wake Forest University School of Medicine Winston-Salem NC*

Abstract. Traumatic Brain Injury (TBI) is a common occurrence of modern warfare. It can be accompanied by multiple co-morbidities including Posttraumatic Stress Disorder (PTSD) and chronic pain. Most brain injuries are mild with complete recovery. However, residual symptoms may remain in some cases, making post-injury adjustment challenging. A thorough understanding of the physics of injury mechanisms, knowledge of neuroanatomy and pathways, and available assessment tools is necessary for optimal clinical management of a brain-injured patient. Clinical treatment guidelines and consensus findings are now available to assist the clinician in caring for these complex patients.

Keywords. neuropsychiatry, neuroanatomy, brain injury, Veteran, Posttraumatic Stress Disorder, chronic pain

Author notes: The views expressed in this paper are those of the authors and do not reflect the official policy of the Veterans Health Administration or United States Government.

Introduction

Traumatic brain injury (TBI) has been labeled a "signature" injury of the current wars in Afghanistan and Iraq. Current evidence indicates that many Veterans have experienced one or more brain injuries during deployment. Although the vast majority of individuals who experience a mild TBI attain a complete recovery, some will have residual cognitive or emotional symptoms. These symptoms can affect adjustment to civilian life and family relationships. This is particularly challenging if multiple conditions are present. Posttraumatic Stress Disorder (PTSD), substance misuse, depression, and chronic pain are commonly reported after return from service and can occur as co-morbidities to TBI. Clinical practices guidelines (CPGs) and expert consensus summaries are available to guide clinical management of these complex cases. The Veteran Health Administration's (VA's) unique Polytrauma System of Care, treatment guidelines for mild TBI and Consensus findings are setting new medical practice standards for screening and assessment of mild TBI in large populations.

---

[1] Corresponding Author. Katherine H. Taber, W.G. Hefner VAMC, 1601 Brenner Ave, Salisbury North Carolina, USA 28144; E-mail: katherine.taber@va.gov.

1. Brain Injury Basics

A TBI occurs when an external force physically disturbs the brain sufficiently to cause at least an alteration in consciousness. TBI severity is defined primarily by the nature and duration of changes in cognition experienced by the patient at the time of injury and shortly thereafter. The joint VA/Department of Defense (DoD) CPG classification scheme, which is based on the American College of Rehabilitation Medicine (ACRM) definitions, is summarized in Table 1 [1]. Note that the presence/absence or duration of each type of symptom defines the severity level. Key symptoms indicating a TBI are: a period of loss of consciousness or alteration in consciousness (e.g., confusion, disorientation); loss of memory (amnesia) for events immediately before or after the injury; neurological deficits (e.g., weakness, loss of balance, change in vision); intracranial lesion.

Table 1. Veterans Health Administration/ Department of Defense Severity Classification for Traumatic Brain Injury (adapted from [1]).

Symptoms	Mild	Moderate	Severe
Alteration of consciousness	Instant to 24 hours	> 24 hours	> 24 hours
Loss of consciousness	0 to 30 minutes	> 30 minutes but < 24 hours	> 24 hours
Amnesia	0 to 1 day	> 1 day but < 7 days	> 7 days
Structural imaging	Normal	Normal or abnormal	Normal or abnormal

Forces sufficient to injure the brain can come from many sources. These include rapid acceleration or deceleration, rotation, blunt trauma, and impact trauma, with rotational acceleration causing the greatest shear stress. The forces present following an explosion (blast) are more complex. An explosion generates a pressure wave (shockwave), an electromagnetic field, loud sound, chemical fumes, and heat [2-8]. These forces can potentially interact with objects (including people) both externally and internally in multiple ways, some of which may result in brain injury. If sufficiently strong, the wind evoked by the changes in pressure can put both objects and people into motion. There is no question that objects put in motion by the blast wind can impact people with sufficient force to injure the brain (secondary blast injury). Similarly, when people are put in motion by the blast wind the impact when they come to an abrupt halt can injure the brain (tertiary blast injury). Other conditions generated by the explosion (e.g., heat, chemical fumes) might also injure the brain (quaternary blast injury).

1.1. Most Common Types of Injury

Both diffuse and focal injuries can occur in TBI [2,9,8]. Diffuse axonal injury (DAI), injury to the fibers (axons) that form the connections (white matter) within the brain, is the most common type of injury to occur in nonpenetrating TBI. When physical forces (e.g., shearing, stretching, angular, rotational) pull on axons they are not usually sufficient to cause rupture. Rather, this stretching of the cell membrane triggers events that may eventually lead to rupture. The areas where this type of injury is most likely to occur (Figure 1, left) are places in which the material properties of the brain change abruptly, as happens at the junction between the cortical gray matter (which is softer)

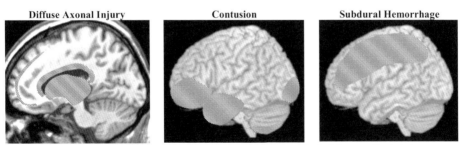

Figure 1. The most common locations for particular types of brain injury are illustrated.

and the underlying white matter (which is quite firm). The frontal and temporal areas of cortex are particularly vulnerable. Areas of highly compacted white matter, such as the corpus callosum and internal capsule, are also more vulnerable. Other common locations for DAI are the deep gray matter and upper brainstem. Areas of injury are usually quite small, and therefore much better visualized by magnetic resonance imaging (MRI) than computed tomography (CT). Gradient echo MR images are the most sensitive to small areas of hemorrhage. If the brain moves sufficiently within the skull to impact bone, a contusion (bruise) may result. The most vulnerable areas (Figure 1, middle) are the undersurfaces of the frontal and temporal lobes. The occipital poles or cerebellum are less often involved. The imaging appearance varies because contusions can contain both edema and hemorrhage. Delayed or progressive hemorrhage is common (~25%) over the initial 48 hours. Movement of the brain within the skull can also tear the veins that bridge from the brain surface to the dural venous sinus, causing a traumatic subdural hemorrhage, most commonly located over the frontal and parietal convexities (Figure 1, right). The preferred imaging modality for this type of hemorrhage is CT. Brain injury can be a dynamic, ongoing process, due to injury cascades (e.g., excitotoxicity, neuroinflammation, oxidative stress) set in motion by the initial injury [8-10]. These can, in turn, lead to the development of secondary injuries (e.g., hypoxia, ischemia).

Visualization of areas of TBI, particularly when the TBI is mild, can be quite challenging [11-13]. As noted above, DAI is the most likely injury to occur in mild TBI. Although clinical MRI is more sensitive than CT in detecting this type of brain injury, even MRI is often negative, particularly in the chronic stage. Functional imaging (e.g., cerebral blood flow, cerebral metabolic rate) may be considerably more sensitive to the presence of TBI than structural imaging. Newer methods of MRI, such as diffusion tensor imaging (DTI), are showing promise for identifying small areas of white matter injury [14-18]. This is important, because such injuries may have devastating functional consequences. Knowledge of the major white matter tracts and the brain areas they interconnect is thus critical for understanding clinical symptoms in the context of TBI [19]. A brief summary is presented in Table 2 of the major association pathways (tracts that connect areas of cortex within a hemisphere). Equally important are the commissural pathways (tracts that connect areas of cortex in one hemisphere with areas in the other hemisphere) and pathways that connect areas of the cortex with subcortical structures.

1.2. Primary Blast Injury

Whether and how the pressure wave generated by the explosion (primary blast forces) injures the brain is a subject for intensive study. Multiple mechanisms by which pressure waves might cause brain injury have been proposed [3-8]. Computer modeling suggests that direct transmission of the pressure wave could produce tissue injury by inducing skull flexure as well as shear stresses, spallation and/or cavitation within the brain [20-24]. Large stresses within the skull may also, through piezoelectric effects, generate electromagnetic fields of sufficient intensity to evoke neurological effects [25]. Indirect modes of injury have also been proposed, such as the formation of gas emboli in the bloodstream that could cause infarction. Transmission of forces from the body into the brain, perhaps via the vasculature, may also occur. Establishment of animal models for studying primary blast exposure is challenging due to the complexity of factors that may influence results (e.g., method of producing blast forces, blast intensity, species, body position relative to explosion, use of protective equipment). However, initial studies in various animal models suggest that the brain is vulnerable to primary blast forces [26-31].

Although still quite limited, there is also a growing clinical literature supporting the vulnerability of the brain to primary blast forces [16-18,32]. In two recent case reports in Operation Enduring Freedom (OEF) and Operation Iraqi Freedom (OIF) veterans, clinically significant symptoms have been documented a considerable time (7-8 months, 3 years) after exposures that appeared to involve only primary blast [16,17]. A study of OIF veterans (n=12) with remote history (2-5 years after the last occurrence) of multiple (3-51) blast exposures found subtle deficits on neurobehavioral testing and areas of decreased metabolism on positron emission tomography (PET) imaging compared to healthy civilians [32]. A study of TBI in OEF/OIF veterans (n=9) in which exposure to explosions was a major injury mechanism reported reduced EEG phase synchrony in lateral frontal sites that correlated with DTI-based measures of frontal white matter integrity but was not associated with neurobehavioral deficits [18]. Studies in civilians of more serious blast exposures indicate that these injuries clearly evolve over time. A case report of probable primary blast injury noted that mental status was normal on initial examination, but declined precipitously shortly thereafter [33]. A minimally depressed linear petrose bone fracture, mild cerebral edema, and intracranial hemorrhage (epidural and subarachnoid) were present on CT. A retrospective case series of blast injury in civilians reported a similar pattern of initially normal mental status that later declined [34]. Of note, several patients with negative admission CT developed imaging findings indicative of TBI within 48 hours. Another study documented development of a hyperinflammatory state associated with blast exposure [35].

Table 2. Summary of major long tracts connecting cortical areas within each hemisphere (adapted from [19])

Pathway	Areas Connected	Common Functional Deficits
Superior longitudinal fasciculus 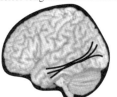	Long fibers (medial) connect lateral Frontal to dorsolateral Parietal, Temporal & Occipital cortex Short fibers (lateral) connect Frontal to Parietal, Parietal to Occipital, Parietal to Temporal cortex	Left injury- conduction aphasia; ideational apraxia; depression; anomia; Right injury- left hemispatial neglect
Inferior longitudinal fasciculus 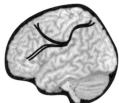	Long fibers connect Temporal to Lingula, Cuneus, Occipital cortex Short fibers connect Temporal to Temporal, Occipital to Occipital, Occipital to Parietal cortex	Disruption of information transfer between visual and limbic/memory areas; impaired visual recent memory; visual object agnosia; contralateral visual field hemiachromatopsia; Bilateral injury-prosphagnosia; Left injury- alexia; tactoverbal dysfunction; Right injury- visual hypoemotionality
Superior fronto-occipital fasciculus 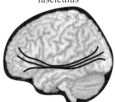	Dorsolateral Prefrontal to superior Parietal cortex; (classic Occipital & Temporal connections now in question)	Left injury- akinetic mutism; disordered initiation & preparation of speech movements; transcortical motor aphasia; anomia & reduction in spontaneous speech with normal articulation
Inferior fronto-occipital fasciculus 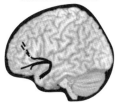	Dorsolateral & ventrolateral Prefrontal to Posterior Temporal & Occipital cortex; (classic Occipital connections now in question)	Seldom injured alone; based on anatomy, injury might cause visuospatial abnormalities; visual recognition abnormalities; topographagnosia
Uncinate fasciculus 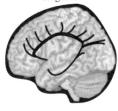	Orbital & inferior Frontal to Temporal Pole, Uncus, Hippocampus & Amygdala	Important for retrieval of past information; Left injury- impaired retrieval of general knowledge of facts; Right injury- impaired retrieval of episodic (autobiographical) memory
Cingulum	Long fibers connect subgenual Frontal cortex & Paraolfactory area to Uncus & Parahippocampal gyrus Short fibers interconnect portions of Frontal, Parietal & Temporal cortex	Lesion/deficit literature provides no way to distinguish between injury to the Cingulum and injury its cortex; Anterior injury: lack of emotional response to pain; depression; anxiety; akinetic mutism; impaired saccades; Posterior injury: Left- loss of verbal memory; blurring of right sides of objects; Right- loss of memory for spatial relationships; topographical disorientation

2. Deployment Related TBI

There is increasing evidence that TBI is a relatively frequent occurrence in the current conflicts [36]. It is becoming clear that OEF/OIF wounding patterns and mechanisms of injury are different from previous conflicts [37]. Among other changes, there are fewer thoracic injuries (OEF/OIF 5.9%, Vietnam 13.4%, World War II 13.9%) and more injuries to the head and neck region (OEF/OIF 30.0%, Vietnam 16.0%, World War II 21.0%). The widespread use of Kevlar armor has been cited as an important factor (38). Changes to injury mechanisms include fewer gunshot wounds (OEF/OIF 19%, Vietnam 35%, World War II 27%) and more explosion-related injuries (OEF/OIF 81%, Vietnam 65%, World War II 73%) [37]. Studies indicate that the majority (75-97%) of injuries treated at forward deployed medical facilities involved exposure to explosions (e.g., improvised explosive device [IED], grenade, rocket-propelled grenade [RPG], mortar) [39-41]. Several studies have utilized the Expeditionary Medical Encounter Database (EMED, previously name Navy-Marine Corps Combat Trauma Registry) to study combat-related TBI [41-44]. One reported that at least 16% of those receiving treatment met criteria for TBI based on retrospective review of the clinical records [41]. The mechanism of injury was explosion-related in 92% of these TBI cases compared to 75% overall. Two found that 88-96% of combat-related TBIs involved exposure to explosions [42,43]. Another reported that TBI occurred in 37% of blast-related combat injuries [44]. All of the EMED studies that reported severity indicated that most (68-89%) were mild TBIs. An early study of soldiers at Walter Reed Army Medical Center who were injured by an explosion while deployed found that almost 60% had a TBI (44% mild) [38]. A recent study of hospitalizations involving deployment-related TBI reported that overall 51% were battle-related, and more than 65% of the more serious injuries involved explosions [45]. These studies support the view that TBI, particularly mild TBI, is a common type of injury during deployment. However, they provide only part of the picture as all are based on military personnel receiving medical care.

It is challenging to determine the overall rate of deployment-related TBI, as this requires capturing information about all military personnel. The present "gold standard," a full assessment by an experienced TBI clinician, is not practical on such a large scale. Published estimates have commonly been based on brief screening questions, sometimes followed by a clinical assessment. Several studies have reported on TBI screening of specific military populations (e.g., Brigade) soon after return from deployment [46-50]. Reported rates ranged from 9.0-15.8% (brief screen alone) to 22.8% (confirmed by clinical interview). A similar rate of 19.5% (brief screen alone) was found by the single population-based survey [51]. Several studies including an assessment of TBI severity reported that the majority (59 - 70%) were mild TBI (concussion) as indicated by alteration of consciousness (e.g., dazed, confused) rather than a loss of consciousness or post-traumatic amnesia [46-48,50,52]. One study assessed common post-concussion symptoms at the time of injury (retrospective self-report) and found a much greater rate of symptoms (65% versus 9%) in those whose injuries included TBI [48]. Reporting of symptoms was lower in both groups by return from deployment.

Studies in VA patient populations capture symptom reporting at a much later time after return from deployment. The largest study to date (n=13,201) reported that 17% were positive on the VA's brief TBI screen, indicating a probable historic TBI while deployed and possible persistent post-concussive symptoms (PPCS) [53]. Veterans that screen positive are referred for a full evaluation by experienced clinicians as part of the VA's polytrauma program. Reports indicate that 67-85% are confirmed to have TBI [54,55]. In veterans with injury to more than one area (polytrauma), mild TBI, chronic pain, and PTSD often occur together (polytrauma clinical triad) [55]. Similar findings have been reported in combat-injured service members receiving inpatient care at a VA Polytrauma Rehabilitation Center [56,57]. All had issues related to pain (headache 52%, musculoskeletal 48%, neuropathic 14%, other 23%), almost all (97%) had a TBI, and many had issues related to mental health (symptoms of depression 36% PTSD 35%). The presence of psychiatric illness (e.g., PTSD, depression) and physical conditions (e.g., chronic pain) with symptom domains that overlap with TBI complicates both symptom attribution and clinical care [58-60].

3. Clinical Management

Although the vast majority of individuals who experience a mild TBI attain a complete recovery, some will have longer term symptoms (i.e. cognitive and/or emotional) [61-63]. Such symptoms can affect adjustment to civilian life and family relationships. This is particular challenging if multiple conditions are present. Presence of other conditions in addition to TBI also increases the risk of suicide [64]. Co-morbid conditions can also influence symptom presentation and so must be considered in both research studies and clinical treatment [65-67]. At this time neuropsychological testing cannot reliably discriminate between mild TBI and PTSD, nor can it be used to differentiate the effects of blast-induced from other causes of TBI [68-70]. It is quite useful for identifying cognitive strengths and weaknesses. Strengths can be capitalized upon by clinicians providing interventions and weaknesses can be targets for remediation. Expert consensus and CPGs are available to guide clinical management of these complex cases [8,71]. A multidisciplinary integrated approach to assessment and treatment, as presented in the joint VA/DoD CPG for mild TBI, is encouraged [1].

There is not sufficient evidenced-based literature to fully guide assessment and treatment of these complex cases [72]. Recently, the National Center for PTSD convened a consensus conference of experts in this area to address this need. A summary of their recommendations has been posted on the National Center for PTSD website (http://www.ptsd.va.gov/professional/pages/traumatic-brain-injury-ptsd.asp). In general, the Conference Panel recommended that providers follow the current CPG for each of the diagnoses for treatment of particular symptoms. If contraindications or problems arise, adjust accordingly. Key recommendations include: (1) provide education to the patient and family on all diagnoses and prognoses; (2) develop a comprehensive treatment plan that includes measuring and monitoring for success (3) maintain full access to treatment teams so that all conditions are addressed simultaneously (e.g. do not wait to treat TBI until PTSD is treated or vice versa); (4) have a coordinated care team that included all disciplines necessary to provide a comprehensive treatment experience for the patient (e.g. PT, OT, cognitive rehabilitation, PTSD cognitive behavioral therapy). Refer to best practice models or consult the expert polytrauma centers when needed. There are no currently FDA-approved medications for the long-term treatment of psychiatric symptoms due to brain injury [73,74]. Opinions of experts in the field suggest that clinicians follow the guidelines for other neuropsychiatric populations with "organic" brain injuries, as detailed in the CPG. Areas to be particularly mindful of include observation/ evaluation for "partial responders" and need to adjust medications, avoidance when possible of polypharmacy or giving contradictory medications from a neurotransmitter view (i.e. agent that enhances dopamine and another that inhibits), as well as discontinuing medications that are not working.

References

[1]   Management of Concussion/mTBI Working Group, VA/DoD Clinical Practice Guideline for Management of Concussion/Mild Traumatic Brain Injury. *J Rehabil Res Dev* **46** (2009) CP1-CP68.

[2]   K.H. Taber, Blast-related traumatic brain injury: what is known? *J Neuropsychiatry Clin Neurosci* **18** (2006) 141-145.

[3]   D.F. Moore, Blast physics and central nervous system injury. *Future Neurology* **3** (2008) 243-250.

[4]   S.J. Wolf, Blast injuries. *Lancet* **374** (2009) 405-415.

[5]   G.A. Elder, Blast-induced mild traumatic brain injury. *Psychiatr Clin North Am* **33** (2010) 757-781.

[6]   R.R. Hicks, Neurological effects of blast injury. *J Trauma* **68** (2010) 1257-1263.

[7]   I. Cernak, Traumatic brain injury: an overview of pathobiology with emphasis on military populations. *J Cereb Blood Flow Metab* **30** (2010) 255-266.

[8]   T.W. McAllister, Effects of psychological and biomechanical trauma on brain and behavior. *Ann NY Acad Sci* **1208** (2010) 46-57.

[9]   T.M.J.C. Andriessen, Clinical characteristics and pathophysiological mechanisms of focal and diffuse traumatic brain injury. *J Cell Mol Med* **14** (2010) 2381-2392.

[10]   B.J. Zink, Emerging concepts in the pathophysiology of traumatic brain injury. *Psychiatr Clin North Am* **33** (2010) 741-756.

[11]   H.G. Belanger, Recent neuroimaging techniques in mild traumatic brain injury. *J Neurospychiatry Clin Neurosci* **19** (2007) 5-20.

[12]   T.H. Le, Neuroimaging of traumatic brain injury. *Mt Sinai J Med* **76** (2009) 145-162.

[13]   R.W. Van Boven, Advances in neuroimaging of traumatic brain injury and posttraumatic stress disorder. *J Rehabil Res Dev* **46** (2009) 717-756.

[14]   D.R. Rutgers, White matter abnormalities in mild traumatic brain injury: A diffusion tensor imaging study. *AJNR AM J Neuroadiol* **29** (2008) 514-519.

[15]   M. Huang, Integrated imaging approach with MEG and DTI to detect mild traumatic brain injury in military and civilian patients. *J Neurotrauma* **26** (2009) 1213-1226.

[16]   A. Rosen, Radiology corner. Case 41. Arcuate fasciculus damage seen on DTI in a blast-exposed soldier with mild traumatic brain injury (mTBI) with associated conduction aphasia. *Mil Med* **174** (2009) v-vi.

[17]   D.L. Warden, Case report of a soldier with primary blast brain injury. *Neuroimage* **47** (2009) T152-T153.

[18]   S.R. Sponheim, Evidence of disrupted functional connectivity in the brain after combat-related blast injury. *Neuroimage* **54** (2011) S21-S29.

[19]   K.H.Taber, Traumatic axonal injury: atlas of major pathways. *J Neuropsychiatry Clin Neurosci* **19** (2007) 100-104.

[20]   D.F. Moore, Computational biology - Modeling of primary blast effects on the central nervous system. *Neuroimage* **47** (2009) T10-T20.

[21]   W.C. Moss, Skull flexure from blast waves: a mechanism for brain injury with implications for helmet design. *Phys Rev Lett* **103** (2009) 108702.

[22]   P.A. Taylor, Simulation of blast-induced early-time intracranial wave physics leading to traumatic brain injury. *J Biomech Eng* **131** (2009) 061007.

[23]   M.S. Chafi, Biomechanical assessment of brain dynamic responses due to blast pressure waves. *Ann Biomed Eng* **38** (2010) 490-504.

[24]   M.D. Alley, Experimental modeling of explosive blast-related traumatic brain injuries. *Neuroimage* **54** (2011) S45-S54.

[25]   K.Y.K. Lee, Blast-induced electromagnetic fields in the brain from bone piezoelectricity. *Neuroimage* **54** (2011) S30-S36.

[26]   R.A. Bauman, An introductory characterization of a combat-casualty-care relevant swine model of closed head injury resulting from exposure to explosive blast. *J Neurotrauma* **26** (2009) 841-860.

[27]   S.I. Svetlov, Morphologic and biochemical characterization of blast injury in a model of controlled blast overpressure exposure. *J Trauma* **69** (2010) 795-804.

[28]   I. Cernak, The pathobiology of blast injuries and blast-induced neurotrauma as identified using a new experimental model of injury in mice. *Neurobio Dis* **41** (2011) 538-551.
[29]   A.D. Leonardi, Intracranial pressure increases during exposure to a shock wave. *J Neurotrauma* **28** (2011) 85-94.
[30]   M. Risling, Mechanisms of blast induced brain injuries, experimental studies in rats. *Neuroimage* **54** (2011) S89-S97.
[31]   A. Saljo, Mechanisms and pathophysiology of the low-level blast brain injury in animal models. *Neuroimage* **54** (2011) S83-S88.
[32]   E.R. Peskind, Cerebrocerebellar hypometabolism associated with repetitive blast exposure mild traumatic brain injury in 12 Iraq war Veterans with persistent post-concussive symptoms. *Neuroimage* **54** (2011) S76-S82.
[33]   S. Yilmaz, An unusual primary blast injury. Traumatic brain injury due to primary blast injury. *Am J Emerg Med* **25** (2007) 97-98.
[34]   G.V. Bochicchio, Blast injury in a civilian trauma setting is associated with a delay in diagnosis of traumatic brain injury. *Am Surg* **74** (2008) 267-270.
[35]   Y. Kluger, The quinary pattern of blast injury. *Am J Disaster Med* **2** (2007) 21-25.
[36]   K.H. Taber, OEF/OIF deployment-related traumatic brain injury. *PTSD Research Quarterly* **21** (2010) 1-7.
[37]   B.D. Owens, Combat wounds in Operation Iraqi Freedom and Operation Enduring Freedom. *J Trauma* **64** (2008) 295-299.
[38]   S. Okie, Traumatic brain injury in the war zone. *N Engl J Med* **352** (2005) 2043-2047.
[39]   J.S. Gondusky, Protecting military convoys in Iraq: an examination of battle injuries sustained by a Mechanized Battalion during Operation Iraqi Freedom II. *Mil Med* **170** (2005) 546-549.
[40]   R.T. Gerhardt, Out-of-hospital combat casualty care in the current war in Iraq. *Ann Emerg Med* **53** (2009) 169-174.
[41]   A.J. MacGregor, Prevalence and psychological correlates of traumatic brain injury in Operation Iraqi Freedom. *J Head Trauma Rehabil* **25** (2010) 1-8.
[42]   M.R. Galarneau, Traumatic brain injury during Operation Iraqi Freedom: findings from the United States Navy-Marine Corps Combat Trauma Registry. *J Neurosurg* **108** (2008) 950-957.
[43]   A.J. MacGregor, Injury-specific correlates of combat-related traumatic brain injury in Operation Iraqi Freedom. *J Head Trauma Rehabil* (in press)
[44]   A.L. Dougherty, Visual dysfunction following blast-related traumatic brain injury from the battlefield. *Brain Inj* **25** (2011) 8-13.
[45]   B.E. Wojcik, Traumatic brain injury hospitalizations of U.S. army soldiers deployed to Afghanistan and Iraq. *Am J Prev Med* **38** (2010) S108-S116.
[46]   K.A. Schwab, Screening for traumatic brain injury in troops returning from deployment in Afghanistan and Iraq: Initial investigation of the usefulness of a short screening tool for traumatic brain injury. *J Head Trauma Rehabil* **22** (2007) 377-389.
[47]   C.W. Hoge, Mild traumatic brain injury in U.S. soldiers returning from Iraq. *N Engl J Med* **358** (2008) 453-463.
[48]   H. Terrio, Traumatic brain injury screening: Preliminary findings in a US Army Brigade Combat Team. *J Head Trauma Rehabil* **24** (2009) 14-23.
[49]   A.I. Drake, Routine TBI screening following combat deployments. *NeuroRehabilitation* **26** (2010) 183-189.
[50]   J.E. Wilk, Mild traumatic brain injury (concussion) during combat: lack of association of blast mechanism with persistent postconcussive symptoms. *J Head Trauma Rehabil* **25** (2010) 9-14.
[51]   T.L. Schell, Survey of individuals previously deployed for OEF/OIF. *Invisible wounds of war: psychological and cognitive injuries, their consequences, and services to assist recovery*, RAND Center for Military Health Policy Research, Santa Monica, 2008.
[52]   A.I. Schneiderman, Understanding sequelae of injury mechanisms and mild traumatic brain injury incurred during the conflicts in Iraq and Afghanistan: Persistent postconcussive symptoms and posttraumatic stress disorder. *Am J Epidemiol* **167** (2008) 1446-1452.
[53]   K.F. Carlson, Psychiatric diagnoses among Iraq and Afghanistan war veterans screened for deployment-related traumatic brain injury. *J Trauma Stress* **23** (2010) 17-24.
[54]   J.J. Hill, Separating deployment-related traumatic brain injury and posttraumatic stress disorder in veterans: preliminary findings from the Veterans Affairs traumatic brain injury screening program. *Am J Phys Med Rehabil* **88** (2009) 605-614.
[55]   H.L. Lew, Prevalence of chronic pain, posttraumatic stress disorder, and persistent postconcussive symptoms in OIF/OEF veterans: polytrauma clinical triad. *J Rehabil Res Dev* **46** (2009) 697-702.
[56]   N.A. Sayer, Characteristics and rehabilitation outcomes among patients with blast and other injuries sustained during the Global War on Terror. *Arch Phys Med Rehabil* **89** (2008) 163-170.

[57] N.A. Sayer, Rehabilitation needs of combat-injured service members admitted to the VA Polytrauma Rehabilitation Centers: The role of PM&R in the care of wounded warriors. *PM&R* **1** (2009) 23-28.
[58] L.A. Brenner, Assessment and diagnosis of mild traumatic brain injury, posttraumatic stress disorder, and other polytrauma conditions: burden of adversity hypothesis. *Rehabil Psychol* **54** (2009) 239-246.
[59] L.L.S. Howe, Giving context to post-deployment post-concussive-like symptoms: blast-related potential mild traumatic brain injury and comorbidities. *Clin Neuropsychol* **23** (2009) 1315-1337.
[60] G.L. Iverson, Challenges associated with post-deployment screening for mild traumatic brain injury in military personnel. *Clin Neuropsychol* **23** (2009) 1299-1314.
[61] R.D. Vanderploeg, Long-term neuropsychological outcomes following mild taumatic brain injury. *J Int Neuropsychol Soc* **11** (2005) 228-236.
[62] R.D. Vanderploeg, Long-term morbidities following self-reported mild traumatic brain injury. *J Clin Exp Neuropsychol* **29** (2007) 585-598.
[63] R.A. Bryant, The psychiatric sequelae of traumatic injury. *Am J Psychiat* **167** (2010) 312-320.
[64] L.A. Brenner, Suicidality and veterans with a history of traumatic brain injury: precipitating events, protective factors, and prevention strategies. *Rehabil Psychol* **54** (2009) 390-397.
[65] J.F. Benge, Postconcussive symptoms in OEF-OIF veterans: factor structure and impact of posttraumatic stress. *Rehabil Psychol* **54** (2009) 270-278.
[66] N.A. Sayer, Veterans with history of mild traumatic brain injury and posttraumatic stress disorder: challenges from provider perspective. *J Rehabil Res Dev* **46** (2009) 703-716.
[67] M.A. Sandberg, Beyond diagnosis: Understanding the healthcare challenges of injured veterans through application of the International Classification of Functioning, Disability and Health (ICF). *Clin Neuropsychol* **23** (2009) 1416-1232.
[68] H.G. Belanger, Cognitive sequelae of blast-related versus other mechanisms of brain trauma. *J Int Neuropsychol Soc* **15** (2009) 1-8.
[69] L.A. Brenner, An exploratory study of neuroimaging, neurologic, and neuropsychological findings in veterans with traumatic brain injury and/or posttraumatic stress disorder. *Mil Med* **174** (2009) 347-352.
[70] L.A. Brenner, Neuropsychological test performance in soldiers with blast-related mild TBI. *Neuropsychology* **24** (2010) 160-167.
[71] L.M. French, Military traumatic brain injury: an examination of important differences. *Ann NY Acad Sci* **1208** (2010) 38-45.
[72] K.F. Carlson, Prevalence, assessment, and treatment of mild traumatic brain injury and posttraumatic stress disorder: a systematic review of the evidence. *J Head Trauma Rehabil* (in press).
[73] T.W. McAllister, Psychopharmacological issues in the treatment of TBI and PTSD. *Clin Neuropsychol* **23** (2009) 1338-1367.
[74] B.W. Writer, Psychopharmacological treatment for cognitive impairment in survivors of traumatic brain injury: a critical review. *J Neuropsychiatry Clin Neurosci* **21** (2009) 362-370.

B.K. Wiederhold (Ed.)
IOS Press, 2011
doi: 10.3233/978-1-60750-797-0-49

Do Persistent Postconcussive Symptoms Exist? Evidence from Epidemiological and Laboratory Studies

James L. SPIRA [a,1]

[a] *National Center for PTSD, Department of Veterans Affairs*

Abstract. There is little doubt as to the existence of persistent post concussive symptoms (PPCSx) more than three months post concussion. However, much controversy exists as to the cause of such persistent symptoms, with some claiming that they are not directly due to concussion per se, but instead from psychological disorders such as Posttraumatic Stress Disorder (PTSD) and depression. Data from 12,000 recently deployed service members reveal that the strongest predictor of PPCSx is indeed PTSD and depression. However, a subset of service members complaining of PPCSx cannot be explained by psychological variables. Additional research revealed that post-deployment service members with PTSD who also suffered from concussion had greater autonomic dysregulation than those with PTSD alone. Together, this research suggests that it is preliminary to discount the possibility that a subset of those complaining of PPCSx have persistent problems due exclusively to PTSD and depression.

Keywords. Posttraumatic Stress Disorder, trauma, mild Traumatic Brain Injury, military, combat

Mild Traumatic Brain Injury (mTBI) has been called the signature wound of the War on Terror (WOT). Due to traditional and innovative explosive devices utilized by modern insurgency, and at the same time improved protection worn by military forces, these factors mean that explosions that once put a soldier out of commission now permit those affected by a blast to more rapidly recover and continue in battle. However, concussion research indicates that subtle neurological dysfunction occurs that is undetected by traditional structural imaging and often goes unnoticed by a cursory examination by non-specialists, or even the concussed person themselves. However, functional imaging and in-depth neuropsychological examination can detect post-concussive impairment in some cases, especially when there have been multiple concussions, or when the subject is asked to perform tasks under increased cognitive and physiological load. There are also indications that concussion due to blast waves may disrupt neurological functioning in a manner different than traditional strikes to the head, and with more diffuse and non-specific neuro-cognitive and somatic effects. The difficulty with diagnosing concussion, along with a reluctance to report and record concussive events in a war zone, result in poor metrics on the real number of those concussed in the field, with estimates ranging from 10-30% of those deployed. However, there may also be a bias against putting resources into an effort to better understand the number of concussed warfighters, since it is believed that the ill effects of concussion wear off within a few hours to a few days. However, such a view may be based on a naive understanding of concussion, since Diffusion Tensor Imaging

---

[1] Corresponding Author: James L. Spira, National Center for PTSD, Department of Veterans Affairs, United States; E-mail: James.Spira@va.gov.

(DTI) and other functional assessments have shown lingering neurological alterations beyond the time that examination and self-report suggest that the concussed person has recovered. In fact, a subsequent concussion, even months later, can lead to far worse effects and longer recovery than would be expected from a single concussion. In addition, although those suffering a concussion may appear to have recovered (to both themselves, as well as their examiners), concussed persons can often temporarily rally their cognitive effort and ignore somatic symptoms in order to complete a task, especially when they are motivated to do so (as in professional sports or military engagement). However, such persons may falter when stressed cognitively (multitasking) and physically (sleep deprivation, heat exposure, exercise) – factors they will face when returning to their normal duties.

Lingering symptoms commonly reported by those with moderate to severe brain injury include cognitive dysfunction, emotional dysregulation, somatic complaints, and behavioral alterations. Those who experienced concussion during combat deployment have reported post-concussive symptoms at record levels. Those who believe that the ill effects of concussion, if they exist at all, resolve completely within hours, days, or at the most, weeks, claim that such symptom reporting is due to psychological problems associated with the stress of combat.

Based on a survey of 384 soldiers with likely concussion versus 435 with other pain, Hoge and colleagues [1] report that soldiers with concussion were significantly more likely to report poor general health, missed workdays, medical visits, and a high number of somatic and post-concussive symptoms than were soldiers with other injuries. They found that Posttraumatic Stress Disorder (PTSD) and depression mediate this effect. Following this report, Hoge and others have argued that treating PPCSx six months following concussion is potentially iatrogenic, worrying and misleading patients unnecessarily, and that it is best to treat the psychological symptoms only [2].

However, this result is based on a covariate analysis of the group, and while the findings reflect a finding for a majority of patients, it may not have picked up a potential minority that may have persistent post-concussive symptoms (PPCSx) not due to psychological factors. Indeed, there are also those who claim that symptoms due to concussion can last many months, and perhaps never completely resolve. This may be a novel situation due to the repeated head trauma that warfighters experience not only from blasts caused by insurgents, but from hitting their head on the ceiling of their vehicle on a daily basis going over large pot holes (and not wearing seat belts), rushing into a room after throwing percussion grenades, and other events that cause multiple stresses to the brain.

Much of this controversy may be due to the similarity in symptoms categories shared by both PTSD and complaints following brain injury. And although a thorough clinical interview can often tease these apart, most questionnaires and non-specialist interviews are unable to do so. Further, there may be a large comorbidity between those complaining of mTBI and those who have developed PTSD. In fact, it may be that concussion reduces the threshold for developing PTSD, depression, and anxiety.

Thus, there has been a great deal of interest in predictors of post-concussive syndrome in order to determine if such complaints months after the index event are purely due to psychological distress or if there is some neurological basis for such complaints. Determining if there is a neurological basis for such complaints is paramount, since consensus reports based on research and practice in patients who suffered a TBI indicate that they improve their functioning much faster and improve their chances for full recovery if they undergo a comprehensive cognitive rehabilitation within months after the trauma. Therefore, if PPCSx truly exist, to only treat their psychological symptoms without a neurocogntive component, and without protecting them from further concussion, may put them at increased risk and reduce their chances of a rapid recovery.

In an attempt to address the question of what predicts PPCSx between six months and a year following deployment, we analyzed data from the U.S. Department of Defense Survey of Health Related Behaviors Among Active Duty Military Personnel (HRB survey). A random sample of 64 military installations worldwide was selected, resulting in 24,690 military personnel across all branches of service, achieving a 70% response rate. Responses were anonymous (in contrast to the PHDA). This study reports on the 13,097 personnel with completed surveys that reported one or more combat deployment since September 11, 2001. Out of these, about 32% had blast exposure, and about 33% of those had neurological sequelae s/p blast (10.7% of the total combat deployed population sampled). Neurological sequelae and postconcussive symptoms were taken from the Postdeployment Health Assessment questions (PDHA). PTSD was assessed from the PTSD Checklist, military version (PCL-m), and depression from a DSM-based depression screen. Service members were asked about PPCSx during and immediately after their last deployment, and also during the last week (6-12 months post combat deployment). Regression analysis, mulitlevel modeling, and path analytic methods were used to analyze the data in order to determine the independent value of potential predictors on PPCSx during or immediately after deployment, and up to one year postdeployment.

Results revealed that PPCSx were not associated with blast exposure alone, but increased with severity of neurological sequelae (dazed and confused, memory loss, LOC). PTSD symptoms similarly increased with degree of neurological sequelae, not simple exposure to blast. Subsequent analysis examined what predicted four or more PPSx. Multilevel modeling revealed that PCS scores were most strongly associated with PTSD, and secondly, by depression, both independent of concussion, supporting the contention of those who argue that PTSD predicts PCS. However, PCS scores were also found to be clearly related to concussion independent of PTSD or depression scores. PCL-m and depression scores were highest for those who reported concussion. Fifteen percent of those were concussed and had low PCL scores (<30) but still reported PPCSx during or immediately after last deployment, and 12% reported symptoms during the prior week. 49% reported moderately elevated but sub-threshold PCL scores (<50) after deployment, with 38% of this group reporting symptoms during the prior week. These rates of PPCSx reporting are between two to three times greater than PPCSx reported by those not blast exposed. Finally, path analysis revealed that although being exposed to a blast predicted PCL and depression scores, blast alone (without associated concussion) did not predict PPCSx scores. Yet, PPCSx scores were independently predicted by concussion, albeit not as strongly as PTSD and depression scores. Results indicate that the best overall predictors of PPSx are PTSD and depression. However, even a year after last deployment, concussion predicts PPCSx for a substantial sub-population of those without evidence of PTSD, depression, or substance dependence.

Thus, there appears to be many combat exposed service members with psychological distress whose symptoms manifest somatically and cognitively, supporting the findings of Hoge and associates. However, in addition, there appears to be a group of concussed service members whose PPCSx cannot be attributed to PTSD, depression, or substance use disorder. Of course, there may be many whose PPCSx are due to concussion, as well as PTSD and/or depression, since PTSD and depression symptoms overlap with the symptoms of concussion. The size of this potentially comorbid group is difficult to determine from the type of epidemiological analysis conducted here. However, it is feasible that one explanation for symptom overlap is that mental health issues increase in those who have been previously concussed since PTSD and depression may more easily activated due to concussion.

Indeed, psychophysiological analysis of a group with PTSD suggests that there is an autonomic dysregulation that occurs due to concussion that makes posttraumatic memories more difficult to control. To determine this possibility, we examined the skin conductance (SC) and heart rate variability in 39 active duty military members with combat-related PTSD due to an event within the prior year. Nineteen out of the sample of 39 reported having been concussed during their recent deployment. At pretreatment assessment, patients' psychophysiology was assessed during a series of five minute conditions: baseline, recall of the most stressful events of their deployment, and instruction to put that out of their minds and rest comfortably. Group x condition analysis of variance and subsequent post-hoc analysis revealed that these two groups reacted differently to stress recall ($p<.001$; effect size $=.48$). Service members with PTSD-only had increased arousal following stress recall ($p<.05$), but stabilized their arousal during recovery ($p<.34$). In contrast, service members who had PTSD and who also reported concussion had a significantly greater arousal upon stress recall ($p<.05$) and continued to increase their arousal significantly during the recovery period ($p<.01$), indicating less ability to control their arousal than non-concussed patients. Moreover, regression analysis revealed that the greater the severity of the concussion (experienced blast but no concussion, dazed or confused, loss of memory, loss of consciousness), the greater the autonomic reactivity ($p<.001$).

Taken together, these studies suggest that more research is required before determining that screenings and treatments for concussion should discontinue.

References

[1]   Hoge, WH, McGurk, D., Thomas, JL., Cox, AL, Engel, C., & Castro, C. Mild Traumatic Brain Injury in U.S. Soldiers Returning from Iraq. NEJM, 2008, vol. 358 no. 5
[2]   USA Today (2009). Military's focus on brain-injury criticized. April 15.

Section III

Treatment

Coping with Blast-Related Traumatic Brain Injury in Returning Troops
B.K. Wiederhold (Ed.)
IOS Press, 2011
© 2011 The authors and IOS Press. All rights reserved.
doi: 10.3233/978-1-60750-797-0-55

Short-Term Intensive Cognitive Rehabilitation in OEF/OIF Veterans – Applying the STEP Model

Joshua B. CANTOR[a,1], Wayne A. GORDON[a], Kristen DAMS-O'CONNOR[a] and Theodore TSAOUSIDES[a]

[a]*Mount Sinai School of Medicine, New York, NY, USA*

Abstract. Among the most common and debilitating cognitive impairments after Traumatic Brain Injury (TBI) is disruption of executive functions and related emotional and behavioral dysregulation. Executive dysfunction after TBI represents one of the most significant barriers to recovery, community reintegration, and return to duty in military personnel with TBI. Investigators at the Brain Injury Research Center of Mount Sinai (BIRC-MS) have developed two theoretically- and empirically-based intensive group cognitive rehabilitation interventions that combine three distinct types of training (attention, emotional regulation and problem solving): Executive Plus and Short Term Executive Plus (STEP). A federally funded randomized controlled trial (RCT) to examine the effectiveness of Executive Plus was recently completed and an RCT of STEP is currently under way at the BIRC-MS. The proposed presentation will describe the methodology of these two RCTs. Preliminary findings from the Executive Plus study will be presented that treatment resulted in lasting benefits in the domains of self-efficacy, problem solving, attention, and quality of life even after treatment was withdrawn. In addition, MIL-STEP, a proposed adaptation of the model for treatment of veterans of OEF/OIF with TBI will be described.

Keywords. Traumatic Brain Injury, cognitive rehabilitation

1. Introduction/Problem

1.1. Overview

Traumatic Brain Injury (TBI) has been described as one of the "signature injuries" of the war in Iraq and Afghanistan [1,2]. The long-term impact of cognitive impairment following TBI for active military personnel, veterans, their families and for society is only now beginning to be appreciated. Among the most common and debilitating cognitive impairments after TBI is disruption of executive functions and related emotional and behavioral dysregulation [3-13]. Because executive functions are essential to the planning and effective execution of all purposeful behavior, including social interactions and productive activity, executive dysfunction after TBI leads to a variety of difficulties in many aspects of daily living. It represents one of the most

---

[1]Corresponding Author: Joshua B. Cantor, Ph.D., Co-Director, Brain Injury Research Center, Associate Professor, Department of Rehabilitation Medicine, Mount Sinai School of Medicine, One Gustave L. Levy Place, Box 1240, New York, NY 10029, Email: joshua.cantor@mountsinai.org.

significant barriers to recovery, community reintegration, and return to duty in injured military personnel [1,4,7,9,14,15,16]. Moreover, since TBI among Operation Enduring Freedom (OEF)/Operation Iraqi Freedom (OIF) veterans commonly co-occurs with combat-related stress, psychiatric disorders (e.g., depression), and medical conditions (e.g., pain, fatigue) that have cumulative detrimental impacts on functioning [17,18], treating either cognitive or emotional symptoms in isolation is likely to be ineffective and result in increased frustration and distress in treatment participants and their families.

Although a few large studies describe the impact of rehabilitation programs on executive dysfunction, most investigations have utilized single-case or small-group designs, and none have focused on military personnel [19-21]. Three small randomized controlled trials (RCTs) of approaches using problem solving training have shown promise, and a federally funded RCT was recently completed and another is currently under way at the Brain Injury Research Center of Mount Sinai (BIRC-MS) to examine their effectiveness [6,15,22,23].

These approaches teach the participant a multi-step process that can be generalized to use across a variety of situations. The steps of the process include: (1) stopping and focusing on the problem at hand; (2) defining the problem; (3) enumerating potential solutions to the problem or steps to solving it; (4) choosing one of the alternatives and implementing it; and (5) evaluating the outcome [24]. Rath and colleagues [22] added cognitive-behavioral training in emotional regulation skills to this intervention to facilitate self-awareness and clear thinking. The model developed at BIRC-MS (the Executive Plus and Short Term Executive Plus [STEP] programs) is a theory-based, short-term, intensive group cognitive rehabilitation program, which combines three distinct types of training (attention, emotional regulation and problem solving). Each of these three types of training has been found to be effective in helping participants compensate for their functional impairments [6,14,15,22,25,26]. This paper will describe the Executive Plus and STEP programs and present preliminary findings from the former. Since there is a pressing need to develop and test effective treatments for military personnel and veterans with TBI that facilitate improved functioning and return to work [1,16,19-21], a proposed version of the STEP model adapted for use with military personnel (MIL-STEP) will also be described. The program combines problem solving training, emotional regulation training, traditional compensatory strategies and remediation, and brain-plasticity-based cognitive training to enhance information processing speed, attention and executive control.

1.2. TBI in the Military

The rate of TBI in veterans deployed in both OEF and OIF is believed to be higher than in any previous war [2]. As advances in both protective body armor and acute care on the battlefield have lowered combat fatalities, they have also resulted in a higher percentage of individuals who survive brain injury [1]. Moreover, the use of improvised explosive devices (IEDs) in the theaters of operation in Afghanistan and Iraq, has resulted in more blast and concussive injuries than in previous conflicts. Estimates of the incidence of TBI in OEF/OIF veterans vary considerably, depending on the population studied and the methods used [27].

For example, in a convenience sample of 596 US Army troops returning from OEF/OIF deployment, estimates of rates of TBI varied from 7% to 16% depending on the screening method used [27]. It is estimated by the Defense and Veterans Brain

Injury Center (DVBIC) at Walter Reed Hospital that of all OEF and OIF veterans returning from their overseas deployments, 30% had experienced a TBI [28]. Of those patients transferred back to the US for treatment, 56% had moderate to severe TBI, while 44% had experienced mild TBI [28].

Veterans with TBI experience a wide array of cognitive, emotional, and physical difficulties. Depending on the nature and severity of their injury, they may struggle with seizures; problems with balance, motor coordination, sleep, attention, concentration, and memory; fatigue; irritability; depression; as well as anxiety and emotional dysregulation. The neural circuitry supporting executive functioning is particularly vulnerable to injury, which can result in impulsivity, disorganization, reduced initiation, poor judgment and ineffective problem solving skills [1]. The impact of TBI and other combat-related cognitive and emotional dysfunction on quality of life, productivity and interpersonal relationships has been well documented [29,30]. Treating cognitive and emotional symptoms in isolation is unlikely to be effective given the tendency for enduring symptoms in one domain to thwart progress in the other domain, due to the functional interconnectedness of thought and emotion in daily living [18]. Therefore, there is a clear need for comprehensive multidimensional treatment programs designed to ameliorate cognitive and emotional sequelae of combat-sustained injuries [29].

1.3. TBI and Executive Functioning

Executive functions are a set of higher-order cognitive abilities that regulate and coordinate other abilities and behaviors. In defining executive functions, Cicerone and Giacino [4] refer to the capacity for anticipation of consequences, goal formation, planning/organization, initiation/execution of activities and self-monitoring, with correction of errors. Rieger and Gauggel [11] cite planning, anticipation, action sequencing, cognitive flexibility, monitoring and inhibition. Lezak [7] divides the executive functions into four components: volition; planning; purposeful action; and effective performance. Sbordone [31] defines executive functioning as "…the complex process by which an individual goes about performing a novel problem solving task, from its inception to its completion" (p. 437). Deficits in executive functioning are among the most disabling consequences of TBI, and they pose the greatest challenge to social and vocational recovery [9,14]. Critical life outcomes following TBI such as vocational success, community reintegration and social autonomy have been associated with executive functioning abilities [9,13,32,33].

Over 40 years ago, Luria [3] described the relationship between executive functioning and problem solving ability and noted that patients with TBI were unable to systematically analyze a problem they were confronted with. These individuals typically had no specific plan to solve the problem, did not appear to engage in a preliminary investigation of its nature and constraints, and evidenced impulsive actions when trying to solve it. He described this phenomenon as an impairment in self-regulation, which results in impairments in anticipation (e.g., unrealistic expectations, failure to appreciate consequences), planning (e.g., impulsivity, poor organization), execution (e.g., perseveration, difficulty maintaining set), and self-monitoring (e.g., emotional dyscontrol, poor error recognition). Engaging in novel situations and problem solving both draw heavily on the use of these functions and, thus, constitute a particularly significant challenge to individuals with TBI [4].

Table 1 presents behavioral manifestations of executive dysfunction commonly observed following TBI. Using Lezak's [7] four-component model of executive dysfunction, Sbordone [31] identified common signs and symptoms associated with impairments in executive functioning.

Table 1. Common Signs and Symptoms Associated with Impaired Executive Functioning.

Volition	Planning	Purposive Action	Effective Performance
• Apathy • Deterioration in personal grooming and hygiene • Lessened curiosity • Lessened self-awareness • Lessened social awareness • Lessened interest in previously enjoyed activities	• Reduced abstract and conceptual thinking • Disorganized behavior and thinking • Inflexible thinking • Poor planning/ organizational skills • Loss of goals or plans for the future • Socially inappropriate behavior	• Distractibility • Lessened initiative • Difficulty performing more than one activity simultaneously • Lessened ability to maintain a set • Disorganized behavior and thinking • Emotional lability • Impatience • Dissociation between expressed verbal intentions and actions • Difficulty maintaining train of thought • Circumstantial or tangential thinking • Difficulty performing novel tasks or tasks in unfamiliar situations	• Perseveration • Cognitive rigidity • Lessened ability to complete or follow through on tasks • Inability to recognize or rectify errors • Poor work habits • Significant problem solving difficulties • Lessened ability to utilize plans or strategies that were effective in the past

1.4. Treatment of Executive Dysfunction

Given the diversity of impairments resulting from executive dysfunction, multiple treatments exist to address deficits in executive functioning, ranging from individual training in planning, sequencing, goal setting, self-monitoring and problem solving, to comprehensive day treatment programs (CDTPs) emphasizing awareness and self-regulation. CDTPs are designed to address a wide range of post-TBI cognitive and behavioral difficulties and have been shown to be effective in improving rehabilitation outcomes [19-21,34-42]. Interventions for executive dysfunction are often embedded in CDTPs to enhance their efficacy. For example, Scherzer [41] found that the effectiveness of a CDTP was significantly enhanced when a problem solving approach was incorporated in the program.

Targeting problem solving deficits has been a primary focus of executive dysfunction interventions [6,15,22,43-45]. Problem solving interventions utilize a "top-down" approach, by teaching the individual metacognitive strategies that are transferable and generalizable. Individuals are taught a strategy of how to complete a task or to solve a problem that can be applied across diverse situations, rather than developing "bottom-up" skills by practicing generic exercises to improve a *specific* lower-order cognitive skill. In order to optimize self-regulation, metacognitive strategies rely on behavioral routines and internalization of "self-talk" to address executive function deficits [4,46-49]. Individuals are trained to consciously use internal verbalization of strategies and self-monitoring procedures whenever they confront situations in which they experience difficulty [8].

A "top-down" problem solving model, presented in the following section, was originally proposed by D'Zurilla and Goldfried [24,50]. This model draws largely on cognitive-behavioral problem solving therapies that originated in the 1960s and early 1970s and is one of the most popular evidence-based approaches to the treatment of executive function found in the rehabilitation literature. This model has been the basis for the development of two evidence-based interventions using problem solving training with individuals with TBI [15,22]. These interventions not only view problem solving from a neuropsychological perspective [6,34,51], but also take into account the motivational, emotional and attitudinal factors that affect the problem solving process as it unfolds in "real life" [22].

1.5. Problem Solving

D'Zurilla and Goldfried define effective problem solving as "a behavioral process, whether overt or cognitive in nature, which: a) makes available a variety of potentially effective response alternatives for dealing with the problematic situation; and b) increases the probability of selecting the most effective response from among these various alternatives" (p. 108) [24]. They assume that problem solving skills can be learned, and emphasize providing a global approach to training. The goal is to ensure that the pervasive problem solving deficits of day-to-day life are addressed, rather than to provide the individual with discrete, situation-bound learning strategies.

The authors divide problem solving into two distinct processes: problem-orientation; and use of problem solving skills [24]. Problem-orientation includes thoughts and beliefs held about problems, as well as the impact of these beliefs on one's ability to recognize problems and act on them [50]. Problem-orientation is critical to facilitating an adaptive problem solving process and, under optimum conditions, consists of the following attitudinal factors:

- A broad-based definition of problems as "any situation involving the need to plan, make a decision, or respond to distress"
- Acceptance of problems as part of life and belief in one's ability to cope with them
- Recognition of problems when they occur
- Inhibition of impulsive reactions or "do nothing" responses to problems that are recognized
- The disruption of any one of these attitudinal factors can impede the initiation and completion of an appropriate problem solving response [50]

D'Zurilla and Goldfried [24] describe four steps in successful problem solving: (1) defining and formulating the problem; (2) generating a list of alternative solutions; (3) decision making; and (4) solution implementation and verification. Problem solving therapy focuses on learning these four steps and integrating all the pieces, with emphasis placed on the application of strategies to real life problems. Throughout this process, therapists provide positive reinforcement and corrective feedback, review positive problem-orientation and facilitate clients' awareness of the applicability of problem solving training. Finally, clients are taught to anticipate obstacles and future problems and to develop corresponding problem solving strategies.

Based on D'Zurilla and Goldfried's [24] model, von Cramon and colleagues [15] developed a problem solving training program, which included exercises in problem identification and problem analysis, selective encoding and comparison, selective combination using different mental representations, self-monitoring, evaluation of solutions and production of problem solutions. Behavioral techniques such as saturation cueing, shaping, facilitating self-instruction, ensuring cognitive activation, minimizing impulsivity and imparting realistic awareness were also used. They compared 20 inpatients with brain injury receiving problem solving training to 17 inpatients receiving memory training of comparable intensity and duration (i.e., six weeks, with an average of 25 sessions per patient). On tasks of reasoning (i.e., the Tower of Hanoi task and a planning test), those who received problem solving training showed more improvements in performance than those receiving memory training. Treatment gains were also noted on an observational rating scale completed by inpatient staff.

Levine et al. [6] took another approach to the remediation of problem solving difficulties, which they refer to as Goal Management Training (GMT). Each of the five stages of GMT was designed to address, in ascending order, levels of the process of goal-directed behavior. These stages parallel quite closely the processes of executive functioning outlined by Luria [3] and the problem solving steps identified by D'Zurilla [50]: (1) stop; (2) define the problem; (3) list the steps to be taken; (4) learn the steps; (5) do it; and (6) self-evaluate performance. Levine and colleagues conducted an RCT in which 60 patients with TBI were randomly assigned to receive either GMT or motor skills training (MST). Two individual sessions of either GMT or MST, each session lasting one hour, were provided to each participant. Improvements were seen on paper-and-pencil tasks corresponding to everyday life problems. Additionally, GMT participants devoted more time to task completion and evidenced a reduced error rate on posttest measures.

In sum, a variety of approaches to problem solving training have been found to be promising interventions for executive dysfunction.

1.6. Emotional Regulation

A crucial element to consider within problem solving training is the role and impact of emotions [50], which may hinder or facilitate problem solving. Individuals with TBI often experience difficulty in modulating their emotions and their reactions to situations, which can reduce the effectiveness of already impaired cognition and result in inaction or impulsivity [4,22,52]. Consequently, helping individuals in treatment reduce emotional "noise" and negative self-talk [22,53] is expected to facilitate problem solving and effective self-talk. Metacognitive strategies in emotional regulation are designed to facilitate inhibition of both impulsive reactions and "do nothing" responses, and to increase acceptance of problems as part of life and foster participants' confidence in their ability to cope with and solve problems [50]. Finally, emotional regulation strategies assist individuals in understanding the ways in which TBI affects their emotional self-regulation and problem solving ability, thereby slowly increasing their awareness of the insidious nature of their cognitive dysfunction. For example, since individuals with TBI often experience "information overload" due to deficits in information processing speed, they need to learn to accept that problem solving and tasks of daily life will require substantially more time than they did in the past [22,54]. Thus, emotional regulation strategies help them accept the paradox that they must "slow down" in order to accomplish more.

Emotions that interfere with problem solving can be generated from several sources: the objective problematic situation; problem-orientation cognitions (as described above); and/or specific problem solving steps. Acknowledging this, Rath and colleagues [22] incorporated cognitive behavioral "emotional regulation" into their treatment program of post-TBI problem solving disorders. They argue that effective emotional regulation is the foundation of the processes that constitute problem solving, and because individuals with TBI are often vulnerable to emotional dysregulation, they advocate providing specific emotional regulation strategies *prior to* initiating problem solving strategies. Their study examined a group of 60 individuals with mild to severe TBI [22], each of whom was enrolled in 24 sessions of either "innovative treatment" or conventional treatment. The former received 12 weeks of "problem-orientation," which focused on emotional self-regulation [24,55] and incorporated elements of cognitive behavioral therapy [56]. This was then followed by 12 weeks of "problem solving skills" treatment, in which the previously learned emotional self-regulation strategies were maintained, while the standard steps of problem solving therapy (outlined above) were taught. Limited improvements were documented in some areas (e.g., in self-appraisal of problem solving abilities, role-play measures, and decreased perseverative performance). Both groups improved on memory tests. No improvement was found on a test of inductive and deductive reasoning. Six-month follow-ups of 31 of the 60 participants showed that the gains achieved were maintained.

1.7. Bottom-Up Approaches to Training Attention and Improving Processing Speed

Executive functioning, problem solving, emotional regulation and learning are mediated by attention and processing speed. Clearly, being able to attend to external and internal events and process information accurately is a prerequisite for intentional learning, emotional regulation, and problem solving. Shallice [58] postulates that regulation and verification of behavior are controlled by an attentional supervisory executive system. Stuss and colleagues [59] view attention and executive functions as intimately related, and Stuss and Benson's [60] hierarchical model of cerebral organization defines attention as the foundation of the hierarchy of functional systems. Several studies [61-64] have demonstrated that individuals with executive dysfunction benefit from interventions to improve attention and that attentional training alone can result in improved anterograde memory. Research has also shown that processing speed is an important determinant of cognitive and executive function. Using structural equation modeling, Rassovsky and colleagues [65] demonstrated that processing speed mediates the relationship between severity of brain injury and everyday function. Indeed, Frencham and colleagues [66] demonstrated that measures of processing speed were the strongest determinants of neuropsychological functioning for individuals after mild TBI. Furthermore, Nelson and colleagues [67] studied a sample of 53 OEF/OIF veterans with TBI and found that processing speed contributed significantly to executive functioning performance. Thus, theory and prior research support the inclusion of attention and processing speed training as a component of remediation of executive dysfunction.

1.8. Treatment of TBI in Military Populations

Military personnel with TBI have access to excellent acute and post-acute care both at military facilities and at major VA centers. However, once patients are discharged from a post-acute rehabilitation facility, they return to their home or base which is often far from a medical facility offering specialized TBI rehabilitation. In response to the increased incidence of TBI in the current wars, the VA issued a directive on April 1, 2007, to screen all OEF/OIF veterans for TBI [68]. As this directive is implemented, many individuals with previously unrecognized TBI are now being identified. However, a standardized, comprehensive and effective program of cognitive rehabilitation treatment services for individuals identified as having TBI has not been established. Thus, the need is clear for establishing effective, affordable service delivery strategies for delivering cognitive rehabilitation to the many service members who are in need of help. As recommended by Helmick [69], group interventions may be one way of maximizing cost-effectiveness while maintaining quality.

The Defense and Veterans Brain Injury Center (DVBIC) has outlined guidelines for the post-acute management of mild TBI [70]. It is not clear to what extent these guidelines are currently implemented in military facilities where TBI is treated. In any case, the guidelines are general in nature and provide very limited information on cognitive rehabilitation. Thus, there is no detailed standard of care for cognitive treatment of post-acute TBI in the military or among veterans. Indeed, the DVBIC guidelines state explicitly that "further investigation regarding the timing and components of cognitive rehabilitation are warranted."

2. Method/Tools

2.1. Executive Plus

The Brain Injury Research Center of Mount Sinai (BIRC-MS) recently completed a randomized controlled trial (RCT) comparing the effectiveness of a 26-week innovative cognitive rehabilitation day program (Executive Plus) to that of a 26-week standard CDTP (Standard Rehab). The study was funded by the National Institute on Disability and Rehabilitation Research of the U.S. Department of Education.

Executive Plus provided attention training followed by concurrent sessions of problem solving training (PST) and emotional regulation training (ERT), that were embedded in the context of a day treatment program [71]. Executive Plus is theory-based (see above) and combines interventions and principles that have individually been found to be effective in the studies cited herein. In both Executive Plus and STEP (described below) training is modular and incorporates a top-down approach, that is embedded within the day-to-day experiences of participants' lives, thereby focusing on the "real life" challenges of participants. Thus the curriculum is not "canned" but draws upon the experiences of those in the groups. Specifically, in both Executive Plus and STEP, problem solving and emotional regulation principles are embedded in all of the treatment groups, providing participants sufficient repetition to learn and practice the rules of problem solving and emotional regulation across a variety of situations, fostering generalization across tasks and contexts.

The Standard Rehab intervention was adopted as a comparison to reflect the current standard of care in CDTPs (it is the current standard of care in day treatment for individuals with TBI at Mount Sinai and is similar to many CDTPs elsewhere). Standard Rehab enrollees participated in a general cognitive skills group and in group psychotherapy, instead of the unique elements of Executive Plus. Although the programs differed, both were CDTPs of equal intensity and duration and employed a range of techniques that are commonly used in group interventions of this kind [15,39]. Groups in both arms included the following: Community Group (daily orientation); Community Access Group (planning and executing community outings); Computer Education Group; Psychoeducation Group; and Life Skills Group. The Standard Rehab program had Cognitive Skills and Psychotherapy Groups instead of PST and ERT, respectively.

2.2. Short-Term Executive Plus (STEP)

STEP is a type of CDTP currently being evaluated in a single-center, wait-list control RCT at the BIRC-MS. This study is funded by the Centers for Disease Control and Prevention. STEP differs from the Executive Plus model in two respects. First, the STEP intervention is delivered in 108 sessions over three months, compared to 467 sessions over six months for Executive Plus. Second, it focuses on the "core ingredients," i.e., problem solving training, emotional regulation, and attention training, with some additional "generic" cognitive remediation techniques.

A pilot study of the core modules of STEP, which included PST and ERT, was conducted in March 2005 to assess feasibility, develop training materials and assess responses to treatment delivery. Changes were made in the program based on feedback from participants and observations by group leaders. Results of the STEP RCT will not be available until the study is completed in late 2012.

3. Results

3.1. Preliminary findings from Executive Plus

Participants in the Executive Plus study were individuals with a medically documented TBI who were at least three months post-injury. The inclusion criteria were presence of executive dysfunction, as determined by scores on the Frontal Systems Behavior Scale (FrSBe) or the Wisconsin Card Sorting Test (WCST), and ability to participate in group treatment and the assessments (e.g. adequate communication skills, IQ of at least 75, sixth grade reading level). Participants were excluded if they presented with active substance abuse, psychosis, suicidality, and disruptive or violent behavior. Fifty two subjects were randomized to either Executive Plus and completed the baseline T1 assessment. A total of 43 subjects completed the treatment and the T3 assessment (EP n = 22, Control n = 21), and a further 32 subjects completed the six-month follow-up T4 assessment (EP n = 17, Control n = 15). Thus, 82.6% of those who began treatment completed it, and 61.5% of subjects who began treatment returned for the six-month follow-up. There were no significant differences between the groups on attrition rates ($\chi 2 (2) = .25$, *ns*).

Those who completed T4 did not differ on gender, ethnicity, marital status, income, age or education from those who only completed T1 or those who completed T3. Within the subjects that completed T4, there were no significant differences between the EP and Control groups on gender, ethnicity, marital status, income, age or education. There was no differential attrition in either group on outcome variables at T4 compared to T1 and T3.

Given the intensity of the program, it was reasonable to expect that treatment would show an effect in both groups. However, for change to be truly meaningful, the effects of treatment should persist beyond the initial "halo effect" period that immediately follows the end of treatment. Thus the analyses focused on T4, the six-month follow-up assessment.

Because the samples were not sufficiently large to conduct between-group, repeated measures comparisons, a single-subject approach was taken. Zhan & Ottenbacher point out that "the difficulty of obtaining large homogeneous samples of subjects with similar disorders...makes group-comparison designs difficult to implement in most rehabilitation settings" [88]. The approach outlined by Beeson & Robey [89] was adapted to the dataset, in which effect sizes were calculated for each subject individually, examining change from baseline to post-treatment to follow-up and using an ipsative pooled standard deviation as the denominator.

At conclusion of treatment the effect sizes were approximately equivalent in the two groups for:

- One neuropsychological measure of executive function (BADS Rule Shift, -.02 vs. -.17)
- Self efficacy (Self Efficacy Questionnaire, 1.11 SR vs. .96 EP)
- Quality of life (Life-3, 1.14 SR vs. .91 EP)
- Self-reported attentional function (Attention Rating and Monitoring Scale, .43 vs. .36)

At conclusion of treatment the SR group had larger effect sizes than the EP group for:

- A neuropsychological measure of attention (Symbol Digit Modality Test, .61 vs. .08)
- A general self-report measure of Executive function (FRSBE, .94 vs. .10)
- A neuropsychological measure of executive function (BADS key search, .44 vs. .05)
- Depression (Beck Depression Inventory-II, .57 SR vs. -.67EP)

At conclusion of treatment the EP group had larger effect sizes than the SR group for:

- A neuropsychological measure of attention (Auditory Consonant Trigrams, .09 vs. .72)
- Three neuropsychological measures of executive function (BADS Zoo map, .52 vs. .72; BADS Modified 6 elements test, .40 vs. .88; BADS Action Programme, 1.25 vs. 1.66)
- Problem solving (Problem Solving Inventory, .53 vs. .90)

At six-month follow-up, the effect sizes were approximately equivalent in the groups for:

- Self efficacy (.64 SR vs. .66 EP)
- Two neuropsychological measure of executive function (BADS key search, .40 SR vs. .47 EP; BADS Modified 6 elements test, .49 SR vs. .30 EP)

At six-month follow-up, the SR group had a larger effect size than the EP group for:

- One neuropsychological measure of executive function (BADS Action Programme, 1.89 SR vs. 1.23 EP)

At six-month follow-up, the EP group had larger effect sizes than the SR group for:

- Self-reported attentional function (Attention Rating and Monitoring Scale, .40 vs. .94)

- Two neuropsychological measures of attention (Auditory Consonant Trigrams, .33 vs. .67, Symbol Digit Modality Test, .33 vs. .68)
- Problem solving (.16 vs. 1.08)
- A general self-report measure of Executive function (FRSBE, .19 vs. .62)
- Two neuropsychological measures of executive function (BADS Rule Shift, .07 vs. .42; BADS Zoo Map, .11 vs. .46)
- Quality of life (.59 vs. 1.02)
- Depression (Beck Depression Inventory, -.14 vs. .23)

In summary:
- Both groups showed meaningful improvements in function during treatment in multiple domains.
- At the end of treatment there was no clear superiority of effect size in any particular domain for either treatment.
- Six months after treatment had ended, effect sizes were larger in the EP group than in the SR group for neuropsychological measures of attention, problem solving, self-reported executive function, and on measures of executive function, quality of life, and depression.

4. Conclusion

These findings suggest that day treatment programs such as EP, employing a combination of top-down meta-cognitive strategies and bottom-up approaches, result in lasting benefits that persist well after treatment is over. The long-term benefits appear to be greater than for patients in standard rehabilitation. Such approaches may be beneficial to veterans with TBI as outlined below:

4.1. MIL-STEP: A Modification of the STEP/Executive Plus Model for Veterans

Given: (a) the dramatic increase in TBI prevalence in the military; (b) the pervasive disability found in individuals with TBI secondary to executive function disorders; (c) the promising success of problem solving-based interventions for executive functions, as reviewed above; and (d) the need for cognitive rehabilitation programs that can facilitate improved function, community integration or return to duty in veteran and military populations, the MIL-STEP program is proposed.

4.2. Program Description

The MIL-STEP program, which is an adaptation of STEP, is characterized as follows:

4.2.1. A Short, Focused, Intensive Program

In the proposed program, participants will receive the proven "key ingredients" of remediation, i.e., training in improving cognitive and emotional functioning, in a brief (12-week), intensive (nine sessions/week) program.

4.2.2. Use of a Top-down Approach

Top-down approaches teach metacognitive processes that can be generalized across situations. This type of approach (which provides the framework for both problem solving and emotional regulation training) will be applied in the MIL-STEP program, for three reasons. First, from a theoretical perspective, the hierarchical organization of cognitive functions – with executive functions controlling subsidiary mental operations – suggests that only top-down approaches are likely to be effective in treating executive dysfunction [60]. Second, top-down approaches, by their very nature, are more likely to generalize across situations and to lead to enduring functional change. Third, empirical findings suggest that metacognitive top-down approaches to cognitive rehabilitation, such as problem solving and emotional regulation, are effective [4,6,19,72].

4.2.3. Problem Solving Training (PST)

PST is the common intervention in the RCTs cited herein and the central component of MIL-STEP. It is an approach that draws on and is consistent with well established models of executive functions [3,34,60]. Participants will receive 36 sessions of group PST.

4.2.4. Emotional Regulation Training (ERT)

ERT is thoroughly integrated into the program, as individuals with TBI often experience difficulty in modulating their emotions and their reactions to situations, which can interfere with cognitive functions that are already compromised secondary to TBI [4,22,52]. The primacy of emotion and personality variables in recovering from cognitive impairments is acknowledged and must be factored into the development of treatment regimens [73]. Participants will receive 36 sessions of group ERT.

4.2.5. Brain-Plasticity-Based Cognitive Training

Brain-plasticity-based cognitive training (BPCT), a methodology developed by Posit Science Corporation, is designed to restore cognitive function. BPCT exercises make use of intact implicit memory and procedural learning abilities, which are largely unaffected by TBI [74,75]. The computerized exercises are designed to gradually improve the speed and accuracy of information processing. The approach is based on well researched principles of brain-plasticity (discussed below) to "teach" the brain to process and record increasingly complex stimuli, more accurately and at a higher speed. As these abilities improve through intensive procedural learning, the encoding of naturalistic information improves. As a result, cognitive functions based on the quality of incoming information (e.g., memory, attentional control, executive functions) are likely to improve as well [76]. The intervention is delivered on a laptop computer, using a game-like interface.

A recent study conducted [77] at the BIRC-MS explored the feasibility of using BPCT with outpatients with TBI and found that individuals were able to learn to use the training program at home and progress through the material. The 10 study participants, all of whom resided in the community, had mild to severe TBI. They were six months to 22 years post injury and, therefore, past the period of spontaneous recovery, i.e., "cognitively stable." Each study participant was given the software to use at home. They were asked to use it for 40 minutes per day, five days per week for six weeks. They received daily reminders to do their training, and progress was monitored by tracking the number of hours spent using the software, which is automatically recorded on the Posit Science website.

Before and after training on the BPCT software, participants were administered the Automated Neuropsychological Assessment Metrics (ANAM-4), a validated computerized neuropsychological battery that tests processing speed, working memory, attention, encoding, spatial processing and accuracy, as well as the Cognitive Failures Questionnaire (CFQ) and Frontal Systems Behavior Scale (FRSBE). Participants also filled out a User Experience Survey (UES) at the end of their participation in the study, which provided feedback on their experiences using the software. We found that all participants were able to use the software. Though eight out of 10 participants reported that the program caused some fatigue, this tended to be relatively mild and decreased over the course of participation. On the UES, participants reported improvements in concentration, executive functioning, visual processing, memory and cognitive stamina. The primary obstacles encountered by participants were technical problems with the software and/or participants' own computers – though seven out of 10 participants reported little or no technical difficulty. Some participants were unable to complete the requested amount of training in the specified time period. Following treatment, improvements were noted on one or more standardized neuropsychological assessment measures for all participants, and all patients reported fewer cognitive "failures" and/or fewer symptoms of executive dysfunction at posttest.

While STEP and Executive Plus use individualized attention training, Posit Science's BPCT was chosen for MIL-STEP for three reasons. First, unlike APT-II, which was used in STEP, the Posit approach does not require constant one-on-one participation of a therapist – the therapist supervises the training but the actual tasks can all be done "solo." Second, it allows for massed practice as the user can do the exercises at home as well as at the rehabilitation center. These factors increase the opportunity for practice and thus, may improve treatment efficiency. Finally, mounting empirical evidence demonstrates the usability and effectiveness of BPCT in improving cognitive functioning in individuals with cognitive impairment [78-83]. Inclusion of BPCT in the proposed RCT is innovative, as it has not been tested in people with TBI in a comprehensive program.

4.2.6. Cognitive Scaffolding

To maximize potential benefits of the program, various standard, empirically validated cognitive remediation approaches will be nested into the program, individualized to each participants' needs [10,84]. These strategies will be provided to each participant by advisors over 36 advising sessions.

4.2.7. Social Scaffolding

Advisors will be members of the MIL-STEP treatment team assigned to work individually with participants over the course of the intervention. They will act as liaisons and advocates for their advisees in treatment team meetings. Advisors will also assist in the use of computerized BPCT and support their advisees' practice of problem solving and emotional regulation strategies. Also, family members and friends will be enlisted in the process of implementing interventions outside of sessions, and progress meetings with members of the participants' social network and the participant will be held twice during the course of the program, led by the advisor.

4.2.8. Ecological Validity

The MIL-STEP program has been designed to resemble as closely as possible a clinical rather than a research program, to ensure that the program can be adopted "as-is" in VA and other military clinical contexts. For example, participants will join the program on the basis of rolling admissions, and sessions will be held in an outpatient setting at a metropolitan medical center. Program staff will be experienced in working with military populations.

4.2.9. Manualization

Whyte and Hart [85-87] describe the importance of rigorously defining and specifying rehabilitation interventions if they are to be disseminated, replicated and ultimately adopted in clinical contexts. Treatment manuals for MIL-STEP will be developed to ensure adherence to the program by MIL-STEP staff over time. The distribution of these manuals (modified as needed) at the end of the program will permit the replication of MIL-STEP in other clinical settings and will facilitate standardization of cognitive rehabilitation received by veterans and military personnel.

References

[1]   McCrea M, Pliskin N, Barth J, Cox D, Fink J, French L, Hammeke T, Hess D, Hopewell A, Orme D, Powell M, Ruff R, Schrock B, Terryberry-Spohr L, Vanderploeg R, Yoash-Gantz R. *Official position of the military TBI task force on the role of neuropsychology and rehabilitation psychology in the evaluation, management, and research of military veterans with traumatic brain injury.* Clin Neuropsychol 2008 Jan;22(1):10-26.
[2]   Warden D. *Military TBI during the Iraq and Afghanistan wars.* J Head Trauma Rehabil 2006 Sep-Oct;21(5):398-402.
[3]   Luria AR. *Higher cortical functions in man.* New York: Oxford University Press; 1966.
[4]   Cicerone K, Giacino J. *Remediation of executive function deficits after traumatic brain injury.* NeuroRehabilitation 1992;2(3):12-22.
[5]   Goldman Rakic PS. Specification of higher cortical functions. *Journal of Head Trauma Rehabilitation* 1993 Mar;8(1):13-23.
[6]   Levine B, Robertson IH, Clare L, Carter G, Hong J, Wilson BA, Duncan J, Stuss DT. Rehabilitation of executive functioning: An experimental-clinical validation of goal management training. *Journal of the International Neuropsychological Society* 2000 Mar;6(3):299-312.
[7]   Lezak MD. *Neuropsychological assessment.* 3rd ed. New York: Oxford University Press; 1995. .
[8]   Mateer CA. *Executive function disorders: Rehabilitation challenges and strategies.* Semin Clin Neuropsychiatry 1999 Jan;4(1):50-9.
[9]   McDonald BC, Flashman LA, Saykin AJ. *Executive dysfunction following traumatic brain injury: Neural substrates and treatment strategies.* NeuroRehabilitation 2002;17(4):333-44.
[10] Prigatano GP. *Principles of neuropsycholgical rehabilitation.* New York: Oxford University Press; 1999 .
[11] Rieger M, Gauggel S. *Inhibition of ongoing responses in patients with traumatic brain injury.* Neuropsychologia 2002;40(1):76-85.
[12] Shallice T, Burgess PW. *Deficits in strategy application following frontal lobe damage in man.* Brain 1991 Apr;114 (Pt 2)(Pt 2):727-41.
[13] Stuss DT, Levine B. *Adult clinical neuropsychology: Lessons from studies of the frontal lobes.* Annu Rev Psychol 2002;53:401-33.
[14] Sohlberg MM, Mateer CA. *Effectiveness of an attention-training program.* J Clin Exp Neuropsychol 1987 Apr;9(2):117-30.

5] von Cramon DY, Matthes-von Cramon G, Mai N. *Problem-solving deficits in brain-injured patients: A therapeutic approach*. Neuropsychol Rehabil 1991;1:45-64.

6] Trudel TM, Nidiffer FD, Barth JT. *Community-integrated brain injury rehabilitation: Treatment models and challenges for civilian, military, and veteran populations*. J Rehabil Res Dev 2007;44(7):1007-16.

7] Vogt DS, Proctor SP, King DW, King LA, Vasterling JJ. *Validation of scales from the deployment risk and resilience inventory in a sample of operation Iraqi freedom veterans*. Assessment 2008;15(4):391.

8] Vanderploeg RD, Belanger HG, Curtiss G. Mild traumatic brain injury and posttraumatic stress disorder and their associations with health symptoms. Arch Phys Med Rehabil 2009 Jul;90(7):1084-93.

9] Cicerone KD, Dahlberg C, Kalmar K, Langenbahn DM, Malec JF, Bergquist TF, Felicetti T, Giacino JT, Harley JP, Harrington DE, Herzog J, Kneipp S, Laatsch L, Morse PA. *Evidence-based cognitive rehabilitation: Recommendations for clinical practice*. Arch Phys Med Rehabil 2000 Dec;81(12):1596-615.

0] Cicerone KD, Dahlberg C, Malec JF, Langenbahn DM, Felicetti T, Kneipp S, Ellmo W, Kalmar K, Giacino JT, Harley JP, Laatsch L, Morse PA, Catanese J. *Evidence-based cognitive rehabilitation: Updated review of the literature from 1998 through 2002*. Arch Phys Med Rehabil 2005 Aug;86(8):1681-92.

1] Cicerone K, Levin H, Malec J, Stuss D, Whyte J. *Cognitive rehabilitation interventions for executive function: Moving from bench to bedside in patients with traumatic brain injury*. J Cogn Neurosci 2006 Jul;18(7):1212-22.

2] Rath JF, Simon D, Langenbahn DM, Sherr RL, Diller L. *Group treatment of problem-solving deficits in outpatients with traumatic brain injury: A randomised outcome study*. Neuropsychological Rehabilitation Sep 2003; Vol 13 (4): 461 488 2003.

3] Gordon WA, Brown M, Bergman AL, Shields RW. "Community integration research: An empowerment paradigm." In: K. Hagglund, A. Heinemann, editors. *Handbook of applied disability and rehabilitation research*. New York: Springer Publishing Company, Inc.; 2006. .

4] D'Zurilla TJ, Goldfried MR. *Problem solving and behavior modification*. J Abnorm Psychol 1971 Aug;78(1):107-26.

5] Palmese CA, Raskin SA. *The rehabilitation of attention in individuals with mild traumatic brain injury, using the APT-II programme*. Brain Inj 2000 Jun;14(6):535-48.

6] Sohlberg MM, McLaughlin KA, Pavese A, Heidrich A, Posner MI. *Evaluation of attention process training and brain injury education in persons with acquired brain injury*. J Clin Exp Neuropsychol 2000 Oct;22(5):656-76.

27] Schwab K, Ivins B, Cramer G, Johnson W, Sluss-Tiller M, Kiley K, Lux W, Warden D. *Screening for traumatic brain injury in troops returning from deployment in Afghanistan and Iraq: Initial investigation of the usefulness of a short screening tool for traumatic brain injury*. J Head Trauma Rehabil 2007;22(6):377.

28] Warden D, Ryan LM, Helmick KM, Schwab K, French LM, Lu W, et al. *War Neurotrauma: The defense and veterans brain injury center (DVBIC) experience at Walter Reed Army Medical Center (WRAMC)* [abstract]. Journal of Neurotrauma 2005;22(10):1178.

29] Halbauer J, Ashford J, Zeitzer J, Adamson M, Lew H, Yesavage J. *Neuropsychiatric diagnosis and management of chronic sequelae of war-related mild to moderate traumatic brain injury*. J Rehabil Res Dev 2009;46(6):757.

30] Monson C, Taft C, Fredman S. *Military-related PTSD and intimate relationships: From description to theory-drive research and intervention development*. Clin Psychol Rev 2009;29(8):707.

31] Sbordone RJ. "The executive functions of the brain." In: Gary Groth-Marnat, editor. *Neuropsychological assessment in clinical practice: A guide to test interpretation and integration*. New York, NY, US: John Wiley and Sons, Inc; 2000.

32] Mazaux JM, Masson F, Levin HS, Alaoui P, Maurette P, Barat M. *Long-term neuropsychological outcome and loss of social autonomy after traumatic brain injury*. Arch Phys Med Rehabil 1997 Dec;78(12):1316-20.

33] Sohlberg M, Mateer CA, Stuss D. *Contemporary approaches to the management of executive dyscontrol*. J Head Trauma Rehabilitation 1993;8:45-58.

34] Ben-Yishay Y, Rattock J, Lakin P, Piasetsky EB, Ross B, Silver Sea. *Neuropsychological rehabilitation: Quest for a holistic approach*. Semin Neurol 1985;5:252-258.

35] Cicerone KD, Mott T, Azulay J, Friel JC. *Community integration and satisfaction with functioning after intensive cognitive rehabilitation for traumatic brain injury*. Arch Phys Med Rehabil 2004 Jun;85(6):943-50.

36] Gordon WA, Zafonte R, Cicerone K, Cantor J, Brown M, Lombard L, Goldsmith R, Chandna T. *Traumatic brain injury rehabilitation: State of the science*. Am J Phys Med Rehabil 2006 Apr;85(4):343-82.

37] Klonoff PS, Lamb DG, Henderson SW, Shepherd J. *Outcome assessment after milieu-oriented rehabilitation: New considerations*. Arch Phys Med Rehabil 1998 Jun;79(6):684-90.

38] Klonoff PS, Lamb DG, Henderson SW. *Milieu-based neurorehabilitation in patients with traumatic brain injury: Outcome at up to 11 years postdischarge*. Arch Phys Med Rehabil 2000 Nov;81(11):1535-7.

39] Malec JF. *Impact of comprehensive day treatment on societal participation for persons with acquired brain injury*. Arch Phys Med Rehabil 2001 Jul;82(7):885-95.

[40] Malec JF, Basford JS. *Postacute brain injury rehabilitation.* Arch Phys Med Rehabil 1996 Feb;77(2):198-207.
[41] Scherzer BP. *Rehabilitation following severe head trauma: Results of a three-year program.* Arch Phys Med Rehabil 1986 Jun;67(6):366-74.
[42] Donnelly K, Donelly J, Dunnam M, Warner G, Kittelson C, Constance J, Bradshaw C, Alt M. *Reliability, sensitivity, and specificity of the VA traumatic brain injury screening tool.* Journal of Head Trauma Rehabilitation in press.
[43] Foxx RM, Martella RC, Marchand Martella NE. *The acquisition, maintenance, and generalization of problem-solving skills by closed head-injured adults.* Behavior Therapy 1989 Win;20(1):61-76.
[44] Luria AR, tsvetkova ld. *The programming of constructive abilities in local brain injuries.* Neuropsychologia 1964;2:95,95.108.
[45] Webb P, Glueckauf R. *The effects of direct involvement in goal setting on rehabilitation outcome in persons with traumatic brain injury.* Rehabilitation Psychology 1994;39(3):179,179-188.
[46] Cicerone KD, Wood JC. *Planning disorder after closed head injury: A case study.* Arch Phys Med Rehabil 1987 Feb;68(2):111-5.
[47] Honda T. *Rehabilitation of executive function impairments after stroke.* Topics in Stroke Rehabilitation 1999 Spr;6(1):15-22.
[48] Hux K, Reid R, Lugert M. *Self-instruction training following neurological injury.* Applied Cognitive Psychology 1994 Jun;8(3):259-71.
[49] O'Callaghan ME, Couvadelli B. *Use of self-instructional strategies with three neurologically impaired adults.* Cognitive Therapy and Research 1998 Apr;22(2):91-107.
[50] D'Zurilla T. "Problem-solving therapies." In: K. Dobson, editor. *Handbook of cognitive behavioral therapies.* New York: The Guilford Press; 1988. .
[51] Luria AR. *Restoration of function after brain injury.* New York: Basic Books; 1963. .
[52] Simon D. *Enhancing emotional control in persons with acquired brain damage* (abstract). Rehabil Psych 2001;46:330.
[53] Meichenbaum D, Cameron R. *The clinical potential of modifying what clients say to themselves.* Psychotherapy: Theory, Research and Practice. 1974 Sum;11(2):103-17.
[54] Fasotti L, Kovacs F, Eling PA, Brouwer WH. *Time pressure management as a compensatory strategy training after closed head injury.* Neuropsychological Rehabilitation Jan 2000; Vol 10 (1): 47 65 2000.
[55] D'Zurilla TJ, Nezu AM. "Problem-solving therapies." In: Keith S. Dobson, editor. *Handbook of cognitive-behavioral therapies.* New York, NY, US: Guilford Press; 2001. FO: Print; AG: Adolescence (13-17-yrs); Adulthood (18-yrs-and-older); PO: Human; AT: Psychology:-Professional-and-Research.
[56] Beck AT. *Cognitive therapy and the emotional disorders.* 1976.
[58] Shallice T. *Neurologic impairment of cognitive processes.* Br Med Bull 1981;37:187-192.
[59] Stuss DT, Shallice T, Alexander MP, Picton TW. *A multidisciplinary approach to anterior attentional functions.* Ann N Y Acad Sci 1995 Dec 15;769:191-211.
[60] Stuss D, Benson D. *The frontal lobes.* New York: Raven Press; 1986. .
[61] Sohlberg, M. & Mateer, C. *Effectiveness of an attention training program.* Journal of Clini & Experim Neuropsych 1987;9:117-30.
[62] Gray JM, Robertson I, Pentland B, Anderson S. *Microcomputer-based attentional retraining after brain damage: A randomised group controlled trial.* Neuropsychological Rehabilitation 1992;2(2):97-115.
[63] Niemann H, Ruff RM, Baser CA. *Computer-assisted attention retraining in head-injured individuals: A controlled efficacy study of an outpatient program.* J Consult Clin Psychol 1990 Dec;58(6):811-7.
[64. Sturm W, Willmes K, Orgass B, Hartje W. *Do specific attention deficits need specific training?* Neuropsychol Rehabil 1997;7:81-103.
[65] Rassovsky Y, Satz P, Alfano MS, Light RK, Zaucha K, McArthur DL, Hovda D. *Functional outcome in TBI II: Verbal memory and information processing speed mediators.* J Clin Exp Neuropsychol 2006 May;28(4):581-91.
[66] Frencham KA, Fox AM, Maybery MT. *Neuropsychological studies of mild traumatic brain injury: A meta-analytic review of research since 1995.* J Clin Exp Neuropsychol 2005 Apr;27(3):334-51.
[67] Nelson L, Yoash-Gantz R, Pickett T, Campbell T. *Relationship between processing speed and executive functioning performance among OEF/OIF veterans: Implications for postdeployment rehabilitation.* J Head Trauma Rehabil 2009;24(1):32.
[68] Mernoff ST, Correia S. *Military blast injury in Iraq and Afghanistan: The veterans health administration's polytrauma system of care.* 2010 Jan:VHA Directive 2007-13.
[69] Helmick K, Members of Consensus Conference. *Cognitive rehabilitation for military personnel with mild traumatic brain injury and chronic post-concussional disorder: Results of april 2009 consensus conference.* NeuroRehabilitation 2010 Jan 1;26(3):239-55.
[70] *Defense and Veterans Brain Injury Center Updated Mild TBI Clinical Practice Guidelines* [Internet]; cMay 8, 2008 [cited 2008 September 24]. Available from: http://dvbic.org/pdfs/mTBI_recs_for_CONUS.pdf.

1] Gordon WA, Cantor J, Ashman T, Brown M. *Treatment of post-TBI executive dysfunction: Application of theory to clinical practice.* J Head Trauma Rehabil 2006 Mar-Apr;21(2):156-67.

2] Ownsworth TL, Mcfarland K. *Memory remediation in long-term acquired brain injury: Two approaches in diary training.* Brain Inj 1999 Aug;13(8):605-26.

3] Sohlberg M, Johnson L, Paule L, Raskin S, Mateer C. *Attention process training (APT-II) manual.* Wake Forest, NC: Lash and Associates; 2001. .

4] Watt S, Shores EA, Kinoshita S. *Effects of reducing attentional resources on implicit and explicit memory after severe traumatic brain injury.* Neuropsychology 1999 Jul;13(3):338-49.

5] Shum D, Jamieson E, Bahr M, Wallace G. *Implicit and explicit memory in children with traumatic brain injury.* J Clin Exp Neuropsychol 1999 Apr;21(2):149-58.

6] Mahncke HW, Connor BB, Appelman J, Ahsanuddin ON, Hardy JL, Wood RA, Joyce NM, Boniske T, Atkins SM, Merzenich MM. *Memory enhancement in healthy older adults using a brain plasticity-based training program: A randomized, controlled study.* Proc Natl Acad Sci USA 2006 Aug 15;103(33):12523-8.

7] *Examining the usability of a computerized cognitive training program in people with traumatic brain injury (TBI): A pilot study.* Poster to be presented at the American Congress of Rehabilitation Medicine, 2009, Denver CO; 2009.

8] Smith GE, Housen P, Yaffe K, Ruff R, Kennison RF, Mahncke HW, Zelinski EM. *A cognitive training program based on principles of brain plasticity: Results from the improvement in memory with plasticity-based adaptive cognitive training (IMPACT) study.* J Am Geriatr Soc 2009 Apr;57(4):594-603.

9] Willis SL, Tennstedt SL, Marsiske M, Ball K, Elias J, Koepke KM, Morris JN, Rebok GW, Unverzagt FW, Stoddard AM, Wright E, ACTIVE Study Group. *Long-term effects of cognitive training on everyday functional outcomes in older adults.* JAMA 2006 Dec 20;296(23):2805-14.

30] Barnes D, Yaffe K, Belfor N, Jagust WJ, DeCarli C, Reed BR, Kramer JH. *Computer-based cognitive training for mild cognitive impairment: Results from a pilot randomized, controlled trial.* Alzheimer Disease & Associated Disorders 2009;24 June:1-6.

31] Fischer D, Stewart AL, Bloch DA, Lorig K, Laurent D, Holman H. *Capturing the patient's view of change as a clinical outcome measure.* JAMA 1999 Sep 22-29;282(12):1157-62.

32] *Improved cognitive function and quality of life in individuals with "chemobrain" after using a brain-plasticity-based training program.* 2008. Poster presented at the American Society of Breast Disease Conference, April 10-12, 2008, San Diego, CA.

33] Cicerone K. Cognitive rehabilitation. In: N. D. Zasler, D. Katz, R. Zafonte, editors. *Neurorehabilitation of traumatic brain injury.* New York: Demos Publishers; 2006. .

34] Whyte J, Hart T. *It's more than a black box; it's a Russian doll. Defining rehabilitation treatments.* Am J Phys Med Rehabil 2003;82:639-652.

35] Hart T, Fann JR, Novack TA. *The dilemma of the control condition in experience-based cognitive and behavioural treatment research.* Neuropsychol Rehabil 2008 Jan;18(1):1-21.

36] *Treatment definition in experience-based rehabilitation research.* [Internet] [cited 2008 3/17]. Available from: http://www.ncrrn.org/papers/methodology_papers/treatment_definition.pdf.

37] Barrett DH, Doebbeling CC, Schwartz DA, Voelker MD, Falter KH, Woolson RF, Doebbeling BN. Posttraumatic stress disorder and self-reported physical health status among U.S. military personnel serving during the gulf war period: A population-based study. Psychosomatics 2002 May-Jun;43(3):195-205.

38] Zhan S, Ottenbacher KJ. *Single subject research designs for disability research.* Disabil Rehabil. 2001 Jan 15;23(1):1-8.

39] Beeson PM, Robey RR. *Evaluating single-subject treatment research: lessons learned from the aphasia literature.* Neuropsychol Rev. 2006 Dec;16(4):161-9.

Coping with Blast-Related Traumatic Brain Injury in Returning Troops
B.K. Wiederhold (Ed.)
IOS Press, 2011
doi: 10.3233/978-1-60750-797-0-72

Traumatic Stress and Injury of the Brain: the Dangerous Liaisons – a Case Study

Radosław TWORUS[a], Stanisław ILNICKI [a, 1] and Maciej ZBYSZEWSKI[a]
[a]Psychiatry and Combat Stress Clinic
of the Military Institute of Medicine in Warsaw

Abstract. We present the case of a soldier evacuated from Iraq because of traumatic stress symptoms with accompanying somatic syndromes. The symptoms occurred after explosion of a rocket that exploded approximately 40 meters away from him. Immediately after evacuation back to Poland, upon admission to the Clinic of Psychiatry and Combat Stress in Warsaw, he reported continuous internal anxiety, as well as many somatic symptoms. Psychological examination showed symptoms suggesting developing Posttraumatic Stress Disorder (PTSD) without any other irregularities including disorders connected with micro-damage of the central nervous system. During a prolonged stay in the clinic, despite medication and applied psychotherapy, the PTSD symptoms remained. With further observation it was found out that the patient suffers from a hearing disorder dissimulated by him by means of lip reading. The examination showed a significant double hearing loss, as well as a deformed nasal septum, and a longitudinal hypodensic area of a scar, located at the base of the left frontal lobe. The case presented shows that there may be comorbidity of PTSD symptoms and mild organic brain damage (mTBI), and disorders of some of the receptors (in this case, hearing).

Keywords. traumatic stress, Posttraumatic Stress Disorder, brain injury, hearing disorders, hyperbaric oxygen therapy, case study

Introduction

Comorbidity of Posttraumatic Stress Disorder (PTSD) symptoms and organic changes in the brain have been confirmed by neuro-imaging functional examination of the central nervous system (CNS). However, the problem of which disorder is of a primary nature and which is of a secondary type has not yet been resolved. Therefore, it is not known whether PTSD is a functional disorder that requires psycho-therapeutical assistance in the first place or it is a biological one that requires other methods of therapy. The answer to the question of whether a traumatic stress results in changes in the CNS or the other way around – changes in the CNS are a factor making PTSD development more likely – extends the scope of possibilities of providing help to those suffering from PTSD.

The explanation of these dependencies is especially important for soldiers. Their participation in combat situations nearly always is connected with exposure to microin-

[1] Corresponding Author: Stanislaw Ilnicki, Psychiatry and Combat Stress Clinic of the Military Institute of Medicine in Warsaw; E-mail: silnicki@wim.mil.pl.

juries of the brain, e.g. through mechanical head injuries including effects of explosion blast, effects of toxic agents released in the combustion process, etc. Moreover, a combat situation predisposes its participants towards developing PTSD [1, 2, 3].

The case we present displays links between PTSD and CNS damage (Traumatic Brain Injury – TBI) as well as sense organs, in our case, hearing. It also shows use of the hyperbaric oxygen therapy (HBOT) as an alternative and more and more frequently used treatment method for people suffering from PTSD and TBI.

1. Method

A 34-year old junior warrant officer was medically evacuated from Iraq due to an acute stress reaction (ASR). He had been married for 12 years with two children, a son of 10 and daughter of 12, and was a career soldier serving in the army for 14 years. The traumatic event occurred in a military base, in his third month of stay in the war operations area. When the soldier was on his way back from the place of duty to the accommodation area a 240-mm rocket (carrying 26 kg of explosive, fragmentation radius of approx. 600 m) exploded at a distance of some 40 m from him. He remembered the blast throwing him to the ground. The patient regained consciousness in the hospital of the Polish Medical Support Group MND CS – Iraq. He was conscious but no contact could be established with him. He does not remember the moment of admission but remember the pain of injections given to him. During the 24-hour observation he reported stabbing pain in the heart area, headache, hand tremor and tinnitus. Examination of his somatic condition revealed no irregularities. Serious acute stress reaction (ASR) was diagnosed and it was urgently recommended to evacuate the patient at the Clinic of Psychiatry and Combat Stress of the Military Institute of Medicine in Warsaw.

At the time of the traumatic event the patient was perceived as an exceptionally energetic person, quick and efficient in action, cheerful, sociable and self-confident. In the opinion of his colleagues, after discharge from the hospital, he was completely different. The patient was permanently anxious and frightened that something wrong would happen to him, crying and helpless, with a visible tremor through his whole bod. He was concerned about the change in his behavior and the symptoms. He said, "I have been in Iraq for such a long time and I experienced so many shelling attacks on the base; the latest one happened just a couple of days ago. It was similar. A projectile exploded close to my accommodation. I heard the explosion in my container and nothing wrong happened to me. But the current event caused such a strange reaction." During the next base-shelling alert he ran very fast to the shelter. When the alert was called off he had to urinate and a powerful fear of dying occurred.

The patient was admitted to the Clinic of Psychiatry and Combat Stress of the Military Institute of Medicine in Warsaw on the seventh day after the traumatic event. Upon admission he reporting having heartache and stabbing pain in the heart area, continuous anxiety, which became more intense when he was talking about or thinking about what had happened. "When I'm thinking or telling about [the event] I feel a ball in my throat, a shortage of air and my ears are clogged. When I was over there then from the moment of this accident I was continuously afraid that something wrong might happen, I was vigilant, I could not sleep at night and I was listening out for approaching artillery shells, and the alert sound." Examination of the mental condition showed a worsening in mood, weepiness, increased speech difficulties – faltering and stuttering, increased manipulation and movement anxiety, inconsistent and chaotic speaking, and high level of fear. Neither psychotic symptoms nor conscience disorder was found. No deviations from regular status were found in examination of both somatic and neurological condition.

Interviews with the patient in the first days of his stay in the clinic revealed he had never undergone psychiatric treatment or had any other health problems. He had never experienced any faints, petit or grand mals or poisoning with toxic substances. He said the following about his stay in the hospital: "I'm glad I was evacuated directly to the hospital because I'm completely different after that event - I am getting upset more about everything. I have little children and now I'm concerned about my behaviour at home, in relation to my family. So far I was energetic and I even had a nickname Speedy because everything had to be made ahead of time. Now I'm so slow and ponderous. It is hard to speak for me, I falter. After the event they were not able to interview me - I was faltering so much. I just cannot think about what happened over there - in Iraq. When I think about that or about my colleagues who stayed there then immediately I feel fear and anxiety inside."

Psychological and neuro-psychological examinations showed symptoms of a developing PTSD syndrome; organic CNS microinjuries, depression and psychotic disorders, as well as personality disorders were excluded. The patient was qualified for both individual and group psychotherapy and also medication adjusted to the clinic symptoms was applied – fluvoxamine 200 mg/24h, propranolol 120 mg/24h, alprazolam 1 mg/24h.

During the prolonged stay of the patient in the clinic, despite the medications and psycho-therapeutical treatment administered, the PTSD symptoms remained and functioning of the patient in the therapeutical community was poor. Self-isolation, as well as permanent restlessness and fear were observed.

During further observation it was found that the patient suffered from a hearing impairment, dissimulated unconsciously by him by means of lip reading. Audiometric and tympanometric examination was conducted, as well as head tomography; a laryngologist and audiologist consulted the patient. A significant double hearing loss of the receiving type was found, as well as a deformed nasal septum, and a longitudinal hypodensic scar, located at the base of the left frontal lobe. All these changes have been qualified as an outcome of a combat injury resulting from effects of explosion blast. The patient qualified for treatment in the hyperbaric chamber. In addition, pro-cognitive therapy was applied, as well as improving brain circulation, along with a steroid therapy.

Treatment of the acoustic injury in the hyperbaric chamber resulted in speedy hearing stabilization. After 15 sessions in the hyperbaric chamber hearing loss symptoms were almost completely eliminated; the improvement was confirmed by an audiometric examination. Along with a modification of the medication and introduction of the hypobaric therapy, also, the buzzing in the ears reported by the patient was eliminated, and a slow stabilization of the mental condition began.

The patient left the clinic after 61 days of therapy, in the condition of a full improvement of the symptoms. He returned to military service and continued the recommended medication (fluvoxamine, propranolol, piracetam) for six months. He needed neither further therapy nor psycho-therapeutical support.

2. Discussion

The case described presents a connection between occurrence of PTSD symptoms and damage to CNS and sense organs (in this case, hearing) that are a kind of brain "satellites." This suggests the necessity of extending the diagnostics towards CNS and sense organs injuries in each soldier who experienced combat injuries, both mental and somatic. This diagnostics should cover not only soldiers with possible TBI, but also every soldier receiving medical care after a combat injury.

In the case described it is not possible to determine unambiguously what affected the improvement of the patient's mental condition, i.e. abatement of the PTSD symptoms. Certainly this improvement was associated in time with the HBOT treatment administered to the patient. However, some questions of diagnostic and therapeutic nature remain unanswered: Did the spectacular hearing improvement alone affect the withdrawal of mental disorder? Should HBOT be the therapy applied in each case of TBI and PTSD co-occurrence? Is HBOT the method that can be applied in treatment of PTSD without concurrent TBI? [4]

Research from the recent several years indicate that HBOT can be a new alternative method of PTSD treatment, especially in patients with co-occurring TBI [5]. The case described confirms these observations and indicates necessity of conducting further research in this direction.

References

[1] J.D. Bremner, P. Randall, T.M. Scott, et al, MRI-based measurement of hippocampal volume in patients with combat-related posttraumatic stress disorder, *Am J Psychiatry* **152** (1995), 973–981.

[2] A.G. Harvey, R.A. Bryant, Two-Year Prospective Evaluation of the Relationship Between Acute Stress Disorder and Posttraumatic Stress Disorder Following Mild Traumatic Brain Injury, *Am J Psychiatry* **157** (2000), 626-628.

[3] L.M. Shin, S.P.Orr, M.A.Carson, et. al, Regional cerebral Blood flow in the amygdala and medial prefrontal cortex during traumatic imagery in male and female Vietnam veterans with PTSD, *Arch. Gen. Psychiatry* **61** (2004), 168 – 176.

[4] **S.** Rockswold, G, : Rockswold, A. Defillo, Hyperbaric oxygen in traumatic brain injury, *Neurological Research* **29** (2007), 162-172.

[5] www.hbot.com

Coping with Blast-Related Traumatic Brain Injury in Returning Troops
B.K. Wiederhold (Ed.)
IOS Press, 2011
doi: 10.3233/978-1-60750-797-0-76

Traumatic Brain Injury due to Landmine Explosions

Yusuf İZCI[a, 1], Ilker SOLMAZ[a], Halil I. SECER[a] and Cemil CELIK[b]
[a]*Department of Neurosurgery, Gulhane Military*
Medical Academy, Ankara, Turkey
[b]*Department of Psychiatry, Gulhane Military Medical Academy, Ankara, Turkey*

Abstract. Landmine explosions cause most of the war injuries on the battlefield and pose a substantial public health risk. Although the lower limbs are usually affected, head injuries may also occur. The aim of this study is to describe the types of head injuries caused by the explosion of landmines, along with the management of the victims. Twenty patients who sustained a head injury due to a landmine explosion were treated in the Department of Neurosurgery between 2000 and 2010. The average age of the patients was 23.5 (range between 20 and 33). Shrapnel, stone and earth were the wounding agents. Six patients underwent neurosurgical treatment and 14 had simple scalp closure and conservative treatment. Twelwe patients had associated lesions in the other parts of the body including thorax, upper and lower limbs, and the abdomen. Three patients died due to massive brain damage. Infection was observed among 6 patients. Five patients were treated by the psychiatry department for memory and cognitive problems. Landmines occasionally cause traumatic brain injury. Surgical intervention is seldom required and survival is likely unless the patient is in a deep coma. Multidisciplinary approaches are required for these patients.

Keywords. landmine, brain injury, surgery

Introduction

Landmines are destructive and lethal weapons. The blast and thermal effects of the landmines produce injuries on the lower extremities [1]. They may also affect the craniofacial region, although there are few reports in the literature [2]. Research is insufficient, and knowledge is limited about the management of head injuries due to landmine explosions [2, 3]. In this study, we tried to present our experience on traumatic brain injury due to landmine explosions and show a management strategy for these rare injuries.

1. Method

The data of 20 patients who sustained head injuries due to landmines explosions were reviewed retrospectively. The mean age was 23.5 years and all of them were male.

---

[1]Corresponding Author: Yusuf Izci MD, Department of Neurosurgery, Gulhane Military Medical Academy, 06018 Etlik-Ankara, Turkey; E-mail: yizci@gata.edu.tr; yusufizci@yahoo.com.

None of the patients had stood on the pressure plate and detonated the landmine. All had been beside the person who detonated the mine and were injured by the consequent explosion. The wounding agents were shrapnel, stone (Fig. 1) and earth. The patients were initially evaluated by military paramedics at the time of injury, and wide spectrum antibiotics were given intravenously. They were transferred to our hospital following first aid. Neurological and radiological examinations were performed at the time of admission. The Glasgow Coma Scale (GCS), the cause of injury and the wounding agent were recorded. The patients were also examined for multiple injuries such as limb, abdominal or thoracic wounds.

Plain X-rays and computed tomography (CT) of the head were obtained. The entrance and exit points and the track of missiles were determined using CT scans and intraparenchymal fragments identified radiologically. The patients who had multiple bone fragments and necrotic brain tissue associated with hemorrhage underwent neurosurgical procedure. If there were no active bleeding, depressed skull fracture or severe brain damage, conservative treatment was applied including simple wound closure. Dural repair was performed for all patients. Wide-broad antibiotics were given to all patients and the antibiotic therapy was continued for 5 days after operation. If evidence of infection was observed, treatment was tailored according to the pathogens isolated. The number of deaths and their causes were recorded. Rehabilitation was planned for patients who had neurological deficits after neurosurgical treatment. The patients who had memory disturbance, cognitive functional disorders or attention disorders were managed by the department of psychiatry after the neurosurgical treatment. All patients followed-up with a neurological examination and CT scan at three-month intervals after discharge.

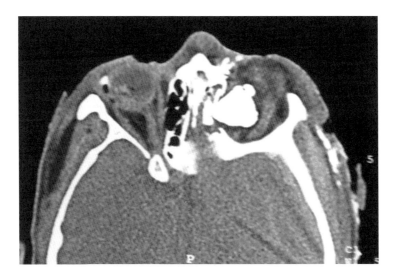

Figure 1. CT scan of a patient who was injured by a landmine shows left intraorbital stone that compresses the left optic nerve. The patient underwent left frontal craniotomy and the stone was removed from the orbit.

2. Results

Twenty armed forces personnel who had a head injury due to landmine explosion were transferred to our department from the field medical facilities. Of these patients, 12 were injured in a zone of conflict and 8 were injured on the road. A metal fragment was the wounding agent in 12 patients and stones associated with soil in 8 patients. The GCS score of the patients on admission ranged between 3 and 15. Six patients who had GCS score of 8 or less were considered as having a "severe brain injury." Fourteen patients who had GCS score higher than 8 were considered 'moderate' and 'mild' brain injuries. Associated wounds, such as orbital injury, thoracic and abdominal injuries were detected in 12 patients. Six patients underwent surgical intervention including craniectomy (Fig. 2), debridement of necrotic brain tissues and dural repair. Wound cleaning, simple closure and conservative treatment was performed for the others. Infection was observed in 6 patients and treated with antibiotics. Three patients died due to massive brain damage while 5 patients underwent treatment for memory disturbance, attention difficulties, and cognitive function disorders in the department of psychiatry.

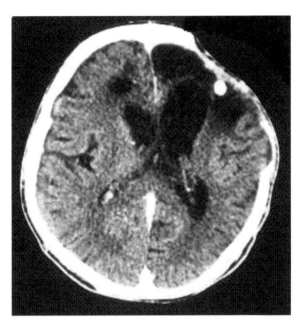

Figure 2. CT scan of a patient with left frontal injury due to landmine explosion. The patient underwent left frontal craniectomy just after the injury and cranioplasty one year after the first surgery. Please note that bone fragment in the necrotic brain tissue did not removed during the surgery.

3. Discussion

We reviewed a series of 20 patients suffering from brain injuries following landmine explosions. We described the widespread prevalence of these anti-personnel weapons and the large number of yearly casualties that are caused by them. Brain injuries are a relatively uncommon injury pattern in this setting, and our description is of interest for the neurosurgical community. By this retrospective study, we shared our experience on the traumatic brain injury due to landmine explosion and we found that these injuries are less invasive than the other types of head injuries and seldom required neurosurgical intervention.

Landmines are weight-triggered explosive devices that are intended to damage a target by blast effect or impact [4]. The target is usually humans but sometimes military or civilian vehicles. The use of landmines is controversial because they are indiscriminate weapons, harming soldiers and civilians alike [5]. But the military personel are the usual targets for terrorist attacks in Turkey.

Anti-personnel mines are designed to kill or injure enemy soldiers as opposed to destroying vehicles. They are often designed to injure rather than kill in order to increase the logistical support (evacuation, medical) burden on the opposing force [3,6,7]. Landmines are usually buried and are detonated by foot pressure. The detonation of a blast mine produces a transient pressure wave and an overpressure of hundreds of pounds per square inch [7]. The blast and thermal effects of the landmine cause injuries that usually involve the lower limbs, the perineum and the upper half of the body. The upper extremities are seldom affected, as well as the head. But if head injury occurs it may cause devastating clinical course and results. The causes of head injury following a landmine explosion are metal fragments, stones or bone fragments. These materials cause low-velocity gunshot wounds and carries high risk of infection for the victims. The kinetik energy transferred to the head from the fragments and cause brain damage.

The management of brain injuries demands the dedication of expensive and limited intensive care resources for considerable lengths of time. Brain injuries caused by landmine explosions result in various radiological lesions such as contusions, intracerebral hematomas, epidural and subdural hematomas [2]. Most of these lesions required neurosurgical intervention. Shrapnels are metal fragments and low-velocity agents to cause brain injury. Because of low-velocity, they transfered low kinetic energy to the brain and do not cause massive brain damage. In our series, 20 patients had brain injury due to landmine explosions in a period of 10 years and 6 of them underwent neurosurgical procedures for hematomas or depressed skull fractures. Fourteen patients underwent only simple closure. Psychiatric findings were observed in 5 patients. Some changes occur in memory, perception, understanding, attention, problem solving, and reasoning functions of the patients who underwent head injuries after landmine explosions. The most common cognitive disorder is shot term memory lost. These patients can remember the events which occcured before the explosion but they have difficulty learning new informations. The treatments used are methods to improve the cognitive functions, skill courses and homeworks that improve memory capacity.

Three patients died despite the surgical and medical treatment. Diffused brain damage associated with injuries in other parts of the body resulted to the death of these patients. Mortality rate was 15%. But, there were no deaths resulting from infections in our patients. Mortality is high among people with a missile injury of the posterior fossa or in the ventricular system. A low GCS score at admission is also an adverse prognostic factor. In our series, 6 patients had a GCS score below 8 and 3 of these patients died.

4. Conclusion

TBI caused by landmine explosions is a rare but important problem affecting military personel. Appropriate neurosurgical management associated with multidisciplinary approaches may improve the quality of life of patients who sustained these injuries.

References

[1]   Bilukha OO, Brennan M, Woodruff BA. Death and injury from landmines and unexploded ordnance in Afghanistan. JAMA 290   (2003), 650-653.
[2]   Secer HI, Gonul E, Izci Y. Head injuries due to landmines. Acta Neurchir (Wien) 149 (2007), 777-781.
[3]   Coupland RM, Korver A. Injuries from antipersonnel landmines: the experience of the international committee of the Red Cross. BMJ 303 (1989), 1509-1512.
[4]   Hayda RH, Harris RM, Bass CD. Blast injury research: modeling injury effects of landmines, bullets and bombs. Clin Orthop Relat 422 (2004), 97-108.
[5]   Kinra S, Black ME. Landmine related injuries in children of Bosnia and Herzegovina 1991-2000: comparisons with adults. J Epidemiol Community Health 57 (2003), 264-265.
[6]   Hanevik K, Kvale G. Landmine injuries in Eritrea. BMJ 321 (2000), 1189.
[7]   http://en.wikipedia.org/wiki/Anti-personnel_mine. (Accessed on February 9, 2011).

Coping with Blast-Related Traumatic Brain Injury in Returning Troops
B.K. Wiederhold (Ed.)
IOS Press, 2011
doi: 10.3233/978-1-60750-797-0-81

Molecular Mechanisms of Traumatic Brain Injury

Nela PIVAC [a, 1], Gordana NEDIC [a], Matea NIKOLAC [a], Maja MUSTAPIC [a],
Dubravka SVOB STRAC [b], Maja JAZVINSCAK JEMBREK [b],
and Dorotea MUCK-SELER [a]

[a]*Rudjer Boskovic Institute, Division of Molecular Medicine, Laboratory of Molecular Neuropsychiatry, Bijenicka 54, HR-10000 Zagreb, Croatia*
[b]*Rudjer Boskovic Institute, Division of Molecular Medicine, Laboratory of Molecular Neuropharmacology, Bijenicka 54, HR-10000 Zagreb, Croatia*

Abstract. Traumatic Brain Injury (TBI) is a frequent head injury, one of the leading causes of disability worldwide and a global health issue. TBI is defined as a direct physical impact to the head, and it elicits physical, cognitive, psychological, psychosocial and functional impairments. TBI can be associated with a fatal outcome. In addition, TBI is related to high healthcare costs, long term rehabilitations, prolonged sick-leaves, and social and functional disability. The conflicts around the globe have facilitated the development of complications after TBI, especially in combat veterans, but also in civilians affected by conflicts and combat situations. The severity of TBI might vary from mild to moderate and severe forms of TBI. The complications of TBI include cognitive dysfunctions, posttraumatic epilepsy, headaches and other motor and sensory neurological impairments. There are two phases of TBI: primary (a head injury) and secondary (a biological response to primary TBI). The understanding of the pathophysiology of the secondary TBI is still unclear. Biological processes that develop after TBI are the result of the organism response to the primary TBI, and they include activation of the inflammatory mediators and secretion of neurotransmitters, the development of apoptosis or necrosis, regenerative processes and altered synaptic plasticity. The main goal in TBI research is to improve the understanding of the underlying molecular mechanisms leading to the secondary TBI, to develop biomarkers that would be used to monitor the severity of injury, to find new targets (new molecules) for treatment and to have biomarkers that would follow the treatment response to reduce mortality and physical, cognitive, psychological, psychosocial and functional impairments after TBI, and to improve the clinical outcome.

Keywords. Traumatic Brain Injury, immune and biochemical mediators, genes, treatment

1. Traumatic Brain Injury

Traumatic Brain Injury (TBI) is a frequent head injury, one of the leading causes of disability worldwide and a global health issue [1-3]. TBI is a complex disease with multiple primary and secondary etiologies. After TBI a series of complex secondary

---

[1] Corresponding Author: Nela Pivac, Rudjer Boskovic Institute, Division of Molecular Medicine, Laboratory of Molecular Neuropsychiatry, Bijenicka 54, HR-10000 Zagreb, Croatia; E-mail: npivac@irb.hr.

molecular events are triggered that are both degenerative and regenerative. The conflicts around the globe have facilitated the development of treatments for complications after TBI, especially in combat veterans, but also in civilians affected by conflicts and combat situations. TBI occurs when a sudden physical assault on the head causes damage to the brain. The damage can be focal (confined to one area of the brain) or diffuse (involving more than one area of the brain).

TBI is one of the leading causes of disability worldwide, a global health issue problem that is related to high healthcare costs, long term rehabilitations, prolonged sick-leaves and social and functional disability. TBI is a consequence of a direct physical impact to the head resulting in physical, cognitive, psychological, psychosocial and functional impairments. TBI can be associated with a fatal outcome. The severity of TBI is an important determinant of the outcome. The patient outcome after TBI depends on the age, Glasgow coma scale, pupil response, and computed tomography characteristics [4]. According to the severity grades, TBI can be mild, moderate or severe. It can also be open or closed. An open head injury, or a penetrating head injury, is a consequence of a gunshot wound, a blow to the head or a result of an object penetrating the skull (i.e. when an object pierces the skull and enters the brain tissue). A closed head injury happens where there are no obvious external signs, resulting from motor vehicle crashes, falls, child abuse and violence, or domestic violence. Closed injuries result from the damage or destruction of brain tissue that occurs due to a blow to the head or a consequence of the head suddenly and violently hitting an object without the object breaking through the skull.

These injuries are the result of the harmful effects of the forces of acceleration, deceleration or rotation, which are responsible for diverse brain lesions [3].

1.1. Primary and Secondary Brain Injury

Immediate result of the TBI or primary brain injury is the injury of all components of the central nervous system (CNS) (damage of the neuronal cell bodies, dendrites, axons, glial cells, and brain vasculature) due to the deformation or compression of the brain tissue. Biological processes that develop after TBI are the result of the response of the organism to the primary TBI [5]. The first biological responses that develop after TBI are the subarachnoid or intracranial hemorrhage, increased intracranial pressure and cerebral volume, decreased cerebral blood flow, consequent cerebral hypoxia and ischemia, hypoperfusion, brain swelling and edema and dysfunction of the blood-brain barrier [3]. These biological processes might lead to seizures, respiratory depression, apnea, ischemia, hypoxic damage and ischemic stroke [3, 6, 7]. The understanding of the pathophysiology of the secondary TBI is still unclear. Secondary processes might worsen primary damage and lead to activation of a cascade of neuronal and axonal pathologies, which in turn determine the patient's overall clinical outcome. Secondary processes, that are possible due to the breakdown of the blood-brain barrier, include the cascade of pathophysiological and molecular events: activation of the inflammatory mediators (cytokines, chemokines, nitric oxide (NO), prostaglandins, matrix metalloproteines, phosphatases, phospholipases and xanthin-oxidases), excessive release of excitotoxines (excitatory amino acids glutamate and aspartate), excessive production of free radicals, release of growth factors and catecholamines, altered calcium homeostasis [3], activation of microglia, astrocytes and neurons, activation and recruitment of systemic neutrophils and macophages, activation of the complements, the development of apoptosis or necrosis, regenerative processes and altered synaptic plasticity (see Figure 1). All these mediators, such as reactive oxygen species, proinflammatory cytokines, vascular endothelial growth factor, and matrix metalloproteinases, are believed to facilitate the increased permeability of the blood-brain barrier observed after TBI [3, 5, 8].

As shown in Figure 2, the inflammatory response is most prominent in the early phase (days), while additional neural cell death, occurring either through apoptosis or necrosis, is an ongoing process over a longer time span (weeks). In time (months), brain tissue remodeling occurs through synaptic plasticity and possible stem cell differentiation.

The secondary brain changes, which appear immediately after TBI or in the following hours or days, include cellular, neurochemical and molecular responses to TBI: inflammatory infiltration, excitotoxicity, oxidative stress, amyloid β-peptide deposition, disruption of calcium homeostasis, neuronal cell death, apoptosis, cytoskeletal dysfunction and mitochondrial dysfunction (see Figure 3).

Apoptosis and the recovery or impairment of cognitive and behavioral functions are also regulated by the complex biochemical cascades and by the different genes. Up- or down-regulation of the genes encoding for growth factors, transcription and signal transduction factors and nuclear proteins, cell cycle, apoptosis, metabolism, inflammation-related factors and others are found after TBI. Specifically, different gene polymorphisms may be involved in the pathological changes after TBI or in processes of healing [9].

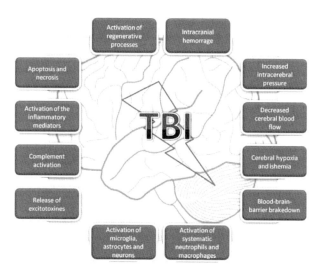

Figure 1. The cascade of events following TBI

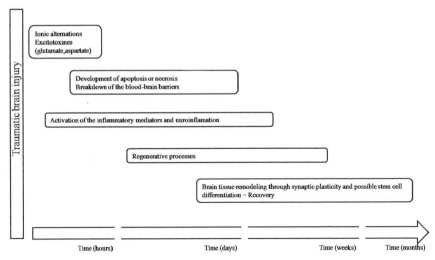

Figure 2. Time course of events following TBI

Neurometabolic cascade after traumatic injury includes cellular and axonal events [10, 11]. Cellular events are nonspecific depolarization and initiation of action potentials, release of excitatory neurotransmitters, altered glucose metabolism and mitochondrial effects, massive efflux of potassium, increased activity of membrane ionic pumps to restore homeostasis, hyperglycolysis to generate more adenosine triphosphate (ATP), lactate accumulation, calcium influx and sequestration in mitochondria, leading to impaired oxidative metabolism, decreased energy production and initiation of apoptosis. Axonal events include axonal disruption and calcium influx, neurofilament compaction via phosphorylation or sidearm cleavage, microtubule disassembly and accumulation of axonally transported organelles, axonal swelling and eventual axotomy, axonal injury and consequent altered brain activation [10, 11].

Common symptoms occuring after TBI are physical, cognitive, emotional symptoms and symptoms related to sleep and energy. Cognitive difficulties after TBI include: confusion, retrograde amnesia, loss of consciousness, trouble with attention, difficulties in concentration, difficulties in remembering, forgetting or feeling confused about recent events, repeating questions and/or answering them more slowly than usual, learning and executive control dysfunctions and memory deficits. Physical signs of TBI are headaches, dizziness, visual problems or sensitivity to light, sensitivity to noise, numbness, brief seizures, poor coordination – balance, slowed reaction time, poor concentration, vomiting – nausea, vacant stare and slurred speech. Emotional symptoms can be seen as irritability, sadness, nervousness, feeling more emotional than usual, showing less interest in favorite activities, and personality changes. The symptoms related to sleep and energy are: fatigue, drowsiness, sleeping more or less than usual, having trouble falling asleep or staying asleep. Figure 3 shows the pathophysiological events after TBI.

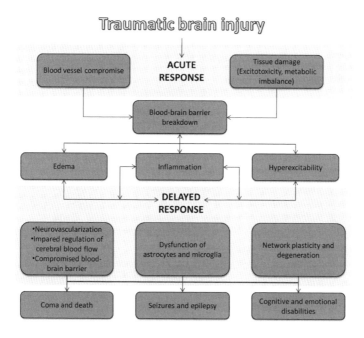

Figure 3. Pathophysiological events after TBI

1.2. Molecular Mechanism in Traumatic Brain Injury

There is accumulating evidence of the various genetic elements in the pathophysiology of brain trauma. It is believed that the extent of brain injury after TBI and possibly the outcome, might be modulated to some degree by genetic variants. The most frequently investigated genes are gene coding apolipoprotein E (ApoE), genes related to dopaminergic system (catechol-o-methyl-transferase /COMT/; dopamine D2 receptor /DRD2/), genes for interleukins (IL), angiotensin converting enzyme (ACE), p53, calcium channel subunit (CACNA1A), neurotrophic factors (brain derived neurotrophic factor /BDNF/) and others. Namely, genes that might have a role in the survival after TBI are genes that regulate inflammatory processes such as *IL-6*, since they have a role in the development of coronary and cerebral aneurysms and the ruptures of these aneurysms. In addition, gene for haemo-oxygenase-1 (HO-1) affects tissue redox homeostasis. The outcome after TBI might also be related to genes regulating the vascular response including hypoxia-inducible factor-1 and -2 (HIF-1 and HIF-2), vascular endothelial growth factor (VEGF), glucose transporter-1 (GLUT-1), transferrin (TRF), transferrin receptor (TRFR). Genes involved in neural, cognitive and behavioral response to TBI are *ApoE*, gene that regulates apoptosis - *p53*, gene that is related to fronto-executive functioning - *COMT*, genes for the caspase family of the cysteine proteases, genes that are homologues to the B-cell leukaemia oncogene-2 (*Bcl-2*). Genes regulating neurotrophic factors such as BDNF, nerve growth factor (NGF), neurotrophin 3, 4 and 5 (NT-3, NT-4 and NT-5) and their receptors are also related to the outcome after TBI. Other genes are genes for neprilysin (NEP), high mobility group protein-1 (HMG-1), the regulator of G-protein signaling 2 (RGS-2), the transforming growth factor B inducible early gene (TIEG), the inhibitor of DNA binding-3 (ID-3), the heterogeneous nuclear ribonucleoprotein H (hnRNP H), transcription factors (c-Jun) and many others that were shown to be associated with a better or poorer outcome after TBI [9, 12].

1.2.1 Cytokines and Brain Injury

As shown in Figure 1, pathological processes after TBI consist of a complex interplay of numerous mechanisms of neuronal injury, including blood-brain barrier breakdown, cerebral edema [13], excitotoxicity [14], altered cerebrovascular reactivity [15] and mitochondrial dysfunction [16]. The brain reacts to TBI or disease by cascades of cellular and molecular responses [17]. One of the responses, as well as key elements in the pathological processes associated with brain injury or damage, are immune-inflammatory processes. Inflammatory processes are not initially detrimental and their pivotal role is to defend organisms from various infections, pathogens or foreign substances. Activation of the immune system by infection triggers neuroendocrine reflexes, induction of plasma proteins cascades (complement, pathways of coagulation, and fibrinolitic systems) and a release of biological mediators of inflammation [18]. When the potential threat no longer exists and homeostasis is restored, the immune response subsides. Brain injury from traumatic and non-traumatic conditions causes long-lasting neurologic dysfunction in survivors. Growing evidence suggests that immuno-inflammatory processes contribute to the damage in neurotrauma, causing secondary damage where cytokines are major mediators [17, 19-27]. It is evident now that the brain is not an immunologically privileged organ as previously thought. Cellular response, including local neuronal cells and peripherally derived immune cells, represents a major element in brain reaction to injury. Direct blows (i.e. blunt or closed impact), deprivation of oxygen and nutrients, transplantation, neurotoxic injury (excitotoxicity), viral attack and immunological activation produce brain response of "gliosis" where resident cells (particularly astrocytes and microglia) undergo activation, hyperthrophy and proliferation [28]. Among the pathological changes of the brain tissue, impairment of the blood-brain barrier occurs in the acute posttraumatic period, allowing the entry of circulating neutrophils, monocytes and lymphocytes to the injured site, directly affecting neuronal survival and death. The significance of this response was originally thought to trigger processes that mediate repair of brain injury by restoration of blood supply, re-establishing the integrity of the blood-brain barrier and promoting general homeostasis. Over time blood-brain barrier leakage becomes sealed by repair mechanisms, however, there is a period during which the endothelium located in the region of damage remains permeable to small molecules, thus sustaining an altered homeostasis of the brain parenchyma and affecting neuronal function by causing edema and intracranial hypertension [29].

Activation of cells, including microglia and astrocytes, invasion of circulating immune cells and local cytokine production, all contribute to the neuroinflammation after TBI. Activated cells thus produce cytokines, chemokines, adhesion molecules, growth factors and other biological mediators that comprise complex intermolecular networks. All those processes causing compromised cerebral oxygenation and blood or nutrient supply with biochemical and metabolic dysregulations, might aggravate initial brain injury by causing secondary brain damage. However, brain responses also include pathways that are involved in reparative processes.

Cytokines, as inflammatory mediators, are not found in the normal CNS. Their levels rapidly increase in response to insult to the brain like infections, ischemia and injury [30-36]. Almost all neural cells can produce these mediators [37-39]. The precise role of the immuno-inflammatory reactions in the dynamics of brain injury and repair is still unclear. Thus, whether cellular activation and their products have either beneficial or detrimental effects leading to reparation after the secondary brain injury is still unclear. In addition, the responsible particular molecular pathways with their complex interactions are still unclear.

Cytokines are glycoproteins synthesized and released by different cells, which act as autocrine and paracrine mediators of the intracellular communication and of the inflammatory response to injury or infection. Cytokines are pleiotropic signaling chemicals whose biological effects depend on the distribution and expression of their receptors. Complex interactions can accentuate or attenuate tissue injury giving the immune system a dual role in brain injury. Activated microglia and astrocytes secrete various pro-inflammatory and anti-inflammatory cytokines in response to TBI. These include IL-1β , tumor necrosis factor α (TNF-α), IL-6 as pro-inflammatory, IL-4 and IL-10 as anti-inflammatory, several chemokines (IL-8), as well as production of reactive oxygen species, proteolytic enzymes, vasoactive substances (prostaglandins and cyclooxygenases) and adhesion molecules. After initial trauma, post-ischaemic response and regeneration depend not only on the cytokines expressed and secreted, but more importantly on the balance between pro-inflammatory and anti-inflammatory cytokines which can determine whether the activation of the immune system is harmful or beneficial to the outcome.

1.2.2. Interleukin-1 System

The IL-1 family includes two agonist proteins, IL-1α and IL-1β, which trigger cell activation upon binding with specific membrane receptors. IL-1 receptor agonist (IL-1ra) is also one of the members of IL-1 family and a naturally occurring inhibitor of IL-1. IL-1 is an important activator of the immune response, playing a key role in the onset and propagation of the complex inflammatory cascade. IL-1β has been detected in the brain parenchyma within the early hours after TBI in both humans and rodents [40, 41]. IL-1β stimulates IL-6 and TNF-α production by microglia and astrocytes and shows other actions in the CNS: it can induce growth factors like nerve growth factor and ciliary neurotrophic factor, stimulate inductible nitric oxide synthase (iNOS) and modify neurotransmitters (gamma-amino butyric acid /GABA/ and glutamate). Action of IL-1 is mediated by two specific cell surface receptors, namely RI and RII. IL-1ra competes with IL-1 for RI receptor but without inducing the signal. Since IL-1ra binds to RI with higher affinity than IL-1, IL-1α or IL1-β, it can be considered an effective inhibitor of IL-1. It has been reported that intracerebroventricular injection of recombinant IL-1ra attenuated neuronal damage [42, 43].

According to a review article by Dardiotis and colleagues [44], few association studies [45-49] have investigated the role of the IL-1 family genes (*IL-1α, IL-1β, IL-1ra*) in patients with TBI (see Figure 4).

1.2.3 Tumor Necrosis Factor α

TNF-α is one of the pro-inflammatory mediators involved in the initiation and regulation of the cytokine cascade during the inflammatory response. It is mostly produced by activated microglia and to a less extent, by neurons [50]. This cytokine was detected in serum and cerebrospinal fluid of patients with TBI [51]. Several TNF-α functions are described. It induces synthesis of other inflammatory mediators (IL-1, IL-6, IL-18), upregulates the production of chemokines and increases metalloproteinase, which contributes to the damage and permeability of the blood-brain barrier. It can also damage myelin and its precursors, induce apoptosis and necrosis, activate complement system, increase activation of astroglia, activate NO synthase and NO production.

Even though IL-1β and TNF-α do not interact with the same receptor and are structurally different, there is a significant synergistic effect of these mediators. The effects of IL-1β are intensified by TNF-α, and both of them have a crucial role in the secondary brain damage. There is evidence that IL-1β and TNF-α, like many other cytokines involved in the pathology of TBI, also have beneficial effects on the clinical outcome after TBI [17, 24, 26].

1.2.4. Interleukin-6

IL-6 is commonly considered as pro-inflammatory cytokine. It has many functions and has both a direct and indirect effect on neurons. Accordingly, elevated IL-6 levels were reported in both the CNS and serum of patients with TBI [52]. Increased IL-6 values were associated with an increase in the acute phase proteins and severe blood-brain barrier dysfunction. On the other hand, administration of recombinant IL-6 in rats showed limited neural damage following ischemia, suggesting its neuroprotective role [27, 53].

Miñambres and colleagues [54] investigated an association between *IL-6* -174 C/G polymorphism and the outcome after TBI and found no association (see Figure 4).

1.2.5 Interleukin-10

IL-10 is secreted peripherally and in the CNS by activated microglia and astrocytes [55-57]. It acts as a neuroprotective agent by suppressing microglia and astrocyte activation, and decreases the expression of pro-inflammatory cytokines [58, 59] and secretion of reactive oxygen species [60]. Although systemic administration of IL-10 improved the recovery after trauma in rats [58], no effect of IL-10 was observed in piglets subjected to hypoxic-ischemic insult [61]. An observed increase in the IL-10 production in subjects with TBI reduced the expression of TNF-α, but had no influence on the outcome [60].

It is evident that increased production of cytokines depends on the upregulation of gene expression that occurs early after TBI, while the activation or inhibition of certain cytokines could influence the outcome.

Contradictory data on the concentration and the role of specific inflammatory mediators might be explained by the time periods when the concentration or expression was measured, indicating that the exact time course and precise mechanism of action are essential for the development of potential treatment. So far, many pieces of the puzzle are still unknown. It is believed that after TBI, the "first wave" is a quick upregulation of transcription factors followed by the "second wave" which consists of an activation of heat shock proteins, and is expressed 1-2h after the initial trauma and then downregulated in 1-2 days. The most investigated is the so-called "third wave," characterized by the elevated cytokine gene expression [62-65], increased chemokines levels [66-68], and increased expression of the adhesion molecules. At this point, aside from detrimental effects, some neuroprotective factors are expressed, including growth factors (NGF and BDNF) and tumor suppressor gene p53. Recently the "fourth wave" was established with the new gene expression associated with inflammatory response in TBI that includes proteolytic enzymes, implicated in the destabilization of extracellular matrix, and related to influx of inflammatory cells and secondary brain injury. The final, "fifth wave" of the new gene expression consists of mediators such as TGF-β [69] and osteopontin (Osteo) [70, 71]. This final wave is involved in the later glial changes and tissue remodeling resulting in scarring that follows the inflammatory brain reaction. Why or when a particular cytokine expresses either a beneficial or detrimental effect depends on the nature of the pathway in which that cytokine is involved at the time of injury.

1.2.6. Chemokines

Chemokines or chemotactic cytokines are small inflammatory mediators influenced by cytokines such as IL-1β and TNF-α. Their RNA is over expressed after TBI [20, 21]. This group includes IL-8, interferon inducible protein-10 (IP-10) and monocyte chemoattractant protein-1 (MCP-1). Chemokines regulate leukocyte activation and migration [72] and are involved in neurogenesis of the nervous system. They are secreted by glia and neurons in the nervous system and they carry out their action through various chemokine receptors. Primarily, they are involved in cellular communication, mediating neuronal growth, repair and survival, but can also act as part of the pathological changes in neurodegenerative diseases [73].

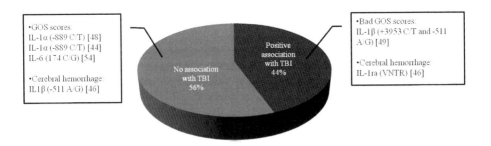

Figure 4. Genes for interleukins and TBI outcome

1.2.7. Excitatory Amino Acids

L-glutamate and L-aspartate are naturally occurring excitatory amino acids (EAA). They are released by neurons and are found in the cortex, cerebellum and spinal cord. Glutamate is the major signalling molecule and the most abundant excitatory neurotransmitter in the mammalian CNS that increases the likelihood of depolarization in the postsynaptic membrane. Although aspartate has been regarded as an excitatory transmitter for many years, the extent of its role as a transmitter is still unclear. Glutamate is important for many vital brain functions such as neuronal development, synaptic plasticity, synaptic transmission, learning and memory [74]. In physiological conditions the extracellular concentration of glutamate is highly regulated by specific, Na^+ and ATP-dependent, transporters in neurons and glia. When the glutamate level in extracellular space rises too high (if excessive amounts of glutamate are released or if glutamate clearance is insufficient), it becomes a toxin that kills neurons [75, 76].

1.2.8. Glutamate Receptors

After release by the presynaptic cells, glutamate activates two types of receptors: ionotropic (ion-channel forming receptors) and metabotropic (G-protein coupled receptors). Ionotropic receptors are pharmacologically subdivided into three classes that are named by their selective agonists: N-methyl-D-aspartate (NMDA), α-amino-3-hydroxy-5-methyl-4-isoxazolepropionic acid (AMPA) and kainate receptors. AMPA and kainate receptors trigger rapid excitatory neurotransmission mostly by promoting the entry of Na^+ ions. NMDA receptors are associated with a high-conductance Ca^{2+} channels that are blocked by Mg^{2+} in a voltage-dependent manner. Influx of Na^+ ions from non-NMDA receptors depolarizes neurons thus allowing the release of Mg^{2+} blockade. After the extrusion of Mg^{2+} ions, binding of glutamate and co-agonist glycine activates NMDA receptors and allows entry of Na^+ and Ca^{2+} ions into the cell. Ca^{2+} ions mediate most of the physiological effects of NMDA receptors activity [76, 77]. Aspartate also stimulates NMDA receptors, though not as strongly as the glutamate. NMDA receptors appear to have a pivotal role in long-term potentiation (the key process responsible for the acquisition of information), long-term depression (activity-dependent reduction in the efficacy of neuronal synapses) and developmental plasticity. Over-activation of NMDA receptors, however, appears to cause brain damage via excitotoxicity. The term was first introduced in 1969 by John Olney in his paper published in *Science* [78] and is defined as a cell death resulting from the toxic actions of excitatory amino acids. Because glutamate is the major excitatory neurotransmitter, neuronal excitotoxicty usually refers to the injury and death of neurons arising from the prolonged exposure to glutamate [75].

1.2.9. Excitotoxicity in Traumatic Brain Injury

Primary brain injury by physical forces causes brain tissue destruction and alteration of function in the early post-injury period. However, clinical outcomes and total volume of injury or lesions largely depend on physiological disturbances caused by molecular and cellular pathophysiological changes that occur after the initial injury and are all related to an increase in extracellular excitatory amino acids, primarily glutamate [79, 80].

Excitotoxicity is the predominant form of glutamate neurotoxicity. It results in the prolonged activation of glutamate receptors and causes an increase of Ca^{2+} influx. Excessive Ca^{2+} is a key factor involved in glutamate-induced neuronal injury [81]. Pathological Ca^{2+} overload triggers many downstream neurotoxic signaling cascade pathways through interactions with cytoplasmic postsynaptic density (PSD) proteins that bind with high specificity to NMDA receptor subunits and physically couple NMDA receptors to downstream signaling enzymes. Calcium-activated enzymes such as proteases, endonucleases and phospholipases contribute to the degradation of different cell components and neuronal death. It was shown that Ca^{2+}-activated proteolytic enzymes, like calpains, can degrade essential proteins and cause microtubule destruction, cytoskeletal breakdown, disruption of axonal transport and axonal disconnection. The loss of axonal function and structure appears to be a major factor in long-term outcome from TBI [82]. Elevated concentration of Ca^{2+} also activates Ca^{2+}-dependent endonucleases which can degrade DNA and Ca^{2+}/calmodulin kinase II (CaM-KII) which in turn phosphorylates a number of enzymes thus modulating their activity.

Massive influx of Ca^{2+} ions also leads to intramitochondrial Ca^{2+} overload, mitochondrial dysfunction and disruption of ATP synthesis [83-85]. Because intracellular concentration of Ca^{2+} ions is energy dependent, these changes further lead to a sustained increase in intracellular Ca^{2+}. Another important mechanism involved in excitotoxic injury is the generation of free radicals (mainly in the form of superoxide) as a consequence of mitochondrial dysfunction and the activation of Ca^{2+}-dependent enzymes such as neuronal nitric oxide synthase (nNOS). Molecular scaffold PSD-95 brings NMDA receptors into close proximity with nNOS thus explaining the preferential activation of nNOS by Ca^{2+} coming through the NMDA receptors over entry through other channels [86]. nNOS activation leads to NO production which in excess can be toxic alone, or when combined with other reactive oxygen species (ROS) such as superoxide to form highly toxic peroxynitrite. Excessive production of ROS and reactive nitrogen species (RNS) mediates detrimental damage to brain cell structures and macromolecules, including lipids, membranes, proteins and DNA via peroxidation and nitration processes [76, 87, 88].

Regulation of cell cycles and cell death following excitotoxicity is also implicated in the pathogenesis of TBI. Apoptosis of neurons and glia contributes to the overall pathology of TBI. Apoptotic cells have been observed alongside degenerating cells exhibiting classic necrotic morphology [89]. Some of the important upstream initiators of apoptosis are release of cytochrome c from the mitochondria [90], tumor suppressor gene p53 [91] and translocation of apoptosis inducing factor-AIF [92].

Besides elevations in extracellular glutamate level, altered glutamate receptor functioning has also been considered as a potential mechanism contributing to brain damage in TBI [93]. Postsynaptic glutamate transporters have altered function and composition and contribute to TBI excitotoxicity as well [14]. The group I family of metabotropic glutamate receptors appears to participate in excitotoxic damage by potentiating NMDA receptors mediated Ca^{2+} influx [94].

In the acute pathologies such as TBI, glutamate excitotoxicity is not considered to be the result of a genetic mutation or structural deficit in the channel, but normal physiological response to a CNS injury [76]. Thus far there is no evidence that genetic alterations in the amino acid sequences of glutamate receptor subunits have any impact on the outcome of TBI.

The cytokine storm (cytokine and glutamate release, the hyper-excitability; decreased ability to induce long term potentiation, the suppressed neurogenesis, reductions in neurotrophic factors and other plasticity-related molecules) after TBI can disrupt all of the beneficial processes of the immune system during normal conditions, resulting in impaired memory, neural plasticity and neurogenesis [95].

1.2.10. Apolipoprotein E and TBI

TBI has a complex etiology and genetic factors might contribute to the brain's susceptibility to injury and capacity to repair damage. ApoE has been implicated in the neuropathology of Alzheimers's disease (AD) [96, 97] but it can also have a role in the pathology of TBI. ApoE is involved in the redistribution and metabolism of cholesterol [98], neuritic extension growth and repair. It also acts as modulator of amyloid beta synthesis. Genetic polymorphism, more precisely allele ε4 of the *ApoE* gene, has been identified as a genetic risk factor for the late onset AD [96].

ApoE polymorphism is a triallelic polymorphism (ε2, ε3, ε4), and these alleles lead to 6 genotypes (E2/2, E2/3, E2/4, E3/3, E3/4, E4/4) and three protein isoforms which differ in single amino acid interchanged at positions 112 and 158; E2 (Cys112-Cys158), E3 (Cys 112-Arg158), E4 (Arg112-Arg158) [99-101].

ApoE is produced primarily by atrocytes, although microglia and neurons have a potential to synthesize ApoE. Apolipoproteins are generally lipid carriers and, as such, have a role in lipid distribution among cells [102, 103]. ApoE has been implicated in the pathology of TBI, but the mechanism of underlying association with disease and injury is unclear. The potential contribution of ApoE could be that different isoforms affect the overall outcome and repair potential after brain injury. Proposed mechanism might have a role in synaptic repair, cytoskeleton stability, oxidative stress, remodeling and neuroprotection and in nervous system plasticity.

ApoE4 isoform might be a contributing factor to outcome after TBI and it might increase the injury severity by: a less efficient transport of lipids [104, 105], an increase of the plaque formation and deposition [102, 106], an exacerbated brain inflammation [107-109], a diminished protection against damaging oxidative injury [110], a decreased brain perfusion [111], growth and branching of neuritis [112, 113] and an increased cytoskeleton susceptibility to damage [113].

On the other hand, several protective effects of ApoE4 have been reported. It has been shown that ε4 allele can activate an extracellular signal-regulated kinase cascade resulting in an activation of cAMP-response element binding protein and induction of many genes (Bcl-2) [114]. Individuals with ε4 allele also have elevated total cholesterol and low density lipoproteins [115], which leads to an increase in g-glutamil-transferase, and enzyme that diminishes protection against excitotoxicity [116]. *ApoE* ε4 allele might have a positive effect on neurogenesis [117-119].

There have been numerous studies which confirmed involvement of ApoE with TBI on several levels. Taesdale et al. [120] and Chiang et al. [121] showed that patients with ApoE4 isoform had an unfavorable outcome after TBI; unfavorable was described as a fatal outcome, or vegetative state or severe disability. In addition to the overall outcome in individuals with ApoE4, ε4 allele in carriers affects various clinical aspects, such as a longer period of unconsciousness [122], poorer recovery of patients with posttraumatic unawareness [123], larger intracranial hematomas following TBI [124] and higher risk of posttraumatic seizures [125]. There are also some contradictory data on the influence of ε4 on the rehabilitation outcome: a strong association with the clinical outcome [122], or a poor outcome [126] was found in ε4 carriers following rehabilitation. ApoE4 has an effect on cognitive function deterioration in patients with ε4 allele [127]. Several studies showed the influence of ApoE on cognitive and/or behavioral functions [128, 129] and memory function [130] after TBI. Even though the majority of the studies reported association of ApoE with the overall outcome after TBI, there were numerous studies reporting a negative association [131-135]. This could be explained by the racial diversity and/or presence of other modifier genes, gene-environment interactions [133], and, one has to consider the possible methodological limitations.

Despite all controversies from the literature [106, 120, 123, 124, 126, 128-130, 132-134, 136-167] (see Figure 5) as described by Dardiotis and colleagues [44], there is a general consensus that the *ApoE* genotype can influence TBI outcome, but the mechanism of ApoE influence is still unknown.

1.2.11. ApoE Gene Promoter

Apart from gene polymorphism in the coding region, there are polymorphisms in the transcriptional regulatory region that can influence the expression of *ApoE* [168]. These polymorphisms are located at position -219 with G/T substitution and A/T substitution at position -491 in the *ApoE* gene promoter. T to G substitution at position -219 results in the 169% increase in the promoter activity. On the contrary, A to T substitution at position -491 results in a 63% decrease [168]. The influence of these polymorphisms on *ApoE* expression could also contribute indirectly to the genetic background, influencing susceptibility and recovery after TBI. The TT genotype of the -219G/T and AA genotype of the -419 A/T promoter polymorphisms have been found to increase risk of AD [169] by affecting the amount of amyloid beta deposition in the AD patients [170, 171]. It has been shown [172] that among carriers of TT genotype of the -219G/T polymorphism, there was a poorer recovery outcome 6 months after TBI. No association was found between the -419A/T promoter polymorphism and the outcome [172].

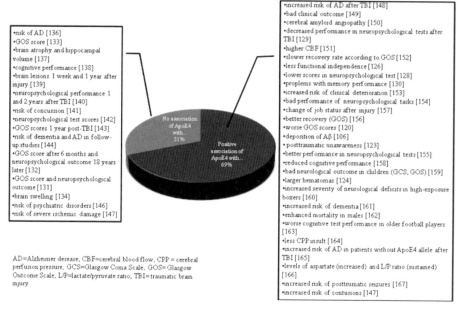

Figure 5. Summary of the risk of ApoE4 isoform and outcome after TBI

1.2.12. Dopaminergic System and TBI

There are eight dopaminergic signaling pathways in the CNS, four of which are presented in Table 1 as the major pathways. TBI disrupts the dopamine system via ascending dopaminergic pathways that are divided into nigrostriatal and mesocorticolimbic pathways [173]. The nigrostriatal dopaminergic system includes substantia nigra innervating striatum, and mesocorticolimbic dopaminergic system or pathway includes ventral tegmental area, projecting to the prefrontal cortex, hippocampus, amygdala, and nucleus accumbens. The disruption of the dopaminergic nigrostriatal system is associated with voluntary movement and this pathway is important for reward processing and acquisition of spatial learning and memory, since dopaminergic system in striatum and dorsolateral prefrontal cortex is important for executive function and working memory. The disruptions of dopaminergic mesocorticolimbic pathways after TBI cause impairments in memory consolidation, motivation, drug reinforcement and addiction, since the dopaminergic mesocorticolimbic pathways modulate arousal, stress response, and addiction. Dopaminergic pathways play an important role in functions of the frontal cortex, striatum and hippocampus [174-180], brain areas critical for cognitive function [181, 182], which are impaired after TBI [176, 183, 184]. Levels of dopamine and glutamate are very strictly controlled by CNS since their oscillations can lead to cellular dysfunction and/or death [185] and because of their potential excitotoxicity [186].

Table 1. Major dopaminergic pathways in CNS.

Dopaminergic pathway	Description	Function	Association
mesolimbic pathway	Transmits dopamine from the ventral tegmental area (VTA) to the nucleus accumbens.	• Memory • Motivation and emotional response • Reward and desire • Addiction	• Neuropsychiatric disorders • Arousal • Stress • Addiction
mesocortical pathway	Transmits dopamine from the VTA to the frontal cortex.		
nigrostriatal pathway	Transmits dopamine from the substantia nigra to the striatum.	• Voluntary movement • Reward processing • Acquisition of spatial learning and memory • Other cognitive functions	Parkinson's disease
tuberoinfudibular pathway	Transmits dopamine from the hypothalamus to the pituitary gland.	• Hormonal regulation • Maternal behavior (nurturing) • Pregnancy • Sensory processes	Hyperprolactinaemia

Dopamine signaling is altered after TBI. One of the alterations in dopaminergic transmission includes initial increase in tissue dopamine, followed by a chronic dopaminergic hypofunction, indicated by the decrease in the evoked dopamine release and total dopamine transporter (DAT) expression [187]. All these changes result in a deficient dopaminergic neurotransmission [173]. Observations by Yan et al. [188] showed increased tyrosine hydroxylase (TH) expression (an enzyme responsible for dopamine synthesis), and no alterations in dopamine beta hydroxylase (DβH) levels (an enzyme that converts dopamine to other catecholamines) after TBI. Alterations in catecholaminergic systems are time- [189-192] and gender-dependent [187]. It has been shown [193] that TBI also stimulates *COMT* gene expression in hippocampus microglia. There are also indications of the alterations in dopaminergic receptor systems following TBI. Dopamine D1 receptor (DRD1) showed a decreased binding capacity immediately following injury [194]. Initially increased dopaminergic levels following TBI could cause excitotoxic and oxidative damage to dopaminergic cellular function, and these alterations later induce decreased dopamine release [195, 196]

TBI is followed by changes in the intracellular calcium release [197, 198], glutamatergic signaling pathways [88, 199], Na/K ATPase functioning [200, 201], metabolic activity [202, 203] and altered levels of excitatory amino acids [79, 204]. It should be noted that dopaminergic signaling pathways play an important role in regulating calcium release [205], cellular metabolism, function of Na/K ATPase [206] and NMDA receptors (through dopamine cAMP regulated phosphoprotein 32 kDa and protein phosphatase-1) [207, 208]. Dopamine also plays a role in inflammatory processes which follow TBI [209].

Polymorphisms in genes that modulate the dopaminergic system could play an important role as mediators of the outcome after TBI by modulating the injury extent, recovery from injury, pre-injury cognitive capacities and reserve and by modulating response to treatment [210]. Studies of the genetic variations that could modulate outcome after TBI are only beginning to gain interest among researches.

1.2.13. Catechol-O-methyltransferase

COMT transfers a methyl group to catecholamines like dopamine, epinephrine and norepinephrine. This enzyme is responsible for their degradation [211]. COMT is important in regulating levels of synaptic dopamine, especially in the prefrontal cortex, which is highly dependent on the action of the COMT in dopamine flux, since it has a lower DAT expression [212, 213]. The prefrontal cortex is responsible for organizing and coordinating information from other parts of the brain and carrying out executive functions [214]. It is involved in planning complex cognitive behavior, personality expression, decision making and moderating correct social behavior, abstract thinking, self-monitoring, emotions and working (short-term) memory [214]. All variations in the *COMT* gene that affect the stability and activity of COMT enzyme alter its ability to break down neurotransmitters in the prefrontal cortex area. The most often studied variation in the *COMT* gene is a single base pair substitution of guanine for adenine resulting in a replacement of the amino acid valine with the amino acid methionine at position 158 (written as Val158Met) in the longer form of the enzyme (membrane-bound COMT or MB-COMT), and at position 108 (written as Val108Met) in the shorter form (soluble COMT or S-COMT). This polymorphism affects COMT activity [215-217]. The methionine variant of COMT has a lower stability and activity, and it is associated with a fourfold decrease in dopamine metabolism. Because of its lower activity, the methionine variant enables a significant increase in dopaminergic stimulation of the post-synaptic neuron. There are few studies that suggest a neuroprotective effect of the Met/Met genotype, especially in preserving executive functioning, among schizophrenics, healthy siblings and relatively healthy subjects [218-222], indicating that higher levels of dopamine in individuals with the Met/Met genotype enhance prefrontal function. Following TBI, patients with Val/Val genotype performed more poorly on the Wisconsin Card Sorting Test (WCST) compared to patients who were homozygotes for low activity Met allele. These results suggest that they had less cognitive flexibility and difficulties in shifting mental state [223]. The Val allele was also associated with poorer performance on a Continuous Performance Test in TBI patients [224].

1.2.14. Dopamine D2 Receptor

McAllister and colleagues [225] hypothesized that the "TaqIA" (rs1800497) polymorphism in the gene for DRD2 could be associated with a poorer performance on memory and attention tasks after TBI. It is well known that the dopaminergic system plays a crucial role in modulating memory, attention and frontal-executive functions in TBI [226]. The T allele of "TaqIA" polymorphism was associated with a 40% reduction in DRD2 expression, but without effects on the receptor affinity [227, 228]. The study showed a correlation between the T allele and poor performance on the California Verbal Learning Test recognition task. There was also a significant interaction of the T allele and slower performance on Continuous Performance Test measures of response latency. The "TaqIA" polymorphism is a non-synonymous coding polymorphism in a functionally unrelated ankyrin repeat and protein kinase domain-containing protein 1 (ANKK1) gene, but it is probably in linkage disequilibrium with a functional *DRD2* polymorphism. A later study by the same group confirmed their previous results and it also showed a great association of a haplo-block of three SNPs in *ANKK1* (rs11604671, rs4938016 and rs1800497) rather than the adjacent *DRD2* gene with cognitive outcome measures [229].

1.2.15. Other Potential Candidate Genes

Polymorphisms in other potential dopaminergic candidate genes like genes coding for dopaminergic D3 receptor (DRD3), dopaminergic D4 receptor (DRD4) and DAT, will be in the focus of the further studies evaluating their association with the outcome after TBI.

1.3. Current and Emerging Treatments of Traumatic Brain Injury

The treatment of individuals after TBI is focused on stabilization of an individual with TBI and prevention of further injury. Further steps are to insure proper oxygen supply to the brain and the rest of the body, to maintain adequate blood flow and to control blood pressure. For moderately to severely injured patients it is important to receive rehabilitation, to receive individually tailored treatment programs in different areas: physical therapy, occupational therapy, speech/language therapy, physiatry, psychology/psychiatry and social support.

The current medical management of TBI mainly includes intensive clinical care and long-term rehabilitation [230]. Besides general supportive care of vital body functions, it consists of various measures including reduction of increased intracranial pressure and cerebral edema, neuroprotection, management of consequences such as seizures and behavioral disorders, as well as rehabilitation for neurological disability (including physical therapy and mental training) [231].

Cerebral edema and associated increased intracranial pressure are the major immediate consequences of TBI. In order to manage these crucial problems which contribute to most early deaths, several treatments are currently applied in the acute phase of TBI including: osmotherapy by the administration of osmotic agents such as hypertonic mannitol or hypertonic saline, hyperbaric oxygen therapy and surgical decompression [232-234].

Moreover, a wide range of neuroprotective strategies for TBI, including different pharmacological and nonpharmacological approaches, have been extensively investigated [231]. Excitotoxicity, perturbation of cellular calcium homeostasis, increased free radical generation and lipid peroxidation, inflammation, mitochondrial damage, apoptosis and diffuse axonal injury, which represent the most important mechanisms of neuronal cell dysfunction and damage associated with TBI, are commonly discussed as possible drug targets for neuroprotective therapy [235-239].

Pharmacological agents investigated for potential neuroprotective effects include: calcium channel blockers (nimodipine, ziconotide, SNX-111, SNX-185) [240], NMDA receptor antagonists (dexanabinol, traxoprodil, aptiganel, eliprodil, memantine, arcain, selfotel, D-CCP-ene, amantadine) [241], non-NMDA antagonists (NBQX), metabotropic glutamate receptor inhibitors (mGluR1 inhibitors - AIDA, CPCCOEt, LY-367385, mGluR5 inhibitors - SIB-1893, MPEP), AMPA-receptor antagonists (zonampanel), corticosteroids (methylprednisolone, dexamethasone, triamincinolone) [242] and aminosteroids (tirilazad mesylate), glucocorticoid receptor antagonists (RU-486), thyrotropin-releasing hormone analogs, human corticotrophin releasing factor, neurosteroids (estrogen, progesterone) [243], modulators of the kinin/kalikrein system (bradykinin beta 2 receptor antagonists-bradycor, anatibant) [244], monoaminergic substances (methylphenidate, amphetamines, bromocriptine) [245], barbiturates (thiopental, pentobarbital) [246], benzodiazepines (diazepam), anesthetics (ketamine, propofol), antiepileptic drugs (topiramate, levetiracetam), cannabinoids (dexanabinol, KN38-7271), opioid receptor antagonists (naloxone), free radical scavengers (polyethylene glycol-conjugated superoxide dismutase (PEG-SOD), lecithinized superoxide dismutase (PC-SOD), alpha-phenyl-*N*-tert-butyl nitrone, second generation nitrone - STAZN, melatonin, superoxide radical scavengers - OPC-14117, poly(ADP-ribose) polymerase (PARP) inhibitors - GPI-6150) [247], NO modulators (inhibitors of NO synthase (NOS) -BN 80933, donors of NO - DETA/NONOate) [248], antioxidants (glutathione, pyruvate, N-acetylcysteine, ebselen, allopurinol), oxygen carriers (oxycyte), necrosis inhibitors (calpain inhibitors), apoptosis and caspase inhibitors (inhibitors of apoptosis proteins, caspase-3-inhibitor - z-DEVD-fmk, caspase-1-inhibitor - mynocycline), necroptosis inhibitors (necrostatin-1), alkalizing agents (tromethamine), anti-inflammatory agents (COX inhibitors, minocycline, celecoxib, nimesulide), immunophilin ligands - immunosuppressants (cyclosporine A, FK506), cytokines (IL-6, IL- 10, TNF-α), erythropoetin (EPO) and carbamylated form of EPO (CEPO) [249], neurotrophic and neurogenesis factors (NGF, BDNF, IGF, inhibitor of extracellular signal-related kinase 1/2 - PD98059, riluzole) and their analogs (NNZ-2566), peroxisome proliferator-activated receptor agonists (fenofibrate, rosiglitazone, pioglitazone), statins (atorvastatin, simvastatin, lovastatin) [250], cholinesterase inhibitors (rivastigmine), inhibitors of complement system (Crry-Ig molecule, monoclonal anti-factor B antibody) [251], recombinant factor VII a [252], low molecular weight heparin (enoxaparin), prostacyclin, citicoline (ceraxon), creatine, magnesium sulfate [253], omega-3 fatty acids, resveratrol, S100B calcium binding protein [254] and many others [231, 235, 237, 255].

In addition to extensive pharmacological investigation, there are also various potential nonpharmacological approaches for neuroprotection in TBI such as: nanobiotechnology-based neuroprotection (cerium oxide or yttrium oxide nanoparticles, PLGA nanoparticles loaded with superoxide dismutase, peptide nanofiber scaffold), antisense approaches (anti-mRNA strategies: antisense oligonucleotides (AS ODNs), small interfering RNA (siRNA)), stem cell therapy (transplantation of bone marrow stromal cells (MSCs) in the brain), gene therapy (transplantation of neural stem cell retrovirally transduced to produce NGF), vaccines (active or passive immunization with CNS-associated self-antigens), inhibition of Nogo-A (growth inhibitory protein) with monoclonal antibody IN -1, modest cooling (35-37.5°C) and hypothermia (32-34°C) [256-260].

Numerous drug compounds and interventions listed here that potentially mediate neuroprotection and/or repair have been tested and identified in preclinical TBI studies over the years. Unfortunately, most of the promising therapeutic approaches developed from experimental animal models of TBI have failed in translation to the clinical application [261-263]. Hence, to date there is no clinically proven effective procedure or treatment with neuroprotective agents to limit secondary brain damage, enhance repair and promote functional recovery [263].

However, as patients in the post-acute phase of TBI often develop disorders of consciousness and arousal, attentional and memory disturbances, disorders of other cognitive domains including executive functions, as well as depression, anxiety, sleep disturbance, fatigue, apathy, limited coping strategies, agitation, irritability, aggression, mania and even psychoses, the pharmacological management of these neurobehavioral disorders following TBI is common practice and includes the use of psychoactive drugs such as neurostimulants (methylphenidate, dextroamphetamine), dopaminergic agents (amantadine, pramipexole, bromocriptine, levodopa), antidepressants (buspirone, doxepin, imipramine, sertraline, fluoxetine, citalopram, carbamazepine, venlafaxine, amitriptyline, desipramine, phenelzine), modafinil, zolpidem, opioid antagonists (naltrexone), cholinesterase inhibitors (physostigmine, donepezil, rivastigmine, galantamine), atomoxetine, antiepileptic agents (phenytoin, topiramate, lamotrigine, gabapentin, pregabalin, valproate, carbamazepine), beta-blockers (propranolol, pindolol), neuroleptics (droperidol, haloperidol, methotrimeprazine, clozapine, quetiapine, ziprasidone, olanzepine), lithium, clonidine and many more [264, 265].

Despite this wide range of therapeutics used as a pharmacological intervention of neurobehavioral consequences in TBI, studies to date have yielded minimal positive evidence for the usage of neurostimulants to improve certain aspects of attention, SSRIs for the treatment of depression and beta-blockers for the control of agitated behavior. Dopaminergic agents were reported to have beneficial effects on attention, arousal and impaired conscious states [265].

1.3.1. Dopaminergic Drugs and Traumatic Brain Injury

The pharmacotherapy of TBI includes the use of drugs acting via dopaminergic system: methylphenidate, amantadine hydrochloride and bromocriptine. These drugs were recommended to be used in acute and rehabilitative phases [196, 264]. Methylphenidate might be used to increase attentional function and speed of processing. Methylphenidate and amantadine hydrochloride might be used to increase general cognitive function after TBI, while bromocriptine might be used to elevate executive function. In eight clinical studies, although including a small number of subjects that were mostly in the chronic phase after TBI, improvements after methylphenidate were noted in memory, attentional recovery, speed of processing, caregiver ratings of attention, cognitive functioning in working memory reaction time, maintaining daytime alertness, increased rate of recovery and reduction in the differences in attentional shifts [173, 264]. These results suggested that methylphenidate had beneficial effects on memory, attention, learning, cognitive processing, disability rating scale scores, behavior, processing speed and visuo-spatial attention. On the other hand, two studies failed to find a significant beneficial effect of methylphenidate on attention, disability rating scale scores, memory or behavior [173]. The other dopaminergic drug that was evaluated for its positive effects in agitation, aggression, arousal, orientation, sequencing skills, processing response time, memory, attention, activities in daily living, cognition, executive function and prefrontal activity is amantadine. Improvement was shown in nine clinical studies with patients in the acute or recovery phase after TBI, while two studies did not confirm its beneficial effects [173]. Bromocriptine was studied in four clinical studies in patients in the recovery phase and resulted in improvements in frontal cognition, reward, motivation, prefrontal function, executive function and reduction in disability rating scale scores, while one study that used higher doses of bromocriptine did not detect effectiveness of bromocriptine in moderate to severe TBI [173].

The limitations in studies using dopaminergic medication to treat consequences of TBI are numerous, including the small patient populations, lack of proper controls, variations in treatment protocols, the absence of randomized clinical trials, a poor definition of TBI, the unknown dose and time period of administration for dopaminergic therapy, the limited understanding of the molecular mechanisms of the disrupted DA signaling and the fact that the treatment differs if dopaminergic disruptions occur after TBI acutely, during recovery, or chronically.

The advantage is that dopaminergic targeted therapies represent a clinical option in the treatment of memory, learning and executive function deficiencies that follow TBI. However, better understanding of the dopaminergic dysfunction after TBI might enable future studies that should include large number of patients and proper control subjects, that should stratify results based upon gender, use genetic markers and better injury profiles. This approach might allow clinicians to recognize which patients should receive drugs acting through dopaminergic pathways [173].

Although physical therapy, exercise, cognitive rehabilitation, deep brain stimulation, environmental enrichment, psychotherapy and other behavioral modification techniques are also applied in the current management of TBI, no strong evidence exists to support that any singular agent or therapeutic intervention is effective in the recovery process from TBI. The explanation might be that pharmacotherapy usually targeted only a single aspect of TBI or a specific pathway of the injury cascade. Multiple mechanisms/pathways involved in the brain damage indicate that strategies combining more than one approach may be required for neuroprotection following TBI. Moreover, combination therapy may be necessary as a series of interventions in the acute or post-acute setting, as well as a longitudinal set of therapies administered over time. These potential combinations include intensive care, surgery, pharmacological intervention, cell replacement therapy, rehabilitation and many other approaches. Finally, many new findings regarding molecular mechanisms of TBI, as well as numerous experimental substances that still await clinical testing, show promise for the future management of TBI.

2. Conclusions

The pathophysiology of the secondary brain injury is still unclear. Although new findings help to reveal some of the underlying mechanisms, there are still a lot of unknown facts regarding molecular mechanisms of the TBI. Therefore, the search for valid and objective biomarkers is important task for reserachers and clinicians worldwide; to find the objective biomarkers, associated either with degenerative or with regenerative processes occurring after TBI, to provide the best possible treatment and to enable the patient prediction outcome. The main goal of the research of TBI is to improve the understanding of the underlying molecular mechanisms leading to the secondary TBI, to develop biomarkers that would be used to monitor the severity of injury, to develop new targets (new molecules) for the treatment, to have biomarkers that would follow the treatment response, to reduce mortality, to reduce physical, cognitive, psychological, psychosocial and functional impairments after TBI and to improve the clinical outcome.

References

[1]   T. Veenith, S. Goon, R.M. Burnstein, Molecular mechanisms of traumatic brain injury: the missing link in management, *World J Emerg Surg* **4** (2009), 7.

[2]   F. Petronilho, G. Feier, B. de Souza, C. Guglielmi, L.S. Constantino, R. Walz, J. Quevedo, F. Dal-Pizzol, Oxidative stress in brain according to traumatic brain injury intensity, *J Surg Res* **164** (2010), 316-320.

[3]   B.J. Zink, J. Szmydynger-Chodobska, A. Chodobski, Emerging concepts in the pathophysiology of traumatic brain injury, *Psychiatr Clin North Am* **33** (2010), 741-756.

[4]   G.D. Murray, I. Butcher, G.S. McHugh, J. Lu, N.A. Mushkudiani, A.I. Maas, A. Marmarou, E.W. Steyerberg, Multivariable prognostic analysis in traumatic brain injury: results from the IMPACT study, *J Neurotrauma* **24** (2007), 329-337.

[5]   M.A. Flierl, W.R. Smith, S.J. Morgan, P.F. Stahel, Molecular mechanisms and management of traumatic brain injury - missing the link?, *World J Emerg Surg* **4** (2009), 10.

[6]   H.M. Bramlett, W.D. Dietrich, Pathophysiology of cerebral ischemia and brain trauma: similarities and differences, *J Cereb Blood Flow Metab* **24** (2004), 133-150.

[7]   M. Gaetz, The neurophysiology of brain injury, *Clin Neurophysiol* **115** (2004), 4-18.

[8]   I.K. Moppett, Traumatic brain injury: assessment, resuscitation and early management, *Br J Anaesth* **99** (2007), 18-31.

[9]   B.D. Jordan, Genetic influences on outcome following traumatic brain injury, *Neurochemical Research* **32** (2007), 905-915.

[10] C.C. Giza, D.A. Hovda, The Neurometabolic Cascade of Concussion, *J Athl Train* **36** (2001), 228-235.

[11] G. Barkhoudarian, D.A. Hovda, C.C. Giza, The molecular pathophysiology of concussive brain injury, *Clin Sports Med* **30** (2011), 33-48, vii-iii.

[12] M. Wilson, H. Montgomery, Impact of genetic factors on outcome from brain injury, *Br J Anaesth* **99** (2007), 43-48.

[13] A.W. Unterberg, J. Stover, B. Kress, K.L. Kiening, Edema and brain trauma, *Neuroscience* **129** (2004), 1021-1029.

[14] J.H. Yi, A.S. Hazell, Excitotoxic mechanisms and the role of astrocytic glutamate transporters in traumatic brain injury, *Neurochem Int* **48** (2006), 394-403.

[15] M. Czosnyka, K. Brady, M. Reinhard, P. Smielewski, L.A. Steiner, Monitoring of cerebrovascular autoregulation: facts, myths, and missing links, *Neurocrit Care* **10** (2009), 373-386.

[16] C.L. Robertson, S. Scafidi, M.C. McKenna, G. Fiskum, Mitochondrial mechanisms of cell death and neuroprotection in pediatric ischemic and traumatic brain injury, *Exp Neurol* **218** (2009), 371-380.

[17] J. Correale, A. Villa, The neuroprotective role of inflammation in nervous system injuries, *J Neurol* **251** (2004), 1304-1316.

[18] M.C. Morganti-Kossmann, M. Rancan, V.I. Otto, P.F. Stahel, T. Kossmann, Role of cerebral inflammation after traumatic brain injury: a revisited concept, *Shock* **16** (2001), 165-177.

[19] B. Arvin, L.F. Neville, F.C. Barone, G.Z. Feuerstein, The role of inflammation and cytokines in brain injury, *Neurosci Biobehav Rev* **20** (1996), 445-452.

[20] G.Z. Feuerstein, X. Wang, F.C. Barone, The role of cytokines in the neuropathology of stroke and neurotrauma, *Neuroimmunomodulation* **5** (1998), 143-159.

[21] R.S. Ghirnikar, Y.L. Lee, L.F. Eng, Inflammation in traumatic brain injury: role of cytokines and chemokines, *Neurochem Res* **23** (1998), 329-340.

[22] S.M. Lucas, N.J. Rothwell, R.M. Gibson, The role of inflammation in CNS injury and disease, *Br J Pharmacol* **147 Suppl 1** (2006), S232-240.

[23] E.G. McKeating, P.J. Andrews, Cytokines and adhesion molecules in acute brain injury, *Br J Anaesth* **80** (1998), 77-84.

[24] P.M. Lenzlinger, M.C. Morganti-Kossmann, H.L. Laurer, T.K. McIntosh, The duality of the inflammatory response to traumatic brain injury, *Mol Neurobiol* **24** (2001), 169-181.

[25] O.I. Schmidt, C.E. Heyde, W. Ertel, P.F. Stahel, Closed head injury--an inflammatory disease?, *Brain Res Brain Res Rev* **48** (2005), 388-399.

[26] O.I. Schmidt, M.C. Morganti-Kossmann, C.E. Heyde, D. Perez, I. Yatsiv, E. Shohami, W. Ertel, P.F. Stahel, Tumor necrosis factor-mediated inhibition of interleukin-18 in the brain: a clinical and experimental study in head-injured patients and in a murine model of closed head injury, *J Neuroinflammation* **1** (2004), 13.

[27] C.D. Winter, A.K. Pringle, G.F. Clough, M.K. Church, Raised parenchymal interleukin-6 levels correlate with improved outcome after traumatic brain injury, *Brain* **127** (2004), 315-320.

[28] V.H. Perry, S. Gordon, Macrophages and the nervous system, *Int Rev Cytol* **125** (1991), 203-244.

[29] H. Tanno, R.P. Nockels, L.H. Pitts, L.J. Noble, Breakdown of the blood-brain barrier after fluid percussive brain injury in the rat. Part 1: Distribution and time course of protein extravasation, *J Neurotrauma* **9** (1992), 21-32.

[30] S. Holmin, B. Hojeberg, In situ detection of intracerebral cytokine expression after human brain contusion, *Neurosci Lett* **369** (2004), 108-114.

[31] H. Kushi, T. Saito, K. Makino, N. Hayashi, IL-8 is a key mediator of neuroinflammation in severe traumatic brain injuries, *Acta Neurochir Suppl* **86** (2003), 347-350.

[32] N.J. Rothwell, G.N. Luheshi, Interleukin 1 in the brain: biology, pathology and therapeutic target, *Trends Neurosci* **23** (2000), 618-625.

[33] T. Shiozaki, T. Hayakata, O. Tasaki, H. Hosotubo, K. Fuijita, T. Mouri, G. Tajima, K. Kajino, H. Nakae, H. Tanaka, T. Shimazu, H. Sugimoto, Cerebrospinal fluid concentrations of anti-inflammatory mediators in early-phase severe traumatic brain injury, *Shock* **23** (2005), 406-410.
[34] F.S. Silverstein, J.D. Barks, P. Hagan, X.H. Liu, J. Ivacko, J. Szaflarski, Cytokines and perinatal brain injury, *Neurochem Int* **30** (1997), 375-383.
[35] M.J. Whalen, T.M. Carlos, P.M. Kochanek, S.R. Wisniewski, M.J. Bell, R.S. Clark, S.T. DeKosky, D.W. Marion, P.D. Adelson, Interleukin-8 is increased in cerebrospinal fluid of children with severe head injury, *Crit Care Med* **28** (2000), 929-934.
[36] J.L. Tchelingerian, L. Vignais, C. Jacque, TNF alpha gene expression is induced in neurones after a hippocampal lesion, *Neuroreport* **5** (1994), 585-588.
[37] S.C. Lee, W. Liu, D.W. Dickson, C.F. Brosnan, J.W. Berman, Cytokine production by human fetal microglia and astrocytes. Differential induction by lipopolysaccharide and IL-1 beta, *J Immunol* **150** (1993), 2659-2667.
[38] G. Sebire, D. Emilie, C. Wallon, C. Hery, O. Devergne, J.F. Delfraissy, P. Galanaud, M. Tardieu, In vitro production of IL-6, IL-1 beta, and tumor necrosis factor-alpha by human embryonic microglial and neural cells, *J Immunol* **150** (1993), 1517-1523.
[39] J.L. Tchelingerian, J. Quinonero, J. Booss, C. Jacque, Localization of TNF alpha and IL-1 alpha immunoreactivities in striatal neurons after surgical injury to the hippocampus, *Neuron* **10** (1993), 213-224.
[40] C.D. Winter, F. Iannotti, A.K. Pringle, C. Trikkas, G.F. Clough, M.K. Church, A microdialysis method for the recovery of IL-1beta, IL-6 and nerve growth factor from human brain in vivo, *J Neurosci Methods* **119** (2002), 45-50.
[41] M.N. Woodroofe, G.S. Sarna, M. Wadhwa, G.M. Hayes, A.J. Loughlin, A. Tinker, M.L. Cuzner, Detection of interleukin-1 and interleukin-6 in adult rat brain, following mechanical injury, by in vivo microdialysis: evidence of a role for microglia in cytokine production, *J Neuroimmunol* **33** (1991), 227-236.
[42] S.A. Loddick, N.J. Rothwell, Neuroprotective effects of human recombinant interleukin-1 receptor antagonist in focal cerebral ischaemia in the rat, *J Cereb Blood Flow Metab* **16** (1996), 932-940.
[43] J.K. Relton, N.J. Rothwell, Interleukin-1 receptor antagonist inhibits ischaemic and excitotoxic neuronal damage in the rat, *Brain Res Bull* **29** (1992), 243-246.
[44] E. Dardiotis, K.N. Fountas, M. Dardioti, G. Xiromerisiou, E. Kapsalaki, A. Tasiou, G.M. Hadjigeorgiou, Genetic association studies in patients with traumatic brain injury, *Neurosurg Focus* **28** (2010), E9.
[45] E. Dardiotis, M. Dardioti, G.M. Hadjigeorgiou, K. Paterakis, Re: Lack of association between the IL-1 gene (-889) polymorphism and outcome after head injury (Tanriverdi T, et al. Surgical Neurology 2006;65 : 7-10), *Surg Neurol* **66** (2006), 334-335.
[46] G. Hadjigeorgiou, E. Dardiotis, K. Paterakis, M. Dardioti, K. Aggelakis, A. Tasiou, G. Xiromerisiou, A. Karantanas, A. Komnos, E. Zintzaras, N. Scarmeas, A. Papadimitriou, Association study of (VNTR) 1L-1RN and (-511) IL-1B gene polymorphisms and cerebral haemorrhagic events in patients with traumatic brain injury, *J Neurol* **252** (2005), 85-85.
[47] G.M. Hadjigeorgiou, K. Paterakis, E. Dardiotis, M. Dardioti, K. Aggelakis, A. Tasiou, G. Xiromerisiou, A. Komnos, E. Zintzaras, N. Scarmeas, A. Papadimitriou, A. Karantanas, IL-1RN and IL-1B gene polymorphisms and cerebral hemorrhagic events after traumatic brain injury, *Neurology* **65** (2005), 1077-1082.
[48] T. Tanriverdi, M. Uzan, G.Z. Sanus, O. Baykara, M. Is, C. Ozkara, N. Buyra, Lack of association between the IL1A gene (-889) polymorphism and outcome after head injury, *Surg Neurol* **65** (2006), 7-10; discussion 10.
[49] M. Uzan, T. Tanriverdi, O. Baykara, A. Kafadar, G.Z. Sanus, E. Tureci, C. Ozkara, O. Uysal, N. Buyra, Association between interleukin-1 beta (IL-1beta) gene polymorphism and outcome after head injury: an early report, *Acta Neurochir (Wien)* **147** (2005), 715-720; discussion 720.
[50] C.D. Breder, M. Tsujimoto, Y. Terano, D.W. Scott, C.B. Saper, Distribution and characterization of tumor necrosis factor-alpha-like immunoreactivity in the murine central nervous system, *J Comp Neurol* **337** (1993), 543-567.
[51] S.A. Ross, M.I. Halliday, G.C. Campbell, D.P. Byrnes, B.J. Rowlands, The presence of tumour necrosis factor in CSF and plasma after severe head injury, *Br J Neurosurg* **8** (1994), 419-425.
[52] E.G. McKeating, P.J. Andrews, D.F. Signorini, L. Mascia, Transcranial cytokine gradients in patients requiring intensive care after acute brain injury, *Br J Anaesth* **78** (1997), 520-523.
[53] M. Penkowa, J. Camats, H. Hadberg, A. Quintana, S. Rojas, M. Giralt, A. Molinero, I.L. Campbell, J. Hidalgo, Astrocyte-targeted expression of interleukin-6 protects the central nervous system during neuroglial degeneration induced by 6-aminonicotinamide, *J Neurosci Res* **73** (2003), 481-496.

[54] E. Minambres, A. Cemborain, P. Sanchez-Velasco, M. Gandarillas, G. Diaz-Reganon, U. Sanchez-Gonzalez, F. Leyva-Cobian, Correlation between transcranial interleukin-6 gradient and outcome in patients with acute brain injury, *Crit Care Med* **31** (2003), 933-938.

[55] F. Aloisi, R. De Simone, S. Columba-Cabezas, G. Levi, Opposite effects of interferon-gamma and prostaglandin E2 on tumor necrosis factor and interleukin-10 production in microglia: a regulatory loop controlling microglia pro- and anti-inflammatory activities, *J Neurosci Res* **56** (1999), 571-580.

[56] B. Mesples, F. Plaisant, P. Gressens, Effects of interleukin-10 on neonatal excitotoxic brain lesions in mice, *Brain Res Dev Brain Res* **141** (2003), 25-32.

[57] Z. Wu, J. Zhang, H. Nakanishi, Leptomeningeal cells activate microglia and astrocytes to induce IL-10 production by releasing pro-inflammatory cytokines during systemic inflammation, *J Neuroimmunol* **167** (2005), 90-98.

[58] S.M. Knoblach, A.I. Faden, Interleukin-10 improves outcome and alters proinflammatory cytokine expression after experimental traumatic brain injury, *Exp Neurol* **153** (1998), 143-151.

[59] S.G. Kremlev, C. Palmer, Interleukin-10 inhibits endotoxin-induced pro-inflammatory cytokines in microglial cell cultures, *J Neuroimmunol* **162** (2005), 71-80.

[60] E. Csuka, M.C. Morganti-Kossmann, P.M. Lenzlinger, H. Joller, O. Trentz, T. Kossmann, IL-10 levels in cerebrospinal fluid and serum of patients with severe traumatic brain injury: relationship to IL-6, TNF-alpha, TGF-beta1 and blood-brain barrier function, *J Neuroimmunol* **101** (1999), 211-221.

[61] K. Lyng, B.H. Munkeby, O.D. Saugstad, B. Stray-Pedersen, J.F. Froen, Effect of interleukin-10 on newborn piglet brain following hypoxia-ischemia and endotoxin-induced inflammation, *Biol Neonate* **87** (2005), 207-216.

[62] J.E. Garcia, Jr., D. Nonner, D. Ross, J.N. Barrett, Neurotoxic components in normal serum, *Exp Neurol* **118** (1992), 309-316.

[63] D. Piani, M. Spranger, K. Frei, A. Schaffner, A. Fontana, Macrophage-induced cytotoxicity of N-methyl-D-aspartate receptor positive neurons involves excitatory amino acids rather than reactive oxygen intermediates and cytokines, *Eur J Immunol* **22** (1992), 2429-2436.

[64] X.K. Wang, F.C. Barone, N.V. Aiyar, G.Z. Feuerstein, Interleukin-1 receptor and receptor antagonist gene expression after focal stroke in rats, *Stroke* **28** (1997), 155-161.

[65] X.K. Wang, T.L. Yue, P.R. Young, F.C. Barone, G.Z. Feuerstein, Expression of Interleukin-6, C-Fos, and Zif268 Messenger-Rnas in Rat Ischemic Cortex, *J Cerebr Blood F Met* **15** (1995), 166-171.

[66] T. Liu, P.R. Young, P.C. McDonnell, R.F. White, F.C. Barone, G.Z. Feuerstein, Cytokine-induced neutrophil chemoattractant mRNA expressed in cerebral ischemia, *Neurosci Lett* **164** (1993), 125-128.

[67] X. Wang, J.A. Ellison, A.L. Siren, P.G. Lysko, T.L. Yue, F.C. Barone, A. Shatzman, G.Z. Feuerstein, Prolonged expression of interferon-inducible protein-10 in ischemic cortex after permanent occlusion of the middle cerebral artery in rat, *J Neurochem* **71** (1998), 1194-1204.

[68] X. Wang, T.L. Yue, F.C. Barone, G.Z. Feuerstein, Monocyte chemoattractant protein-1 messenger RNA expression in rat ischemic cortex, *Stroke* **26** (1995), 661-665; discussion 665-666.

[69] X. Wang, T.L. Yue, R.F. White, F.C. Barone, G.Z. Feuerstein, Transforming growth factor-beta 1 exhibits delayed gene expression following focal cerebral ischemia, *Brain Res Bull* **36** (1995), 607-609.

[70] J.A. Ellison, J.J. Velier, P. Spera, Z.L. Jonak, X. Wang, F.C. Barone, G.Z. Feuerstein, Osteopontin and its integrin receptor alpha(v)beta3 are upregulated during formation of the glial scar after focal stroke, *Stroke* **29** (1998), 1698-1706; discussion 1707.

[71] X. Wang, C. Louden, T.L. Yue, J.A. Ellison, F.C. Barone, H.A. Solleveld, G.Z. Feuerstein, Delayed expression of osteopontin after focal stroke in the rat, *J Neurosci* **18** (1998), 2075-2083.

[72] W. Lu, J.A. Gersting, A. Maheshwari, R.D. Christensen, D.A. Calhoun, Developmental expression of chemokine receptor genes in the human fetus, *Early Hum Dev* **81** (2005), 489-496.

[73] L. Fan, P.R. Young, F.C. Barone, G.Z. Feuerstein, D.H. Smith, T.K. McIntosh, Experimental brain injury induces expression of interleukin-1 beta mRNA in the rat brain, *Brain Res Mol Brain Res* **30** (1995), 125-130.

[74] S.R. Platt, The role of glutamate in central nervous system health and disease--a review, *Vet J* **173** (2007), 278-286.

[75] X.X. Dong, Y. Wang, Z.H. Qin, Molecular mechanisms of excitotoxicity and their relevance to pathogenesis of neurodegenerative diseases, *Acta Pharmacol Sin* **30** (2009), 379-387.

[76] A. Lau, M. Tymianski, Glutamate receptors, neurotoxicity and neurodegeneration, *Pflugers Arch* **460** (2010), 525-542.

[77] G.E. Hardingham, Coupling of the NMDA receptor to neuroprotective and neurodestructive events, *Biochem Soc Trans* **37** (2009), 1147-1160.

[78] J.W. Olney, Brain lesions, obesity, and other disturbances in mice treated with monosodium glutamate, *Science* **164** (1969), 719-721.

[79] A.I. Faden, P. Demediuk, S.S. Panter, R. Vink, The role of excitatory amino acids and NMDA receptors in traumatic brain injury, *Science* **244** (1989), 798-800.

[80] R. Bullock, A. Zauner, J.J. Woodward, J. Myseros, S.C. Choi, J.D. Ward, A. Marmarou, H.F. Young, Factors affecting excitatory amino acid release following severe human head injury, *J Neurosurg* **89** (1998), 507-518.

[81] M. Tymianski, C.H. Tator, Normal and abnormal calcium homeostasis in neurons: a basis for the pathophysiology of traumatic and ischemic central nervous system injury, *Neurosurgery* **38** (1996), 1176-1195.

[82] M.W. Greve, B.J. Zink, Pathophysiology of traumatic brain injury, *Mt Sinai J Med* **76** (2009), 97-104.

[83] A.F. Schinder, E.C. Olson, N.C. Spitzer, M. Montal, Mitochondrial dysfunction is a primary event in glutamate neurotoxicity, *J Neurosci* **16** (1996), 6125-6133.

[84] A. Atlante, P. Calissano, A. Bobba, S. Giannattasio, E. Marra, S. Passarella, Glutamate neurotoxicity, oxidative stress and mitochondria, *FEBS Lett* **497** (2001), 1-5.

[85] Y. Wang, Z.H. Qin, Molecular and cellular mechanisms of excitotoxic neuronal death, *Apoptosis* **15** (2010), 1382-1402.

[86] R. Sattler, Z. Xiong, W.Y. Lu, M. Hafner, J.F. MacDonald, M. Tymianski, Specific coupling of NMDA receptor activation to nitric oxide neurotoxicity by PSD-95 protein, *Science* **284** (1999), 1845-1848.

[87] R. Radi, J.S. Beckman, K.M. Bush, B.A. Freeman, Peroxynitrite-induced membrane lipid peroxidation: the cytotoxic potential of superoxide and nitric oxide, *Arch Biochem Biophys* **288** (1991), 481-487.

[88] M. Arundine, M. Tymianski, Molecular mechanisms of glutamate-dependent neurodegeneration in ischemia and traumatic brain injury, *Cell Mol Life Sci* **61** (2004), 657-668.

[89] R.H. Singleton, J.T. Povlishock, Identification and characterization of heterogeneous neuronal injury and death in regions of diffuse brain injury: evidence for multiple independent injury phenotypes, *J Neurosci* **24** (2004), 3543-3553.

[90] A. Buki, D.O. Okonkwo, K.K. Wang, J.T. Povlishock, Cytochrome c release and caspase activation in traumatic axonal injury, *J Neurosci* **20** (2000), 2825-2834.

[91] J. Lu, S. Moochhala, C. Kaur, E. Ling, Changes in apoptosis-related protein (p53, Bax, Bcl-2 and Fos) expression with DNA fragmentation in the central nervous system in rats after closed head injury, *Neurosci Lett* **290** (2000), 89-92.

[92] X. Zhang, J. Chen, S.H. Graham, L. Du, P.M. Kochanek, R. Draviam, F. Guo, P.D. Nathaniel, C. Szabo, S.C. Watkins, R.S. Clark, Intranuclear localization of apoptosis-inducing factor (AIF) and large scale DNA fragmentation after traumatic brain injury in rats and in neuronal cultures exposed to peroxynitrite, *J Neurochem* **82** (2002), 181-191.

[93] L. Zhang, B.A. Rzigalinski, E.F. Ellis, L.S. Satin, Reduction of voltage-dependent Mg2+ blockade of NMDA current in mechanically injured neurons, *Science* **274** (1996), 1921-1923.

[94] V. Bruno, A. Copani, T. Knopfel, R. Kuhn, G. Casabona, P. Dell'Albani, D.F. Condorelli, F. Nicoletti, Activation of metabotropic glutamate receptors coupled to inositol phospholipid hydrolysis amplifies NMDA-induced neuronal degeneration in cultured cortical cells, *Neuropharmacology* **34** (1995), 1089-1098.

[95] R. Yirmiya, I. Goshen, Immune modulation of learning, memory, neural plasticity and neurogenesis, *Brain Behav Immun* **25** (2011), 181-213.

[96] E.H. Corder, A.M. Saunders, W.J. Strittmatter, D.E. Schmechel, P.C. Gaskell, G.W. Small, A.D. Roses, J.L. Haines, M.A. Pericak-Vance, Gene dose of apolipoprotein E type 4 allele and the risk of Alzheimer's disease in late onset families, *Science* **261** (1993), 921-923.

[97] L.A. Farrer, L.A. Cupples, J.L. Haines, B. Hyman, W.A. Kukull, R. Mayeux, R.H. Myers, M.A. Pericak-Vance, N. Risch, C.M. van Duijn, Effects of age, sex, and ethnicity on the association between apolipoprotein E genotype and Alzheimer disease. A meta-analysis. APOE and Alzheimer Disease Meta Analysis Consortium, *JAMA* **278** (1997), 1349-1356.

[98] U. Beffert, M. Danik, P. Krzywkowski, C. Ramassamy, F. Berrada, J. Poirier, The neurobiology of apolipoproteins and their receptors in the CNS and Alzheimer's disease, *Brain Res Brain Res Rev* **27** (1998), 119-142.

[99] R.W. Mahley, Apolipoprotein E: cholesterol transport protein with expanding role in cell biology, *Science* **240** (1988), 622-630.

[100] R.W. Mahley, T.L. Innerarity, S.C. Rall, Jr., K.H. Weisgraber, Plasma lipoproteins: apolipoprotein structure and function, *J Lipid Res* **25** (1984), 1277-1294.

[101] S.C. Rall, Jr., R.W. Mahley, The role of apolipoprotein E genetic variants in lipoprotein disorders, *J Intern Med* **231** (1992), 653-659.

[102] D.I. Graham, K. Horsburgh, J.A. Nicoll, G.M. Teasdale, Apolipoprotein E and the response of the brain to injury, *Acta Neurochir Suppl* **73** (1999), 89-92.

[103] D.H. Mauch, K. Nagler, S. Schumacher, C. Goritz, E.C. Muller, A. Otto, F.W. Pfrieger, CNS synaptogenesis promoted by glia-derived cholesterol, *Science* **294** (2001), 1354-1357.

[104] A.D. Kay, S.P. Day, M. Kerr, J.A. Nicoll, C.J. Packard, M.J. Caslake, Remodeling of cerebrospinal fluid lipoprotein particles after human traumatic brain injury, *J Neurotrauma* **20** (2003), 717-723.

[105] J. Poirier, A. Baccichet, D. Dea, S. Gauthier, Cholesterol synthesis and lipoprotein reuptake during synaptic remodelling in hippocampus in adult rats, *Neuroscience* **55** (1993), 81-90.

[106] J.A. Nicoll, G.W. Roberts, D.I. Graham, Apolipoprotein E epsilon 4 allele is associated with deposition of amyloid beta-protein following head injury, *Nat Med* **1** (1995), 135-137.

[107] H.P. Grocott, M.F. Newman, H. El-Moalem, D. Bainbridge, A. Butler, D.T. Laskowitz, Apolipoprotein E genotype differentially influences the proinflammatory and anti-inflammatory response to cardiopulmonary bypass, *J Thorac Cardiovasc Surg* **122** (2001), 622-623.

[108] D.T. Laskowitz, S. Goel, E.R. Bennett, W.D. Matthew, Apolipoprotein E suppresses glial cell secretion of TNF alpha, *J Neuroimmunol* **76** (1997), 70-74.

[109] D.T. Laskowitz, W.D. Matthew, E.R. Bennett, D. Schmechel, M.H. Herbstreith, S. Goel, M.K. McMillian, Endogenous apolipoprotein E suppresses LPS-stimulated microglial nitric oxide production, *Neuroreport* **9** (1998), 615-618.

[110] Y. Lee, M. Aono, D. Laskowitz, D.S. Warner, R.D. Pearlstein, Apolipoprotein E protects against oxidative stress in mixed neuronal-glial cell cultures by reducing glutamate toxicity, *Neurochem Int* **44** (2004), 107-118.

[111] D.T. Laskowitz, H. Sheng, R.D. Bart, K.A. Joyner, A.D. Roses, D.S. Warner, Apolipoprotein E-deficient mice have increased susceptibility to focal cerebral ischemia, *J Cereb Blood Flow Metab* **17** (1997), 753-758.

[112] S. Bellosta, B.P. Nathan, M. Orth, L.M. Dong, R.W. Mahley, R.E. Pitas, Stable expression and secretion of apolipoproteins E3 and E4 in mouse neuroblastoma cells produces differential effects on neurite outgrowth, *J Biol Chem* **270** (1995), 27063-27071.

[113] W.J. Strittmatter, A.M. Saunders, M. Goedert, K.H. Weisgraber, L.M. Dong, R. Jakes, D.Y. Huang, M. Pericak-Vance, D. Schmechel, A.D. Roses, Isoform-specific interactions of apolipoprotein E with microtubule-associated protein tau: implications for Alzheimer disease, *Proc Natl Acad Sci U S A* **91** (1994), 11183-11186.

[114] N. Ohkubo, N. Mitsuda, M. Tamatani, A. Yamaguchi, Y.D. Lee, T. Ogihara, M.P. Vitek, M. Tohyama, Apolipoprotein E4 stimulates cAMP response element-binding protein transcriptional activity through the extracellular signal-regulated kinase pathway, *J Biol Chem* **276** (2001), 3046-3053.

[115] C.F. Sing, J. Davignon, Role of the apolipoprotein E polymorphism in determining normal plasma lipid and lipoprotein variation, *Am J Hum Genet* **37** (1985), 268-285.

[116] A.G. Dyker, C.J. Weir, K.R. Lees, Influence of cholesterol on survival after stroke: retrospective study, *BMJ* **314** (1997), 1584-1588.

[117] J. Altman, G.D. Das, Autoradiographic and histological evidence of postnatal hippocampal neurogenesis in rats, *J Comp Neurol* **124** (1965), 319-335.

[118] P.S. Eriksson, E. Perfilieva, T. Bjork-Eriksson, A.M. Alborn, C. Nordborg, D.A. Peterson, F.H. Gage, Neurogenesis in the adult human hippocampus, *Nat Med* **4** (1998), 1313-1317.

[119] E. Gould, A.J. Reeves, M.S. Graziano, C.G. Gross, Neurogenesis in the neocortex of adult primates, *Science* **286** (1999), 548-552.

[120] G.M. Teasdale, J.A. Nicoll, G. Murray, M. Fiddes, Association of apolipoprotein E polymorphism with outcome after head injury, *Lancet* **350** (1997), 1069-1071.

[121] M.F. Chiang, J.G. Chang, C.J. Hu, Association between apolipoprotein E genotype and outcome of traumatic brain injury, *Acta Neurochir (Wien)* **145** (2003), 649-653; discussion 653-644.

[122] G. Friedman, P. Froom, L. Sazbon, I. Grinblatt, M. Shochina, J. Tsenter, S. Babaey, B. Yehuda, Z. Groswasser, Apolipoprotein E-epsilon4 genotype predicts a poor outcome in survivors of traumatic brain injury, *Neurology* **52** (1999), 244-248.

[123] S. Sorbi, B. Nacmias, S. Piacentini, A. Repice, S. Latorraca, P. Forleo, L. Amaducci, ApoE as a prognostic factor for post-traumatic coma, *Nat Med* **1** (1995), 852.

[124] I. Liaquat, L.T. Dunn, J.A. Nicoll, G.M. Teasdale, J.D. Norrie, Effect of apolipoprotein E genotype on hematoma volume after trauma, *J Neurosurg* **96** (2002), 90-96.

[125] R. Diaz-Arrastia, Y. Gong, S. Fair, K.D. Scott, M.C. Garcia, M.C. Carlile, M.A. Agostini, P.C. Van Ness, Increased risk of late posttraumatic seizures associated with inheritance of APOE epsilon4 allele, *Arch Neurol* **60** (2003), 818-822.

[126] S.W. Lichtman, G. Seliger, B. Tycko, K. Marder, Apolipoprotein E and functional recovery from brain injury following postacute rehabilitation, *Neurology* **55** (2000), 1536-1539.

[127] T.W. Teasdale, O.S. Jorgensen, C. Ripa, A.S. Nielsen, A.L. Christensen, Apolipoprotein E and subjective symptomatology following brain injury rehabilitation, *Neuropsychol Rehabil* **10** (2000), 151-166.

[128] J.N. Liberman, W.F. Stewart, K. Wesnes, J. Troncoso, Apolipoprotein E epsilon 4 and short-term recovery from predominantly mild brain injury, *Neurology* **58** (2002), 1038-1044.

[129] A. Sundstrom, P. Marklund, L.G. Nilsson, M. Cruts, R. Adolfsson, C. Van Broeckhoven, L. Nyberg, APOE influences on neuropsychological function after mild head injury: within-person comparisons, *Neurology* **62** (2004), 1963-1966.

[130] F.C. Crawford, R.D. Vanderploeg, M.J. Freeman, S. Singh, M. Waisman, L. Michaels, L. Abdullah, D. Warden, R. Lipsky, A. Salazar, M.J. Mullan, APOE genotype influences acquisition and recall following traumatic brain injury, *Neurology* **58** (2002), 1115-1118.

[131] L. Chamelian, M. Reis, A. Feinstein, Six-month recovery from mild to moderate Traumatic Brain Injury: the role of APOE-epsilon4 allele, *Brain* **127** (2004), 2621-2628.

[132] K. Millar, J.A. Nicoll, S. Thornhill, G.D. Murray, G.M. Teasdale, Long term neuropsychological outcome after head injury: relation to APOE genotype, *J Neurol Neurosurg Psychiatry* **74** (2003), 1047-1052.

[133] N. Nathoo, R. Chetry, J.R. van Dellen, C. Connolly, R. Naidoo, Apolipoprotein E polymorphism and outcome after closed traumatic brain injury: influence of ethnic and regional differences, *J Neurosurg* **98** (2003), 302-306.

[134] T.J. Quinn, C. Smith, L. Murray, J. Stewart, J.A. Nicoll, D.I. Graham, There is no evidence of an association in children and teenagers between the apolipoprotein E epsilon4 allele and post-traumatic brain swelling, *Neuropathol Appl Neurobiol* **30** (2004), 569-575.

[135] G.M. Teasdale, G.D. Murray, J.A. Nicoll, The association between APOE epsilon4, age and outcome after head injury: a prospective cohort study, *Brain* **128** (2005), 2556-2561.

[136] B.L. Plassman, R.J. Havlik, D.C. Steffens, M.J. Helms, T.N. Newman, D. Drosdick, C. Phillips, B.A. Gau, K.A. Welsh-Bohmer, J.R. Burke, J.M. Guralnik, J.C. Breitner, Documented head injury in early adulthood and risk of Alzheimer's disease and other dementias, *Neurology* **55** (2000), 1158-1166.

[137] H. Isoniemi, T. Kurki, O. Tenovuo, V. Kairisto, R. Portin, Hippocampal volume, brain atrophy, and APOE genotype after traumatic brain injury, *Neurology* **67** (2006), 756-760.

[138] J. Ponsford, D. Rudzki, K. Bailey, K.T. Ng, Impact of apolipoprotein gene on cognitive impairment and recovery after traumatic brain injury, *Neurology* **68** (2007), 619-620.

[139] H. Hiekkanen, T. Kurki, N. Brandstack, V. Kairisto, O. Tenovuo, MRI changes and ApoE genotype, a prospective 1-year follow-up of traumatic brain injury: a pilot study, *Brain Inj* **21** (2007), 1307-1314.

[140] M. Rapoport, U. Wolf, N. Herrmann, A. Kiss, P. Shammi, M. Reis, A. Phillips, A. Feinstein, Traumatic brain injury, Apolipoprotein E-epsilon4, and cognition in older adults: a two-year longitudinal study, *J Neuropsychiatry Clin Neurosci* **20** (2008), 68-73.

[141] V.L. Kristman, C.H. Tator, N. Kreiger, D. Richards, L. Mainwaring, S. Jaglal, G. Tomlinson, P. Comper, Does the apolipoprotein epsilon 4 allele predispose varsity athletes to concussion? A prospective cohort study, *Clin J Sport Med* **18** (2008), 322-328.

[142] T.A. Ashman, J.B. Cantor, W.A. Gordon, A. Sacks, L. Spielman, M. Egan, M.R. Hibbard, A comparison of cognitive functioning in older adults with and without traumatic brain injury, *J Head Trauma Rehab* **23** (2008), 139-148.

[143] H. Hiekkanen, T. Kurki, N. Brandstack, V. Kairisto, O. Tenovuo, Association of injury severity, MRI-results and ApoE genotype with 1-year outcome in mainly mild TBI: a preliminary study, *Brain Inj* **23** (2009), 396-402.

[144] K.M. Mehta, A. Ott, S. Kalmijn, A.J. Slooter, C.M. van Duijn, A. Hofman, M.M. Breteler, Head trauma and risk of dementia and Alzheimer's disease: The Rotterdam Study, *Neurology* **53** (1999), 1959-1962.

[145] L. Chamelian, M. Reis, A. Feinstein, Six-month recovery from mild to moderate Traumatic Brain Injury: the role of APOE-epsilon 4 allele, *Brain* **127** (2004), 2621-2628.

[146] S. Koponen, T. Taiminen, V. Kairisto, R. Portin, H. Isoniemi, S. Hinkka, O. Tenovuo, APOE-epsilon4 predicts dementia but not other psychiatric disorders after traumatic brain injury, *Neurology* **63** (2004), 749-750.

[147] C. Smith, D.I. Graham, L.S. Murray, J. Stewart, J.A. Nicoll, Association of APOE e4 and cerebrovascular pathology in traumatic brain injury, *J Neurol Neurosurg Psychiatry* **77** (2006), 363-366.

[148] R. Mayeux, R. Ottman, G. Maestre, C. Ngai, M.X. Tang, H. Ginsberg, M. Chun, B. Tycko, M. Shelanski, Synergistic effects of traumatic head injury and apolipoprotein-epsilon 4 in patients with Alzheimer's disease, *Neurology* **45** (1995), 555-557.

[149] G. Friedman, P. Froom, L. Sazbon, I. Grinblatt, M. Shochina, J. Tsenter, S. Babaey, A. Ben Yehuda, Z. Groswasser, Apolipoprotein E-epsilon 4 genotype predicts a poor outcome in survivors of traumatic brain injury, *Neurology* **52** (1999), 244-248.

[150] P.D. Leclercq, L.S. Murray, C. Smith, D.I. Graham, J.A. Nicoll, S.M. Gentleman, Cerebral amyloid angiopathy in traumatic brain injury: association with apolipoprotein E genotype, *J Neurol Neurosurg Psychiatry* **76** (2005), 229-233.

[151] M.E. Kerr, M.I. Kamboh, Y. Kong, S. Alexander, H. Yonas, Apolipoprotein E genotype and CBF in traumatic brain injured patients, *Adv Exp Med Biol* **578** (2006), 291-296.

[152] S. Alexander, M.E. Kerr, Y. Kim, M.I. Kamboh, S.R. Beers, Y.P. Conley, Apolipoprotein E4 allele presence and functional outcome after severe traumatic brain injury, *J Neurotraum* **24** (2007), 790-797.

[153] Y. Jiang, X. Sun, L. Gui, Y. Xia, W. Tang, Y. Cao, Y. Gu, Correlation between APOE -491AA promoter in epsilon4 carriers and clinical deterioration in early stage of traumatic brain injury, *J Neurotrauma* **24** (2007), 1802-1810.

[154] M. Ariza, R. Pueyo, M.D. Matarin, C. Junque, M. Mataro, I. Clemente, P. Moral, M.A. Poca, A. Garnacho, J. Sahuquillo, Influence of APOE polymorphism on cognitive and behavioural outcome in moderate and severe traumatic brain injury, *J Neurol Neurosur Ps* **77** (2006), 1191-1193.

[155] S.D. Han, A.I. Drake, L.M. Cessante, A.J. Jak, W.S. Houston, D.C. Delis, J.V. Filoteo, M.W. Bondi, Apolipoprotein E and traumatic brain injury in a military population: evidence of a neuropsychological compensatory mechanism?, *J Neurol Neurosur Ps* **78** (2007), 1103-1108.

[156] A.H. Willemse-van Son, G.M. Ribbers, W.C. Hop, C.M. van Duijn, H.J. Stam, Association between apolipoprotein-epsilon4 and long-term outcome after traumatic brain injury, *J Neurol Neurosurg Psychiatry* **79** (2008), 426-430.

[157] S.D. Han, H. Suzuki, A.I. Drake, A.J. Jak, W.S. Houston, M.W. Bondi, Clinical, Cognitive, and Genetic Predictors of Change in Job Status Following Traumatic Brain Injury in a Military Population, *J Head Trauma Rehab* **24** (2009), 57-64.

[158] K. Muller, T. Ingebrigtsen, T. Wilsgaard, G. Wikran, T. Fagerheim, B. Romner, K. Waterloo, Prediction of time trends in recovery of cognitive function after mild head injury, *Neurosurgery* **64** (2009), 698-704; discussion 704.

[159] E. Brichtova, L. Kozak, Apolipoprotein E genotype and traumatic brain injury in children - association with neurological outcome, *Child Nerv Syst* **24** (2008), 349-356.

[160] B.D. Jordan, L.D. Relkin, A.R. Ravdin, A.R. Jacobs, A. Bennett, S. Gandy, Apolipoprotein E epsilon4 associated with chronic traumatic brain injury in boxing, *The journal of the American Medical Association* **278** (1997), 5.

[161] H. Luukinen, J. Jokelainen, K. Kervinen, Y.A. Kesaniemi, S. Winqvist, M. Hillbom, Risk of dementia associated with the ApoE epsilon4 allele and falls causing head injury without explicit traumatic brain injury, *Acta Neurol Scand* **118** (2008), 153-158.

[162] M. Ost, K. Nylen, L. Csajbok, K. Blennow, L. Rosengren, B. Nellgard, Apolipoprotein E polymorphism and gender difference in outcome after severe traumatic brain injury, *Acta Anaesthesiol Scand* **52** (2008), 1364-1369.

[163] K.C. Kutner, D.M. Erlanger, J. Tsai, B. Jordan, N.R. Relkin, Lower cognitive performance of older football players possessing apolipoprotein E epsilon4, *Neurosurgery* **47** (2000), 651-657; discussion 657-658.

[164] T.Y. Lo, P.A. Jones, I.R. Chambers, T.F. Beattie, R. Forsyth, A.D. Mendelow, R.A. Minns, Modulating effect of apolipoprotein E polymorphisms on secondary brain insult and outcome after childhood brain trauma, *Childs Nerv Syst* **25** (2009), 47-54.

[165] Z. Guo, L.A. Cupples, A. Kurz, S.H. Auerbach, L. Volicer, H. Chui, R.C. Green, A.D. Sadovnick, R. Duara, C. DeCarli, K. Johnson, R.C. Go, J.H. Growdon, J.L. Haines, W.A. Kukull, L.A. Farrer, Head injury and the risk of AD in the MIRAGE study, *Neurology* **54** (2000), 1316-1323.

[166] M.E. Kerr, M. Ilyas Kamboh, K. Yookyung, M.F. Kraus, A.M. Puccio, S.T. DeKosky, D.W. Marion, Relationship between apoE4 allele and excitatory amino acid levels after traumatic brain injury, *Crit Care Med* **31** (2003), 2371-2379.

[167] R. Diaz-Arrastia, Y.H. Gong, S. Fair, K.D. Scott, M.C. Garcia, M.C. Carlile, M.A. Agostini, P.C. Van Ness, Increased risk of late posttraumatic seizures associated with inheritance of APOE epsilon 4 allele, *Arch Neurol-Chicago* **60** (2003), 818-822.

[168] M.J. Artiga, M.J. Bullido, I. Sastre, M. Recuero, M.A. Garcia, J. Aldudo, J. Vazquez, F. Valdivieso, Allelic polymorphisms in the transcriptional regulatory region of apolipoprotein E gene, *FEBS Lett* **421** (1998), 105-108.

[169] J.C. Lambert, L. Araria-Goumidi, L. Myllykangas, C. Ellis, J.C. Wang, M.J. Bullido, J.M. Harris, M.J. Artiga, D. Hernandez, J.M. Kwon, B. Frigard, R.C. Petersen, A.M. Cumming, F. Pasquier, I. Sastre, P.J. Tienari, A. Frank, R. Sulkava, J.C. Morris, D. St Clair, D.M. Mann, F. Wavrant-DeVrieze, M. Ezquerra-Trabalon, P. Amouyel, J. Hardy, M. Haltia, F. Valdivieso, A.M. Goate, J. Perez-Tur, C.L. Lendon, M.C. Chartier-Harlin, Contribution of APOE promoter polymorphisms to Alzheimer's disease risk, *Neurology* **59** (2002), 59-66.

[170] J.C. Lambert, D. Mann, L. Goumidi, J. Harris, P. Amouyel, T. Iwatsubo, C. Lendon, M.C. Chartier-Harlin, Effect of the APOE promoter polymorphisms on cerebral amyloid peptide deposition in Alzheimer's disease, *Lancet* **357** (2001), 608-609.

[171] J.C. Lambert, D. Mann, F. Richard, J. Tian, J. Shi, U. Thaker, S. Merrot, J. Harris, B. Frigard, T. Iwatsubo, C. Lendon, P. Amouyel, Is there a relation between APOE expression and brain amyloid load in Alzheimer's disease?, *J Neurol Neurosurg Psychiatry* **76** (2005), 928-933.

[172] C.L. Lendon, J.M. Harris, A.L. Pritchard, J.A. Nicoll, G.M. Teasdale, G. Murray, Genetic variation of the APOE promoter and outcome after head injury, *Neurology* **61** (2003), 683-685.

[173] J.W. Bales, A.K. Wagner, A.E. Kline, C.E. Dixon, Persistent cognitive dysfunction after traumatic brain injury: A dopamine hypothesis, *Neurosci Biobehav Rev* **33** (2009), 981-1003.

[174] P. Seeman, J.L. Tedesco, T. Lee, M. Chau-Wong, P. Muller, J. Bowles, P.M. Whitaker, C. McManus, M. Tittler, P. Weinreich, W.C. Friend, G.M. Brown, Dopamine receptors in the central nervous system, *Fed Proc* **37** (1978), 131-136.

[175] J.C. Baron, D. Comar, E. Zarifian, Y. Agid, C. Crouzel, H. Loo, P. Deniker, C. Kellershohn, Dopaminergic receptor sites in human brain: positron emission tomography, *Neurology* **35** (1985), 16-24.

[176] B.C. McDonald, L.A. Flashman, A.J. Saykin, Executive disfunction following traumatic brain injury: neural substrates and treatment strategies, *NeuroRehabilitation* **17** (2002), 12.

[177] Y. Chudasama, T.W. Robbins, Functions of frontostriatal systems in cognition: comparative neuropsychopharmacological studies in rats, monkeys and humans, *Biol Psychol* **73** (2006), 19-38.

[178] N. Lemon, D. Manahan-Vaughan, Dopamine D1/D5 receptors gate the acquisition of novel information through hippocampal long-term potentiation and long-term depression, *J Neurosci* **26** (2006), 7723-7729.

[179] C.M. O'Carroll, S.J. Martin, J. Sandin, B. Frenguelli, R.G. Morris, Dopaminergic modulation of the persistence of one-trial hippocampus-dependent memory, *Learn Mem* **13** (2006), 760-769.

[180] N. Granado, O. Ortiz, L.M. Suarez, E.D. Martin, V. Cena, J.M. Solis, R. Moratalla, D1 but not D5 dopamine receptors are critical for LTP, spatial learning, and LTP-Induced arc and zif268 expression in the hippocampus, *Cereb Cortex* **18** (2008), 1-12.

[181] M.J. Buckley, The role of the perirhinal cortex and hippocampus in learning, memory, and perception, *Q J Exp Psychol-B* **58** (2005), 246-268.

[182] A. Raz, Anatomy of attentional networks, *The Anatomical Record* **281** (2004), 16.

[183] S. McDowell, J. Whyte, M. DEsposito, Working memory impairments in traumatic brain injury: evidence from a dual task paradigm, *Neuropsychologia* **35** (1997), 1341-1353.

[184] S.R. Millis, M. Rosenthal, T.A. Novack, M. Sherer, T.G. Nick, J.S. Kreutzer, W.M. High, J.H. Ricker, Long-term neuropsychological outcome after traumatic brain injury, *J Head Trauma Rehab* **16** (2001), 343-355.

[185] G.V. Williams, S.A. Castner, Under the curve: Critical issues for elucidating D1 receptor function in working memory, *Neuroscience* **139** (2006), 263-276.

[186] J.W. Olney, C.F. Zorumski, G.R. Stewart, M.T. Price, G.J. Wang, J. Labruyere, Excitotoxicity of L-Dopa and 6-Oh-Dopa - Implications for Parkinsons and Huntingtons Diseases, *Experimental Neurology* **108** (1990), 269-272.

[187] A.K. Wagner, X. Chen, A.E. Kline, Y. Li, R.D. Zafonte, C.E. Dixon, Gender and environmental enrichment impact dopamine transporter expression after experimental traumatic brain injury, *Exp Neurol* **195** (2005), 475-483.

[188] H.Q. Yan, A.E. Kline, X.C. Ma, E.L. Hooghe-Peters, D.W. Marion, C.E. Dixon, Tyrosine hydroxylase, but not dopamine beta-hydroxylase, is increased in rat frontal cortex after traumatic brain injury, *Neuroreport* **12** (2001), 2323-2327.

[189] F.P. Huger, G.A. Patrick, Effects of Concussive Injury on Tyrosine-H-3 Uptake Invitro by Rat-Brain Synaptosomes, *Federation Proceedings* **38** (1979), 524-524.

[190] A. Dunnmeynell, S.J. Pan, B.E. Levin, Focal Traumatic Brain Injury Causes Widespread Reductions in Rat-Brain Norepinephrine Turnover from 6 to 24 H, *Brain Research* **660** (1994), 88-95.

[191] T.K. Mcintosh, T. Yu, T.A. Gennarelli, Alterations in Regional Brain Catecholamine Concentrations after Experimental Brain Injury in the Rat, *Journal of Neurochemistry* **63** (1994), 1426-1433.

[192] J.L. Massucci, A.E. Kline, X.C. Ma, R.D. Zafonte, C.E. Dixon, Time dependent alterations in dopamine tissue levels and metabolism after experimental traumatic brain injury in rats, *Neuroscience Letters* **372** (2004), 127-131.

[193] J.B. Redell, P.K. Dash, Traumatic brain injury stimulates hippocampal catechol-O-methyl transferase expression in microglia, *Neurosci Lett* **413** (2007), 36-41.

[194] J.M. Henry, N.K. Talukder, A.B. Lee, M.L. Walker, Cerebral trauma-induced changes in corpus striatal dopamine receptor subtypes, *J Invest Surg* **10** (1997), 281-286.

[195] M.Y.T. Globus, R. Busto, W.D. Dietrich, E. Martinez, I. Valdes, M.D. Ginsberg, Effect of Ischemia on the Invivo Release of Striatal Dopamine, Glutamate, and Gamma-Aminobutyric Acid Studied by Intracerebral Microdialysis, *Journal of Neurochemistry* **51** (1988), 1455-1464.

[196] J.W. Bales, A.E. Kline, A.K. Wagner, C.E. Dixon, Targeting dopamine in acute traumatic brain injury, *The Open Drug Discovery Journal* **2** (2010), 10.

[197] I. Fineman, D.A. Hovda, M. Smith, A. Yoshino, D.P. Becker, Concussive Brain Injury Is Associated with a Prolonged Accumulation of Calcium - a Ca-45 Autoradiographic Study, *Brain Research* **624** (1993), 94-102.

[198] Y. Shapira, G. Yadidi, S. Cotev, E. Shohami, Accumulation of calcium in the brain following head trauma, *Neurological Research* **11** (1989), 4.

[199] Q.Z. Gong, L.L. Phillips, B.G. Lyeth, Metabotropic glutamate receptor protein alterations after traumatic brain injury in rats, *J Neurotraum* **16** (1999), 893-902.

[200] S.T. Ross, I. Soltesz, Selective depolarization of interneurons in the early posttraumatic dentate gyrus: Involvement of the Na+/K+-ATPase, *J Neurophysiol* **83** (2000), 2916-2930.

[201] F.D. Lima, M.A. Souza, A.F. Furian, L.M. Rambo, L.R. Ribeiro, F.V. Martignoni, M.S. Hoffmann, M.R. Fighera, L.F.F. Royes, M.S. Oliveira, C.F. de Mello, Na+,K+-ATPase activity impairment after experimental traumatic brain injury: Relationship to spatial learning deficits and oxidative stress, *Behav Brain Res* **193** (2008), 306-310.

[202] A. Yoshino, D.A. Hovda, T. Kawamata, Y. Katayama, D.P. Becker, Dynamic Changes in Local Cerebral Glucose-Utilization Following Cerebral Concussion in Rats - Evidence of a Hypermetabolic and Subsequent Hypometabolic State, *Brain Research* **561** (1991), 106-119.

[203] S. Scafidi, J. O'Brien, I. Hopkins, C. Robertson, G. Fiskum, M. McKenna, Delayed cerebral oxidative glucose metabolism after traumatic brain injury in young rats, *Journal of Neurochemistry* **109** (2009), 189-197.

[204] H. Zhang, X.D. Zhang, T.L. Zhang, C. Liren, Excitatory amino acids in cerebrospinal fluid of patients with acute head injuries, *Clin Chem* **47** (2001), 1458-1462.

[205] V. Verma, A. Hasbi, B.F. O'Dowd, S.R. George, Dopamine D1-D2 Receptor Heteromer-mediated Calcium Release Is Desensitized by D1 Receptor Occupancy with or without Signal Activation DUAL FUNCTIONAL REGULATION BY G PROTEIN-COUPLED RECEPTOR KINASE 2, *Journal of Biological Chemistry* **285** (2010), 35092-35103.

[206] A. Nishi, G. Fisone, G.L. Snyder, I. Dulubova, A. Aperia, A.C. Nairn, P. Greengard, Regulation of Na+, K+-ATPase isoforms in rat neostriatum by dopamine and protein kinase C, *J Neurochem* **73** (1999), 1492-1501.

[207] A. Nishi, M. Hamada, H. Higashi, Regulation of DARPP-32 phosphorylation by NMDA and AMPA receptors in neostriatal neurons, *Jpn J Pharmacol* **88** (2002), 189p-189p.

[208] P. Greengard, P.B. Allen, A.C. Nairn, Beyond the dopamine receptor: the DARPP-32/protein phosphatase-1 cascade, *Neuron* **23** (1999), 435-447.

[209] G. Beck, P. Brinkkoetter, C. Hanusch, J. Schulte, K. van Ackern, F.J. van der Woude, B.A. Yard, Clinical review: immunomodulatory effects of dopamine in general inflammation, *Crit Care* **8** (2004), 485-491.

[210] T.W. McAllister, Polymorphisms in genes modulating the dopamine system: do they inf luence outcome and response to medication after traumatic brain injury?, *J Head Trauma Rehabil* **24** (2009), 65-68.

[211] R.M. Weinshilboum, D.M. Otterness, C.L. Szumlanski, Methylation pharmacogenetics: Catechol O-methyltransferase, thiopurine methyltransferase, and histamine N-methyltransferase, *Annu Rev Pharmacol* **39** (1999), 19-52.

[212] D.A. Lewis, D.S. Melchitzky, S.R. Sesack, R.E. Whitehead, S. Auh, A. Sampson, Dopamine transporter immunoreactivity in monkey cerebral cortex: regional, laminar, and ultrastructural localization, *J Comp Neurol* **432** (2001), 119-136.

[213] M.S. Mazei, C.P. Pluto, B. Kirkbride, E.A. Pehek, Effects of catecholamine uptake blockers in the caudate-putamen and subregions of the medial prefrontal cortex of the rat, *Brain Res* **936** (2002), 58-67.

[214] S.W. Anderson, Neuropsychological consequences of dysfunction in human dorsolateral prefrontal cortex, In: *Handbook oh Neurophysiology* 7, Second ed., Edited by J. Grafman, Elsevier, Amsterdam 2002.

[215] R. Weinshilboum, F. Raymond, Variations in catechol-O-methyltransferase activity in inbred strains of rats, *Neuropharmacology* **16** (1977), 703-706.

[216] T. Lotta, J. Vidgren, C. Tilgmann, I. Ulmanen, K. Melen, I. Julkunen, J. Taskinen, Kinetics of Human Soluble and Membrane-Bound Catechol O-Methyltransferase - a Revised Mechanism and Description of the Thermolabile Variant of the Enzyme, *Biochemistry* **34** (1995), 4202-4210.

[217] H.M. Lachman, D.F. Papolos, T. Saito, Y.M. Yu, C.L. Szumlanski, R.M. Weinshilboum, Human catechol-O-methyltransferase pharmacogenetics: Description of a functional polymorphism and its potential application to neuropsychiatric disorders, *Pharmacogenetics* **6** (1996), 243-250.

[218] M.F. Egan, T.E. Goldberg, B.S. Kolachana, J.H. Callicott, C.M. Mazzanti, R.E. Straub, D. Goldman, D.R. Weinberger, Effect of COMT Val108/158 Met genotype on frontal lobe function and risk for schizophrenia, *Proc Natl Acad Sci U S A* **98** (2001), 6917-6922.

[219] R. Joober, J. Gauthier, S. Lal, D. Bloom, P. Lalonde, G. Rouleau, C. Benkelfat, A. Labelle, Catechol-O-methyltransferase Val-108/158-Met gene variants associated with performance on the Wisconsin Card Sorting Test, *Arch Gen Psychiatry* **59** (2002), 662-663.

[220] A.K. Malhotra, L.J. Kestler, C. Mazzanti, J.A. Bates, T. Goldberg, D. Goldman, A functional polymorphism in the COMT gene and performance on a test of prefrontal cognition, *Am J Psychiatry* **159** (2002), 652-654.

[221] A. Rosa, V. Peralta, M.J. Cuesta, A. Zarzuela, F. Serrano, A. Martinez-Larrea, L. Fananas, New evidence of association between COMT gene and prefrontal neurocognitive function in healthy individuals from sibling pairs discordant for psychosis, *Am J Psychiatry* **161** (2004), 1110-1112.

[222] G.E. Bruder, J.G. Keilp, H. Xu, M. Shikhman, E. Schori, J.M. Gorman, T.C. Gilliam, Catechol-O-methyltransferase (COMT) genotypes and working memory: associations with differing cognitive operations, *Biol Psychiatry* **58** (2005), 901-907.

[223] R.H. Lipsky, M.B. Sparling, L.M. Ryan, K. Xu, A.M. Salazar, D. Goldman, D.L. Warden, Association of COMT Val158Met genotype with executive functioning following traumatic brain injury, *J Neuropsychiatry Clin Neurosci* **17** (2005), 465-471.

[224] L.A. Flashman, A.J. Saykin, C.H. Rhodes, T.W. McAllister, Effect of COMT Val/Met genotype on frontal lobe functioning in traumatic brain injury, *The Journal of Neuropsychiatry and Clinical Neurosciences* **16** (2004), 2.

[225] T.W. McAllister, C.H. Rhodes, L.A. Flashman, B.C. McDonald, D. Belloni, A.J. Saykin, Effect of the dopamine D2 receptor T allele on response latency after mild traumatic brain injury, *Am J Psychiatry* **162** (2005), 1749-1751.

[226] T.W. McAllister, L.A. Flashman, M.B. Sparling, A.J. Saykin, Working memory deficits after traumatic brain injury: catecholaminergic mechanisms and prospects for treatment -- a review, *Brain Inj* **18** (2004), 331-350.

[227] J. Thompson, N. Thomas, A. Singleton, M. Piggott, S. Lloyd, E.K. Perry, C.M. Morris, R.H. Perry, I.N. Ferrier, J.A. Court, D2 dopamine receptor gene (DRD2) Taq1 A polymorphism: reduced dopamine D2 receptor binding in the human striatum associated with the A1 allele, *Pharmacogenetics* **7** (1997), 479-484.

[228] T. Ritchie, E.P. Noble, Association of seven polymorphisms of the D2 dopamine receptor gene with brain receptor-binding characteristics, *Neurochem Res* **28** (2003), 73-82.

[229] T.W. McAllister, L.A. Flashman, C. Harker Rhodes, A.L. Tyler, J.H. Moore, A.J. Saykin, B.C. McDonald, T.D. Tosteson, G.J. Tsongalis, Single nucleotide polymorphisms in ANKK1 and the dopamine D2 receptor gene affect cognitive outcome shortly after traumatic brain injury: a replication and extension study, *Brain Inj* **22** (2008), 705-714.

[230] N.A. Carney, J. Ghajar, Guidelines for the management of severe traumatic brain injury. Introduction, *J Neurotrauma* **24 Suppl 1** (2007), S1-2.

[231] K.K. Jain, Neuroprotection in traumatic brain injury, *Drug Discov Today* **13** (2008), 1082-1089.

[232] M.D. Sorani, D. Morabito, G. Rosenthal, K.M. Giacomini, G.T. Manley, Characterizing the dose-response relationship between mannitol and intracranial pressure in traumatic brain injury patients using a high-frequency physiological data collection system, *J Neurotrauma* **25** (2008), 291-298.

[233] N. Plesnila, Decompression craniectomy after traumatic brain injury: recent experimental results, *Prog Brain Res* **161** (2007), 393-400.

[234] G.H. Wang, X.G. Zhang, Z.L. Jiang, X. Li, L.L. Peng, Y.C. Li, Y. Wang, Neuroprotective effects of hyperbaric oxygen treatment on traumatic brain injury in the rat, *J Neurotrauma* **27** (2010), 1733-1743.

[235] A. Verma, Opportunities for neuroprotection in traumatic brain injury, *J Head Trauma Rehabil* **15** (2000), 1149-1161.

[236] H. Bayr, R.S. Clark, P.M. Kochanek, Promising strategies to minimize secondary brain injury after head trauma, *Critical Care Medicine* **31** (2003), 6.

[237] K.K. Wang, S.F. Larner, G. Robinson, R.L. Hayes, Neuroprotection targets after traumatic brain injury, *Curr Opin Neurol* **19** (2006), 514-519.

[238] C. Werner, K. Engelhard, Pathophysiology of traumatic brain injury, *Br J Anaesth* **99** (2007), 4-9.

[239] Y. Xiong, A. Mahmood, M. Chopp, Emerging treatments for traumatic brain injury, *Expert Opin Emerg Drugs* **14** (2009), 67-84.

[240] J. Langham, C. Goldfrad, G. Teasdale, D. Shaw, K. Rowan, Calcium channel blockers for acute traumatic brain injury, *Cochrane Database Syst Rev* (2003), CD000565.

[241] K.W. Muir, Glutamate-based therapeutic approaches: clinical trials with NMDA antagonists, *Curr Opin Pharmacol* **6** (2006), 53-60.

[242] P. Alderson, I. Roberts, Corticosteroids for acute traumatic brain injury, *Cochrane Database Syst Rev* (2005), CD000196.
[243] M. Vandromme, S.M. Melton, J.D. Kerby, Progesterone in traumatic brain injury: time to move on to phase III trials, *Crit Care* **12** (2008), 153.
[244] K. Ker, K. Blackhall, Beta-2 receptor antagonists for acute traumatic brain injury, *Cochrane Database Syst Rev* (2008), CD006686.
[245] R.J. Forsyth, B. Jayamoni, T.C. Paine, Monoaminergic agonists for acute traumatic brain injury, *Cochrane Database Syst Rev* (2006), CD003984.
[246] I. Roberts, Barbiturates for acute traumatic brain injury, *Cochrane Database Syst Rev* (2000), CD000033.
[247] M. Yunoki, M. Kawauchi, N. Ukita, T. Sugiura, T. Ohmoto, Effects of lecithinized superoxide dismutase on neuronal cell loss in CA3 hippocampus after traumatic brain injury in rats, *Surg Neurol* **59** (2003), 156-160; discussion 160-151.
[248] D. Lu, A. Mahmood, R. Zhang, M. Copp, Upregulation of neurogenesis and reduction in functional deficits following administration of DEtA/NONOate, a nitric oxide donor, after traumatic brain injury in rats, *J Neurosurg* **99** (2003), 351-361.
[249] A. Mahmood, D. Lu, C. Qu, A. Goussev, Z.G. Zhang, C. Lu, M. Chopp, Treatment of traumatic brain injury in rats with erythropoietin and carbamylated erythropoietin, *J Neurosurg* **107** (2007), 392-397.
[250] D. Lu, C. Qu, A. Goussev, H. Jiang, C. Lu, T. Schallert, A. Mahmood, J. Chen, Y. Li, M. Chopp, Statins increase neurogenesis in the dentate gyrus, reduce delayed neuronal death in the hippocampal CA3 region, and improve spatial learning in rat after traumatic brain injury, *J Neurotrauma* **24** (2007), 1132-1146.
[251] H. Rus, C. Cudrici, S. David, F. Niculescu, The complement system in central nervous system diseases, *Autoimmunity* **39** (2006), 395-402.
[252] D.M. Stein, R.P. Dutton, M.E. Kramer, C. Handley, T.M. Scalea, Recombinant factor VIIa: decreasing time to intervention in coagulopathic patients with severe traumatic brain injury, *J Trauma* **64** (2008), 620-627; discussion 627-628.
[253] C. van den Heuvel, R. Vink, The role of magnesium in traumatic brain injury, *Clin Calcium* **14** (2004), 9-14.
[254] A. Kleindienst, F. Hesse, M.R. Bullock, M. Buchfelder, The neurotrophic protein S100B: value as a marker of brain damage and possible therapeutic implications, *Prog Brain Res* **161** (2007), 317-325.
[255] N.C. Royo, S. Shimizu, J.W. Schouten, J.F. Stover, T.K. McIntosh, Pharmacology of traumatic brain injury, *Curr Opin Pharmacol* **3** (2003), 27-32.
[256] D. Schubert, R. Dargusch, J. Raitano, S.W. Chan, Cerium and yttrium oxide nanoparticles are neuroprotective, *Biochem Biophys Res Commun* **342** (2006), 86-91.
[257] M. Maegele, U. Schaefer, Stem cell-based cellular replacement strategies following traumatic brain injury (TBI), *Minim Invasive Ther Allied Technol* **17** (2008), 119-131.
[258] F. Shen, L. Wen, X. Yang, W. Liu, The potential application of gene therapy in the treatment of traumatic brain injury, *Neurosurg Rev* **30** (2007), 291-298; discussion 298.
[259] B.T. Ang, G. Xu, Z.C. Xiao, Therapeutic vaccination for central nervous system repair, *Clin Exp Pharmacol Physiol* **33** (2006), 541-545.
[260] J. Sahuquillo, A. Vilalta, Cooling the injured brain: how does moderate hypothermia influence the pathophysiology of traumatic brain injury, *Curr Pharm Des* **13** (2007), 2310-2322.
[261] R.K. Narayan, M.E. Michel, B. Ansell, A. Baethmann, A. Biegon, M.B. Bracken, M.R. Bullock, S.C. Choi, G.L. Clifton, C.F. Contant, W.M. Coplin, W.D. Dietrich, J. Ghajar, S.M. Grady, R.G. Grossman, E.D. Hall, W. Heetderks, D.A. Hovda, J. Jallo, R.L. Katz, N. Knoller, P.M. Kochanek, A.I. Maas, J. Majde, D.W. Marion, A. Marmarou, L.F. Marshall, T.K. McIntosh, E. Miller, N. Mohberg, J.P. Muizelaar, L.H. Pitts, P. Quinn, G. Riesenfeld, C.S. Robertson, K.I. Strauss, G. Teasdale, N. Temkin, R. Tuma, C. Wade, M.D. Walker, M. Weinrich, J. Whyte, J. Wilberger, A.B. Young, L. Yurkewicz, Clinical trials in head injury, *J Neurotrauma* **19** (2002), 503-557.
[262] E.M. Doppenberg, S.C. Choi, R. Bullock, Clinical trials in traumatic brain injury: lessons for the future, *J Neurosurg Anesthesiol* **16** (2004), 87-94.
[263] K. Beauchamp, H. Mutlak, W.R. Smith, E. Shohami, P.F. Stahel, Pharmacology of traumatic brain injury: where is the "golden bullet"?, *Mol Med* **14** (2008), 731-740.
[264] D.L. Warden, B. Gordon, T.W. McAllister, J.M. Silver, J.T. Barth, J. Bruns, A. Drake, T. Gentry, A. Jagoda, D.I. Katz, J. Kraus, L.A. Labbate, L.M. Ryan, M.B. Sparling, B. Walters, J. Whyte, A. Zapata, G. Zitnay, Guidelines for the pharmacologic treatment of neurobehavioral sequelae of traumatic brain injury, *J Neurotrauma* **23** (2006), 1468-1501.
[265] E. Chew, R.D. Zafonte, Pharmacological management of neurobehavioral disorders following traumatic brain injury--a state-of-the-art review, *J Rehabil Res Dev* **46** (2009), 851-879.

Coping with Blast-Related Traumatic Brain Injury in Returning Troops
B.K. Wiederhold (Ed.)
IOS Press, 2011
doi: 10.3233/978-1-60750-797-0-112

Cognitive and Functional Outcome of Terror Victims who Suffered from Traumatic Brain Injury in Jerusalem

Zeev MEINER[a,1], Maya TUCHNER[a], Jeanna TSENTER[a], Shimon SHIRI[a],
Michal KATZ-LEURER[b] and Isabella SCHWARTZ[a]

[a]*Department of Physical Medicine and Rehabilitation,*
Hadassah-Hebrew University Hospital, Jerusalem, Israel
[b]*Physical Therapy Department, School of Health Professions,*
Tel-Aviv University, Ramat-Aviv, Israel

Abstract. Between September 2000 and September 2004, 72 casualties of terror attacks were treated in the rehabilitation department in Jerusalem; among them 17 suffered from Traumatic Brain Injury (TBI). As a control, we evaluated the rehabilitation process and outcome of 39 non-terror TBI patients treated in the same department at the same period. All patients were assessed upon admission and discharged from the rehabilitation department and at the end of their stay in rehabilitation day-care. Clinical data include demographic data, injury severity according to the Injury Severity Scale (ISS), length of stay, imaging results, surgical interventions, and complications. ADL was measured using the Functional Independence Measurement (FIM); cognitive and memory functions were measured using specific evaluation batteries. Terror TBI patients were significantly younger than the non-terror group (29 ± 9.5 versus 39.5 ±21, p=0.05). ISS score was significantly higher among terror victims and they had a higher rate of intracerebral hemorrhage, brain surgery and penetrating brain injuries with foreign bodies. The mean total length of stay of terror TBI patients in rehabilitation was 201± 88 days as opposed to 167± 148 days of non-terror victims (not significant). There was no difference in the mean FIM values of terror and non-terror TBI patients and both groups improved similarly reaching a mean FIM score of 119 upon discharge. In both groups, cognitive and memory tests improved significantly during rehabilitation without differences between the groups. Terror victims suffered from a higher percentage of posttraumatic epilepsy (35% versus 10% p=0.05). The rate of PTSD was similar in both groups as well as the rate of return to previous occupation. Although TBI terror victims had more severe injuries, they gained backmost ADL functions and their rehabilitation outcomes were similar to non-terror TBI patients.

Keywords: terror victims, TBI, cognitive, functional, outcome

---

[1] Corresponding Author: Zeev Meiner, Department of Physical Medicine and Rehabilitation, Hadassah-Hebrew University Hospital, Jerusalem, Israel; E-mail: meiner@hadassah.org.il.

Introduction

Terror attacks are one of the major threats to human society in our generation. Terror attacks have a severe impact on the lives of the casualties themselves and their family members [1]. Surprisingly, only a few articles regarding the rehabilitation treatment and functional outcome of terror victims were found in the literature [2]. At least 30% of terror victims suffered from a Traumatic Brain Injury (TBI) and this injury had a severe impact on their outcome [3, 4]. However, the rehabilitation process and outcomes of terror victims with TBI were not described in the literature.

The state of Israel has one of the highest rates of terror attacks in the world. In the period of four years extending from 29 September2000 until 1 September 2004 there were more than 1,000 deaths and more than 7,000 wounded due to terror attacks in Israel, mostly civilians [5]. The attacks include suicide bombing, drive-by shootings, intrusions into homes, knife or gun attacks, missiles and mortars.

A number of published articles have compared terror casualties with non-terror patients regarding the severity, outcome, and service utilization in acute care management in Israel [6,7]. According to recent data, terror victims sustain more severe injuries and experience higher mortality when compared to any other form of trauma, with ever-increasing demands on healthcare resources. Their resource utilization is higher in terms of duration of hospitalization, procedures carried out in operating rooms, intensive-care treatment, and so on, especially when penetrating wounds occur, elevating the cost of their treatment [8]. Sixty percent of terror victims underwent operating procedures and a third were admitted to intensive care units [9].

According to the national trauma registry in Israel, in general, 30% of terror victims suffered from any head injury [3]. In the pediatric population of terror victims, the rate of TBI was 22% [7]. In comparison, between blast and gunshot injuries, the rate of TBI was 18% in blast injuries versus 10% in gunshot injuries. TBI due to terror attacks is usually severe due to the combined aspects of closed head injuries due to blast effects with penetrating injuries from shrapnel [10]. In a recent study regarding terror victims due to gunshot injuries alone, the overall percentage of head injury was 9.3% and was more frequent among civilian patients then in soldiers. Patients with TBI were more severely injured then terror victims without TBI. The rate of death and ICU admission was also higher in terror victims with TBI [11].

In this article, we will focus on the rehabilitation outcome of terror victims with TBI in comparison to the rehabilitation outcome of non-terror TBI patients treated in the same facility at the same period.

1. Method

This study is a historical prospective chart review of people injured through terrorist acts who were treated in a Department of Physical Medicine and Rehabilitation of Hadassah University Hospital in Jerusalem from 29 September 2000 until 1 September 2004. We extracted relevant data from a database containing information about patients discharged from the rehabilitation department and rehabilitation day-care department over this period.

1.1. Participants

During the study period, 72 casualties of terror attacks were treated in the rehabilitation department. All patients were screened for CNS involvement using brain and spine CT at admission to acute care departments. Of them, 17 patients suffered from TBI. At the same time period, 39 patients were hospitalized in the same rehabilitation department because of non-terror-related TBI and served as controls.

1.2. Data Collection and Measures

Medical data of the hospitalized patients were collected from the trauma registry records and from the rehabilitation records. The data included: age, gender, injury mechanism, type of injury, severity of injury according to Injury Severity Scale (ISS) [12, 13], Glasgow Coma Scale (GCS) on admission, coma duration, length of stay in the acute care departments, surgical interventions, and complications. Additional data included length of stay in the rehabilitation departments, functional outcome according to Functional Independence Measurement (FIM^{TM}) [14], occupational outcome evaluated by returning to previous occupation, psychological outcome estimated by a Revised PTSD Inventory [15] based on Brief Symptoms Inventory questionnaire [16], Glasgow outcome scale (GOS) [17] and the post traumatic epilepsy rate. Cognitive and memory evaluation was performed using the Loewenstein Occupational Therapy Cognitive Assessment (LOTCA) battery and the Rivermead Battery Memory test (RBMT) respectively [18,19]. CT scan results including type of injury, location of injury, presence of foreign bodies and intra-ventricular rupture of blood was evaluated for the terror and non-terror groups.

All patients were assessed upon admission and upon discharge from the rehabilitation department and at the end of their stays as outpatients in rehabilitation day care in the same center.

1.3. Statistical Evaluation

Data were collected and compared between terror patients and non-terror patients. Statistical tests included χ^2 for categorical data, t-tests for continuous variables, and to test differences between groups over time, repeated measures ANOVA with a between-subjects variable of group (terror vs. non-terror) and a within-subjects variable of time (rehabilitation entry time, end of in- and outpatient rehabilitation periods). SPSS statistical software was used for data analysis. A value of $p < 0.05$ was considered statistically significant.

2. Results

2.1 Demographic Data

During the study period 17 terror and 39 non-terror TBI patients were treated in the department of rehabilitation in Hadassah University Hospital in Jerusalem. The demographic data of the terror and non-terror patients is presented in Table 1. In the terror victim group there were 58.8% men with a mean age of 29.0 ± 9.5 years, whereas in the non-terror group there were 71.8 % men with mean age of 39.5 ± 21 years

(P<0.05). There were no other differences in demographic variables including familial status, education, and employment between the groups.

Table 1. Socio-Demographic characteristics by groups: Terror versus Non-Terror.

	Terror N=17 (%)	Non-terror N=39 (%)	p value
Gender			
Male	10 (58.8)	28 (71.8)	0.33
Age group	29.0 ± 9.5	39.5 ± 21.0	
< 29	12 (70.6)	17 (43.6)	0.05
30-44	4 (23.5)	3 (7.7)	
45-59	1 (5.9)	10 (25.6)	
>60	0 (0)	9 (23.1)	
Familial status			
Married	7 (41.2)	17 (43.6)	0.70
Education 12 yrs. and above	11 (64.7)	19 (48.7)	0.20
Employment^			
Pupil/Student	2 (12.5)	9 (27.3)	
Soldier	2 (12.5)	2 (6.1)	
* Blue collar	5 (31.3)	10 (30.3)	0.48
* White collar	7 (43.8)	9 (27.3)	
Unemployed/ Pensioner	0 (13.3)	3 (9.1)	

Values in the table are means±SD, number (percentage)
+p value obtained by t-test, χ^2 test.
* blue color- agents, sales workers and service workers, skilled agricultural workers, manufacturing, construction and other skilled workers, and unskilled workers.
* white color- academic professionals, associate professionals and technicians, managers, clerical workers

2.2 Injury Mechanisms and Severity

The most common mechanism of injury in the terror group was explosion (13 persons, 70.6%), other mechanisms include gunshot and stabbing. Many of the blast injury patients also suffered from penetrating brain damage due to a variety of objects which were placed in these bombs to maximize the damage and the penetration to the skull, including ball bearings, metal bolts, hexagonal nuts, segments of metal rods, and nails (Figure 1). In the non-terror group the main mechanism was motor vehicle crash (25 persons, 64.1%) (Table 2). The trauma severity as measured by the ISS score was significantly higher among terror TBI victims as compared to control TBI group (32.0±11.8 versus 24.3±11.7, P< 0.03). Although more patients (53% versus 33%) of the terror group were classified as having a severe brain injury (GCS≤8), the difference did not reach statistically significance (P=0.23). The mean coma duration was similar in both groups. More patients in the terror TBI group suffered from vascular lesions (35% versus 7.6%, p=0.01) mainly pseudo-aneurisms in brain vessels, whereas more patients in the non-terror group suffered from long bone fractures (35% versus 74% p<0.01) (Table 2).

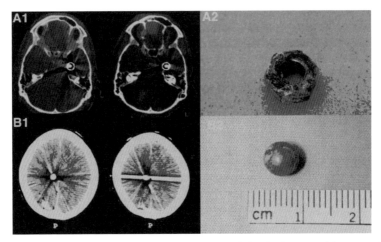

Figure 1. Different objects that were placed in the bombs to maximize the damage and the penetration to the skull. A1-Hexagonal nut located at the left hippocampus of a terror victim that was removed surgically. A2: following elective surgical removal. B1: Metal bolt penetrated to the right frontal area, B2 – following elective surgical removal.

Table 2. Injury cause and severity by groups: Terror versus Non-Terror.

	Terror N=17 (%)	Non-terror N=39 (%)	p value
Mechanism of injury			<0.01
Explosions	13 (70.6)		
Gunshot injuries	3 (17.6)		
Stone/knife	2(11.8)	5 (12.9)	
MVA		25 (64.1)	
Fall from Height		9 (23.1)	
GCS 3-8	9 (52.9)	13 (33.3)	0.23
9-12	2 (11.8)	4 (30.8)	
13-15	6 (35.3)	16 (35.9)	
ISS	32.0±11.8	24.3±11.7	0.03
Coma duration (days)	6.6±8.5	11.0±15.0	0.29
Long bone fractures	6 (35.3)	29 (74.3)	<0.01
Vascular lesions	6 (35.3)	3 (7.6)	0.01
Traumatic amputation	1 (5.9)	0 (0)	0.20
Peripheral nerve injury	4 (23.5)	7 (17.9)	0.97
Abdominal injury	2 (11.8)	6 (15.3)	0.72
Chest injury	7 (41.1)	12 (30.7)	0.45

Values in the table are means±SD, number (percentage)
*Percentage of total care time
+p value obtained by t-test, $\chi 2$ test.

2.3 Characteristics of Brain Injury According to Imaging

None of the terror victims had normal CT scans as opposed to 28.2 % of the non-terror group (P=0.002). Most of the terror victims had intra-cerebral hemorrhages (70.1%) with a high rate of intra-ventricular extension (41.2%) as opposed to only 53.8% of ICH in the non-terror group with only 5.1% intra-ventricular extension (P=0.05) (Table 3). Most terror victims were injured in explosions resulting from explosion of suicide bombings in which the mechanisms of the injury includes blast injury and penetrating trauma resulting from bomb fragments and nails, bolts, and steel pellets embedded in the bomb (Figure 1). Therefore, in 37.5% of terror victims, foreign bodies were found in brain tissues and 70.6% of them underwent at least one brain surgery for removal of foreign bodies and/or evacuation of associated hematomas, if indicated as opposed to only 25.6% in the non-terror group (P=0.006).

Table 3. Imaging findings in terror victims and control.

		Terror N=17	Control N=39	p-value
CT side	Rt	6 (35.3)	7 (17.9)	0.002
	Lt	10 (58.8)	8 (20.5)	
	Rt+Lt	1 (5.9)	13 (33.3)	
	normal	0(0)	11(28.2)	
CT type	ICH	8 (47.1)	7 (17.9)	0.05
	SDH	0 (0)	1 (2.6)	
	EDH	1 (5.9)	1 (2.6)	
	SAH	2 (11.8)	1 (2.6)	
	DAI	2 (11.8)	3 (7.7)	
	combined	4 (23.5)	26 (66.7)	
CT place	Frontal	6(35.3)	4 (10.3)	0.08
	Parietal	2 (11.8)	1 (2.6)	
	Temporal	1 (5.9)	5 (12.8)	
	Occipital	1 (5.9)	1 (2.6)	
	Infra	1 (5.9)	1 (2.6)	
	Diffused	6(35.3)	27 (69.5)	
Intra-ventricular bleeding	N	10 (58.8)	37 (94.9)	0.001
	Y	7 (41.2)	2 (5.1)	
Brain surgery	N	5 (29.4)	29 (74.4)	0.006
	One	9 (52.9)	7 (17.9)	
	More	3 (17.6)	3 (7.7)	

Values in the table are means$\pm$SD, number (percentage) . +p value obtained by t-test, $\chi 2$ test.

2.4 Length of Stay

The mean total length of stay of terror TBI patients in rehabilitation was 201± 88 days as opposed to 167± 148 days of non-terror victims. The main difference was in LOS in out-patient rehabilitation facility, 120 ± 79 versus 87 ± 55. However, no significantly differences was found in LOS, neither total nor in any of treatment facilities, acute care, inpatient and outpatient rehabilitation departments (Figure 2).

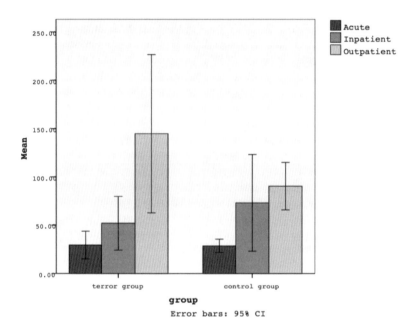

Figure 2. Mean length of stay (LOS) in acute care, inpatient and outpatient rehabilitation departments. Terror vs. Non- terror*.

2.5 ADL and General Cognitive Functions

FIM score was obtained at the end of each treated facility. The mean FIM values upon admission to rehabilitation were 76.8±36.9 in terror TBI victims as compared to 78±31.1 in non-terror victims. At the end of rehabilitation period, both groups improved significantly reaching a mean FIM score of 119.5 ±13, however there was no different between the groups (Table 4). A similar pattern was found for motor FIM and cognitive FIM, no difference was found between the two groups at the entry and discharge from each rehabilitation facilities, inpatient as outpatient departments (Table 4). The FIM score gain (ΔFIM) was 42.7 points in the terror victims and 41.5 points in the other TBI patients without difference between groups. The rate of FIM improvement over time was also similar between both groups (F $_{2,56}$=0.02 p=0.99).

Table 4. The FIM values – Total, Motor , Cognitive in different rehabilitation periods by groups: Terror versus Non-Terror.*

Evaluation	Admission to Rehabilitation Department		Discharge from inpatient Rehabilitation Department		Discharge from outpatient Rehabilitation Department	
	Terror	Non-terror	Terror	Non-terror	Terror	Non-terror
Total FIM	76.8±36.9	78.0±31.1	108±17.9	105±20.2	119.5±13.9	119.5±6.3
Motor FIM	55.3±29.6	60.4±18.9	80.8±9.6	82.2±8.2	86.8±11.0	87.8±3.9
Cognitive FIM	23.8±11.0	24.5±7.1	29.8±5.6	26.7±5.5	32.7±3.1	31.4±3.9

* There was a significant improvement ($P<0.01$) in all FIM values , total FIM, motor FIM and cognitive FIM between all the different time points in both groups, terror and non-terror without difference between the groups.

2.6 Specific Cognitive Evaluations

The cognitive performance was evaluated according to the specific five domains of the LOTCA battery [18]: orientation (max= 16), visual and spatial perception (max = 28), visual motor organization (max=28), thinking operation (max=35), and praxis (max = 12). There was no difference in the mean value of each of these domains between terror and non-terror TBI groups in the first evaluation done in rehabilitation. Both groups improved significantly in all cognitive functions except of praxis during rehabilitation period, without difference between terror and non-terror TBI groups in the rate of improvement and the final cognitive values at discharge (Figure 3). Memory evaluation according to the RBMT [19] was similar between terror and non-terror TBI groups upon admission and both groups improved significantly during rehabilitation period without any difference between groups.

2.7 Clinical, Psychological and Occupational Outcomes

We compared the clinical outcomes of terror TBI patients with non-terror patients at the end of the rehabilitation process. According to the GOS, 53% of terror victims had good recovery, 35.6% had moderate disability and 11.8% were left with severe disability. This distribution was similar with the non-terror group (Table 5). The prevalence rate of post-traumatic epilepsy (PTE) in the terror victims was found to be significantly higher than the prevalence of PTE in the non-terror group (35.2% vs. 10%, $P=0.05$, Table 5). As expected, there was a strong correlation between the existence of PTE and the presence of foreign bodies in the brains of terror TBI patients. The rate of patients diagnosed as suffering from PTSD according to Revised PTSD Inventory [15] was high in both groups (47% and 51.2% respectively) without significant differences between the groups. One of the important rehabilitation outcomes is the returning to previous occupation. Surprisingly, although terror victims suffered from more severe TBI, almost half (47%) of them succeeded in returning to their previous work or education setting similar or even better than the non-terror TBI group (28.2%, $P=0.32$, Table 5).

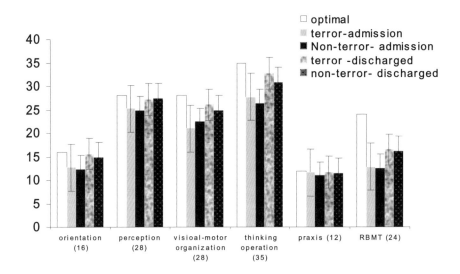

Figure 3. LOTCA[a] and RBMT[b] mean values at entry and discharged of rehabilitation facilities, Terror vs. Non-Terror*.

a. LOTCA- Loewenstein Occupational Therapy Cognitive Assessment (18)
b. RBMT- Rivermead Battery Memory Test (19)
c. In the terror group, there were LOTCA and RBMT data for 12 and 9 out of 17 patients. respectively. In the non-terror group there were LOTCA and RBMT data for 26 and 13 out of 39 patients.
*Both groups improved significantly (P <0.05) in all cognitive functions except of praxis during rehabilitation period, without difference between terror and non-terror groups.

Table 5. Clinical, psychological and occupational outcomes: Terror versus Non-Terror.

		Terror N=17 (%)	Non-terror N=39 (%)	p value
GOS	2		1 (2.8)	0.50
	3	2 (11.8)	4 (11.1)	
	4	6 (35.3)	19 (52.8)	
	5	9 (52.9)	12 (33.3)	
Epilepsy		6 (35.2)	4 (10.0)	0.05
PTSD		8 (47.0)	20 (51.2)	0.77
Return to previous occupation		8 (47.0)	11 (28.2)	0.32

PTSD-Post Traumatic Stress Disorder
GOS- Glasgow Outcome Scale
Values in the table are means+SD, number (percentage)
+p value obtained by t-test, $\chi 2$ test.

3. Discussion

To our knowledge, this is the first study comparing the rehabilitation outcomes of terror TBI patients with non-terror TBI counterparts. Our study showed that terror TBI victims are younger and suffered from more severe injuries than the non-terror TBI group according to ISS and imaging findings. In addition, the rate of long-term complications such as PTE was significantly higher among terror TBI victims. Nevertheless they spent similar time in rehabilitation and reached similar ADL functions and 47% of them succeed to return to their previous occupation similar to non-terror TBI patients.

As shown in previous studies terror victims tend to be younger in age and male in gender [2, 3, 6]. The same parameters were found in our study. Terror TBI victim are younger than non-terror TBI controls (29 versus 39.5, P=0.05) and mostly men (58.8%). Seventy percent of our patients, (total terror- 56.9%), were between the ages of 15-29, similar to data reported by Peleg et al. [3], in which 62% of all terror victims in Israel were between the ages of 15-29. This difference reflects the paucity of children and elderly in the terror TBI group and may be explained by the location of many of the terrorist acts in restaurants, discos or other social meeting places of young people. It is known that younger people with TBI have better rehabilitation outcomes than older individuals, presumably due to a better regeneration capacity of the younger brain [20-24], which can influence the overall better outcome of our terror TBI victims. No other demographic parameters were different between terror and non-terror TBI patients.

One of the important findings of our study is the fact that terror TBI patients suffered from more severe injuries than non-terror TBI controls. The severity of the TBI was determined by the higher ISS score of terror TBI patients (32.0 ± 11.8 versus 24.3 ± 11.7, P< 0.03). The ISS [12, 13] is used to quantify the severity of injury and allows comparison of severity among dissimilar types of injury and therefore, was chosen to quantify the diverse effects of injury due to terrorism. Numerous studies have used the ISS to measure injury severity among different types of injury confirming the validity of this measure and extending its potential usefulness [25, 26]. Similar to our findings, it was previously found that general terror victims in Israel had a high ISS (30% >16), a high rate of intensive care unit admission (22.8% in Israel), and have a more prolonged hospital course and higher mortality than victims of any other form of trauma [3, 4, 6, 7].

Another important finding is the extent of the intra-cerebral lesions as measured by brain imaging in the terror TBI patients. The severity of the lesion is augmented due to the mechanisms of injuries in terrorism including penetrating trauma resulting from bomb fragments and nails, bolts, and steel pellets embedded in the bomb and blunt trauma sustained when the victim is propelled against an object by the blast wind [27, 28]. The severity of the injuries is further increased when the blast occurs in confined spaces as opposed to open air as happened in many of the suicide attacks, especially in buses [29]. We suggest that the penetration of brain tissues by these objects was the reason for the higher percentage of ICH, higher rate of operations, higher complication rate and higher rate of PTE in terror TBI patients in our study.

Surprisingly, although they suffered from severe injury, the rehabilitation outcomes of terror TBI patients were not worse than non-terror counterparts. Both groups spent comparable time in rehabilitation and achieved similar FIM gain (ΔFIM) and final FIM values. The ΔFIM of our TBI patients, terror as well as non-terror, was similar to the reported ΔFIM of TBI patients in previous studies [30-32]. The LOS as in-patients in rehabilitation of our TBI patients, terror as well as non-terror, was similar to the LOS of TBI patients in some older studies but longer than the LOS of TBI patients in a recent study [33, 34]. This elongated rehabilitation period was possible because the rehabilitation process of terror victims in Israel is financed by the government through the National Insurance Institute. The factors that can contribute to the success of the rehabilitation of terror TBI victims are their young age as discussed previously [23], the relative longer stay in rehabilitation day care and the unique features of their rehabilitation treatment that will be discussed later [35].

Another unexpected finding in our study was the relatively good cognitive outcome of our terror TBI victims. Although the extent of intra-cerebral damage and the rate of required surgery were higher in terror TBI patients, their cognitive performance as evaluated by the Cognitive FIM, LOTCA and RBMT batteries at the beginning and at the end of rehabilitation was similar to the non-terror TBI controls. The LOTCA battery is primarily used to assess cognitive functions after stroke and other brain injuries and it has been shown to have adequate psychometric properties in persons with brain damage [18, 36]. The RBMT is a standardized, validated and reliable test for everyday memory [19]. It is ecologically valid, using tasks similar to activities of everyday life; it tests both short-term and long-term memory for verbal and spatial information as well as prospective memory, visual memory and memory of faces [37,38]. The cognitive functions of both groups improved significantly during rehabilitation without significant differences between them. On the contrary, in other studies of TBI patients, a correlation was found between the severity of brain lesions on CT or MRI or neurosurgical intervention and worse neuropsychological outcomes [39, 40]. The reason for this difference may be due to the different instruments used for cognitive evaluations in these studies although one of them used cognitive FIM as primary outcome like us [39]. Another possibility is in the unique rehabilitation process of terror TBI patients as discussed previously.

One of the important outcomes after any multiple traumas, and especially following terror attacks, is the developing of chronic psychological disorders such as PTSD [41-43]. According to a prospective study of post-traumatic stress in 70 victims of terrorist attacks that occurred in a Paris subway in December 1996, 41% of participants met PTSD criteria at six months; 34.4% still had PTSD at 18 months [44]. In a prospective evaluation of prevalence of PTSD in terror victims in Israel, 39 survivors of terrorist attacks had higher rates of PTSD in comparison with 354 survivors of motor vehicle accidents (37.8% versus 18.7%) [45]. Similarly, in our study, 47% of terror TBI victims suffered from signs of PTSD, however, in opposed to previous studies, also the control non-terror TBI victims suffered from high percentage (51%) of PTSD. This can be explained by higher rate of PTSD in general TBI patients as compared to general multiple trauma patients [46].

However, this high rate of PTSD did not influence the rate of return to previous occupation or integration into society of terror TBI victims. On the contrary, the rate of return to previous occupation was high in terror TBI patients (47%), although not significantly higher than non-terror TBI controls (28%). This rate was similar to or even higher than other studies which showed that less than 30% of TBI patients returned to work [47-50]. These unexpected and encouraging findings in our terror TBI patients have been achieved maybe due to the special attention given to social and psychological issues in rehabilitation of terror victims. Another important factor is the fact that, as mentioned before, terror victims in Israel are supported by the government and the process of occupational rehabilitation is started early already during their stay in out-patient rehabilitation facilities.

One of the main reasons for the success of the rehabilitation process of terror TBI victims in our study is the unique support of many official and voluntary organizations in these patients. These patients were treated from the outset by psychologists and social workers, including close support for their families and relatives. We also think that due to the sensitivity of Israeli citizens to the problem of terrorism, even our rehabilitation teams subconsciously pay more attention to and give them more quality treatment. Another important reason is that the treatment of terror victims in Israel is financed by the National Insurance Institute, which allows an adequate period of rehabilitation treatment and sufficient resources as needed.

4. Conclusions

Although TBI terror victims had more severe injuries, they gained most of their ADL functions back and their rehabilitation outcomes were similar to non-terror TBI patients. This was probably achieved due to a multidisciplinary rehabilitation approach including intensive psychological and social support. Our study emphasizes the importance of a multidisciplinary approach to the rehabilitation of terror TBI victims and allowing an adequate period for rehabilitation and recovery.

References

[1]   Arnold JL, Halpern P, Tsai MC, Smithline H. Mass casualty terrorist bombings: a comparison of outcomes by bombing type. Annals of Emergency Medicine 2004;43:263-273.

[2]   Schwartz I, Tsenter J, Shochina M, Shiri S,Kedary M, Katz-Leurer M, Meiner Z. Rehabilitation Outcome of Terror Victims with Multiple Trauma. Archives of Physical Medicine and Rehabilitation 2007;88:440-448.

[3]   Peleg K, Aharonson-Daniel L, Michael M, Shapira SC, Israel Trauma Group. Patterns of injury in hospitalized terrorist victims. The American Journal of Emergency Medicine 2003; 21:258-262.

[4]   Mintz Y, Shapira SC, Pikarsky AJ, Goitein D, Gertcenchtein I, Mor-Yosef S, Rivkind AI. The Experience of one institution dealing with terror: The El Aqsa Intifada riots. Israel Medical Assiciation Journal 2002;4:554-556.

[5]   Israel Defence Force official web site. Available at: (http://www1.idf.il/SIP_STORAGE/DOVER/files/7/21827.doc) Accessed October 2007.

[6]   Kluger Y, Peleg K, Daniel-Aharonson L, Mayo A; Israeli Trauma Group. The special injury pattern in terrorist bombings. Journal of the American College of Surgeons 2004;199:875-879.

[7]   Aharonson-Daniel L, Waisman Y, Dannon YL and Peleg K. Epidemiology of terror-related versus non-terror-related traumatic injury in children. Pediatrics 2003;112:280-284.

[8]   Einav S, Aharonson-Daniel L, Weissman C, Freund HR, Peleg K; Israel Trauma Group. In-hospital resource utilization during multiple casualty incidents. Annals of Surgery 2006;243:533-540.

[9]   Singer P, Cohen J. D, Stein M. Conventional terrorism and critical care. Critical Care Medicine 2005;33(suppl):S61-S65.

[10] Peleg K, Aharonson-Daniel L, Stein M, et al; Israeli Trauma Group (ITG). Gunshot and explosion injuries: characteristics, outcomes and implications for care of terror-related injuries in Israel. Annals of Surgery 2004;239:311-318.

[11] Peleg K, Rivkind A, Aharonson-Daniel L; Israeli Trauma Group. Does body armor protect from firearm injuries? Journal of the American College of Surgeons 2006;202:643-648.

[12] Baker SP, O'Neill B, Haddon W, Long WB. The injury severity score: A method for describing patients with multiple injuries and evaluating emergency care. Journal of Trauma, Injury, Infection & Critical Care 1974; 14:187-196.

[13] Baker SP, O'Neill B. The injury severity score: An update. Journal of Trauma, Injury, Infection & Critical Care 1976;16:882-885.

[14] Granger CV, Hamilton BB, Sherwin FS. Guide for the use of the uniform data set for medical rehabilitation. Buffalo: Uniform Data System for Medical Rehabilitation Project Office, Buffalo General Hospital; 1986.

[15] Solomon Z, Benbenishty R, Neria Y, Abramowitz M, Ginzburg K, and Ohry A.. Assessment of PTSD: Validation of the Revised PTSD Inventory. Israel Journal of Psychiatry and Related Sciences 1993;30:110-115.

[16] Derogatis LR, Spencer PM. Administration and procedures: BSI manual I. Baltimor: Clinical Psychometric Research; 1982

[17] Jennett B, Snoek J, Bond MR, Brooks N. Disability after severe head injury: observations on the use of the Glasgow Outcome Scale. Journal of Neurology, Neurosurgery and Psychiatry 1981;44:285–293.

[18] Katz N, Itakovitch M, Averbuch S, Elazar B . Loewenstein Occupational Therapy Cognitive Assessment (LOTCA) battery for brain-injured patients: reliability and validity. The American Journal of Occupational Therapy 1989;43:184-192.

[19] Wilson BA, Cockburn J, Baddeley AD, Hiorns R. The development and validation of a test battery for detecting and monitoring everyday memory problems. Journal of Clinical and Experimental Neuropsychology 1989;11: 855–870.

[20] Testa JA, Malec JF, Moessner AM, Brown AW. Outcome after traumatic brain injury: effects of aging on recovery. Archives of Physical Medicine and Rehabilitation 2005;86:1815-1823.

[21] Katz DI, Alexander MP. Predicting course of recovery and outcome for patients admitted to rehabilitation. Archives of Neurology 1994;51:661-670.

[22] Mosenthal AC, Lavery RF, Addis M, Kaul S, Ross S, Marburger R, Deitch EA, Livingston DH. Isolated traumatic brain injury: Age is an independent predictor of mortality and early outcome. Journal of Trauma, Injury, Infection & Critical Care 2002;52:907-911.

[23] Hukkelhoven CW, Steyerberg EW, Rampen AJ, Farace E, Habbema JD, Marshall LF, Murray GD, Ai M. Patient age and outcome following severe traumatic brain injury: An analysis of 5600 patients. Journal of Neurosurgery 2003;99:666-673.

[24] Vollmer DG, Torner JC, Jane JA, Sadovnic B, Charlebois D, Eisenberg HM, Foulkes MA, Marmarour A, Marshall LF. Age and outcome following traumatic coma: Why do older patients fare worse. Neurosurgery 1991;75:37-49.

[25] Maurer A, Morris JA. Injury severity scoring. In: Moore EE, Feliciano DV, Mattox LK, editors. Trauma (5th ed), McGraw-Hill, New York 2004. p 87-92.

[26] Osler T, Baker SP, Long W. A modification of the injury severity score that both improves accuracy and simplifies scoring. Journal of Trauma, Injury, Infection & Critical Care 1997;43:922-925.

[27] Kluger Y. Bomb explosion in act of terrorism- detonation, wound ballistics, triage and medical concerns. Israel Medical Assiciation Journal 2003;5:235-240.

[28] Kluger Y, Kashuk J, Mayo A. Terror bombing- mechanism, consequences and implications. Scandinavian Journal of Surgery 2004;93:11-14.

[29] Katz E, Ofek B, Adler I, Abramowitz HB, Krausz MM. Primary blast injury after a bomb explosion in a civilian bus. Annals of Surgery, 1989;209:484-488.

[30] Novack TA, Bush BA, Meythaler JM, Canupp K. Outcome after traumatic brain injury: pathway analysis of contributions from premorbid, injury severity, and recovery variables. Archives of Physical Medicine and Rehabilitation, 2001;82:300-305.

[31] Cope DN. The effectiveness of traumatic brain injury rehabilitation: a review. Brain Injury 1995;9:649-670.

[32] Corrigan JD, Smith-Knapp K, Granger CV. Validity of the functional independence measures in persons traumatic brain injury. Archives of Physical Medicine and Rehabilitation 1997;12:14-26.

[33] Heinemann AW, Linacre JM, Wright BD, Hamilton BB, Granger C. Prediction of rehabilitation outcomes and disability measures. Archives of Physical Medicine and Rehabilitation 1994;75:133-143.

[34] Bode RK, Heinemann AW. Course of functional improvement after stroke, spinal cord injury, and traumatic brain injury. Archives of Physical Medicine and Rehabilitation 2002;83:100-106.

[35] Spivak G, Spettel CM, Ellis DW, Ross SE. Effects of intensity of treatment and length of stay on rehabilitation outcomes. Brain Injury 1992;6:419-434.

[36] Katz N, Hartman-Maeir A, Ring H, Soroker N. Relationships of cognitive performance and daily function in patients following right hemisphere stroke: Predictable and ecological validity of the LOTCA Battery. Occupational Therapy Journal of Research 2000;20:3–17.

[37] Cockburn J,Wilson BA, Baddeley AD, Hiorns R. Assessing everyday memory in patients with perceptual deficits. Clinical Rehabilitation 1990;4:129–135.

[38] Cockburn, J. The pragmatic and ecological perspective: Evaluation of memory disorders. European Review of Applied Psychology 1996;46:201–205.

[39] De Guise E, Leblanc J, Feyz M, Lamoureux J. Predictors of the level of cognitive functional independence in acute care following traumatic brain injury. Brain Injury 2005;19:1087-1093.

[40] Dikmen SS, Machamer JE, Winn HR. Neuropsychological outcome at 1 year post head injury. Neuropsychology 1995;9:80-90.

[41] Silver RC, Holman EA, McIntosh DN, Poulin M, Gil-Rivas V. Nationwide longitudinal study of psychological responses to September 11. Journal of the American Medical Association 2002;288:1235-1244.

[42] Schlenger WE, Caddell JM, Ebert L, Jordan BK, Rourke KM, Wilson D, Thalji L, Dennis JM, Fairbank JA, Kulka RA. Psychological reactions to terrorist attacks: Findings from the National Study of Americans' Reactions to September 11. Journal of the American Medical Association 2002;288:581–588.

[43] Gidron Y, Kaplan Y, Velt A, Shalem R. Prevalence and moderators of terror-related post-traumatic stress disorder symptoms in Israeli citizens. Israel Medical Association Journal 2004;6:387-391.

[44] Jehel L, Duchet C, Paterniti S, Consoli SM, Guelfi JD. Prospective study of post-traumatic stress in victims of terrorist attacks. Encephale 2001;27:393-400.

[45] Shalev AY, Freedman S. PTSD following terrorist attacks: a prospective evaluation. American Journal of Psychiatry 2005;162:1188-1191.

[46] Frenisy MC, Benony H, Chahraoui K, Minot D, d'Athis P, Pinoit JM, Freysz M. Brain injury patients versus multiple trauma patients: Some neurobehavioral and psychopathological aspects. Journal of Trauma, Injury, Infection & Critical Care 2006;60:1018-1026.

[47] Avensani R, Salvi G, Rigoli G, Gambini MG. Reintegration after severe brain injury: A retrospective study. Brain Injury 2005;19:933-939.

[48] Yasuda S, Wehman P, Targett P, Cifu DX, West M. Return to work after spinal cord injury: a review of recent research. Neurorehabilitation 2002;17:177-186.

[49] Brooks N, McKinlay W, Symington C, Beattie A, Campsie L. Return to work within the first seven years of severe head injury. Brain Injury 1987;1:5-19.

[50] Rao N, Rosenthal M, Cronin-Stubbs D, Lambert R, Barnes P, Swanson B. Return to work after rehabilitation following traumatic brain injury. Brain Injury 1990;4:49-56.

Coping with Blast-Related Traumatic Brain Injury in Returning Troops
B.K. Wiederhold (Ed.)
IOS Press, 2011
© *2011 The authors and IOS Press. All rights reserved.*
doi: 10.3233/978-1-60750-797-0-126

Evaluation of Post-deployment Screening for Traumatic Brain Injury and Blast Exposure in a Sample of High-Risk Sailors Deployed to Iraq

Justin S. CAMPBELL [a], Jeffrey H. GREENBERG [a], Mikias WOLDE [a]
and Jack W. TSAO [a,1]
[a] *Wounded, Ill, and Injured Directorate*
United States Navy Bureau of Medicine & Surgery

Abstract. Mild Traumatic Brain Injury (mTBI) is a common injury from combat. Detecting persistent symptoms is important in the care for returning service members. Retrospective self-reports were collected in a sample of 63 U.S. Navy Sailors who served a tour in Iraq while engaged in a high-risk mission for blast exposure. The sample fell into three injury exposure categories: no-injury (n = 17), blast only (n = 40), and blast plus blow-to-the-head (n = 6). Consistent with expectations, blast plus blow exposure resulted in greater symptom prevalence within category.

Keywords. Traumatic Brain Injury, mTBI, blast exposure, concussion symptoms, improvised explosive device, Iraq

Disclaimer: The opinions or assertions contained herein are the private views of the authors and are not to be construed as official or as reflecting the views of the Department of the Navy or the Department of Defense.

Introduction

Mild Traumatic Brain Injury (mTBI) is one the primary injuries United States service members encounter serving in combat zones. Early detection, treatment by rest, and education about clinical outcomes and expectations is of great clinical importance. Treating persistent symptoms and identifying service members who may need treatment upon return from deployment is also important. The current methods used to identify service members with mTBI are routine post-deployment surveillance surveys which are not 100% sensitive or specific. In order to improve identification of service members with clinical symptoms, a performance improvement project was undertaken utilizing retrospective self-report surveys, with clinician confirmation of symptoms, to evaluate blast exposure and related neurological symptoms associated with concussion/mTBI in a sample of U.S. Navy Sailors assigned to two Weapons Intelligence Teams (WITs) who were frequently exposed to improvised explosive devices as a part of their daily duties during a six-month tour in Iraq during 2009.

---

[1] Corresponding Author. Jack W. Tsao, Wounded, Ill, and Injured Directorate, United States Navy Bureau of Medicine & Surgery; E-mail: Jack.Tsao@med.navy.mil.

1. Rationale for the Study

According to the Defense and Veteran's Brain Injury Center (DVBIC), mild brain injury/concussion sustained through blast exposure is complex, often mixing elements of injury due to a wave of over-pressurization that dissipates through neural soft-tissue resulting in axonal shearing, as well as more traditional blunt force trauma and rapid brain acceleration/deceleration within the cranial cavity [1].

DVBIC also notes that mTBI can occur not just in the face of blast exposure, but also during the course of daily occupational and recreational activities [1]. Not surprisingly, many military samples may report symptoms of mTBI both for blast exposure as well as for other blows to the head. In the current analysis, we attempted to evaluate whether clinical symptom severity and patterns differed according to whether or not a blow to the head was also experienced along with blast exposure.

2. Sample

The sample consisted of two distinct WITs (team 1, n = 27; team 2, n = 36) deployed to Iraq in 2009, which will be treated as a single sample for the remainder of the discussion, who received post-deployment surveys in the first two days after return from deployment. A clinician evaluated each person to confirm the presence or absence and nature of the symptoms reported on the survey. Almost all Sailors had completed prior combat tours in Iraq (76.2%), while only 3.2% of the sample reported a prior deployment to Afghanistan. The total sample consisted of three officers, eight Senior enlisted (E7 or above), and a wide range of junior enlisted Sailors. The mean (M) age of the sample was 36 years old (Standard Deviation [SD] = 7.44, range: 20 to 48 years). WITs consist of service members from many occupational specialties, including photography, intelligence analyst, explosive ordnance disposal, master-at-arms, and administration.

3. Results

To test the hypothesis that blast exposure head injury will result in a different severity of mTBI/concussion symptoms than a blow-induced head injury, we first conducted a cross-tabulation to determine whether distinct blast or blow injury groups (from the most recent deployment) existed. The resulting head injury exposure categories were observed: no injury (n = 17); blast only (n= 40); and blast plus blow (n = 6). No Sailors reported only an isolated blow to the head.

The mean total mTBI/concussion symptoms increased from the no injury (M = .12, SD = .48) to blast only (M = .58, SD = 1.00) group and further to the blast plus blow group (M = 1.5, SD = 1.64). Due to the small and heterogeneous between-groups sample sizes, the Kruskal-Wallis non-parametric test of group differences was applied to determine whether ordinal group differences in mTBI/concussion symptoms were significantly different, with p<0.05 considered significant. The result (χ^2 = 8.76, p < .05) confirmed significant differences in mTBI/concussion symptoms between groups.

Table 1: Endorsement of mTBI/concussion Symptoms by Exposure Categories.

Symptom	No Injury (n = 17)	Blast Only (n = 40)	Blast plus Blow (n = 6)
	n (%)	n (%)	n (%)
Memory loss	0	0	0
Headaches	0	3 (8%)	2 (33%)
Ringing in the ears	0	3 (8%)	1 (17%)
Trouble sleeping	1 (6%)	6 (15%)	2 (33%)
Balance problems, dizziness, or vertigo	0	1 (3%)	1 (17%)
Irritability (short temper)	1 (6%)	9 (23%)	2 (33%)
Sensitivity to bright light or noise	0	1 (3%)	1 (17%)
Nausea/vomiting	0	0	0

Note: Column values represent number of individuals endorsing the symptom. Percentages are within exposure group.

4. Discussion

Although our analysis focused on a small group of service members, there were distinct findings in the number of mTBI/concussion symptoms reported at the time of re-deployment from the combat environment. The average total symptom number (we did not assess for severity) significantly increased from the no blast, to blast only, and then to blast plus head blow groups.

The absence of individuals reporting only blows to the head on their deployment to Iraq prevented a true comparison of blast versus blow mTBI/concussion symptoms and symptom patterns. Nevertheless, it was observed that blast exposure plus head blow leads to a significantly greater number of mTBI/concussion symptoms, thus emphasizing the need to consider both sources of trauma when evaluating the potential for mTBI/concussion in combat-deployed service members.

Further, the prevalence of sleep disturbance and irritability symptoms across all categories begs consideration of the notion that these two symptoms, known to be associated also with psychological disorders, may prove to confound attempts to evaluate the relative impact of different sources of mTBI/concussion symptoms. In particular, it may be necessary to identify a baseline of sleep and irritability symptoms that occurs outside of head trauma. Larger sample sizes will be needed to confirm whether these initial findings are borne out and would alter the post-deployment screening process for service members returning from combat deployments.

References

[1] http://www.dvbic.org/TBI---The-Military/Blast-Injuries.aspx,

IOS Press, 2011
doi: 10.3233/978-1-60750-797-0-129

Generic Brain-computer Interface for Social Networks and Rehabilitation Assistance

Christoph GUGER[a,1], Christoph HINTERMÜLLER[a] and Günter EDLINGER[a]

[a] *g.tec medical engineering GmbH and Guger Technologies OG*
Austria

Abstract. After suffering from a severe disease like spinal cord injury or stroke, patients are often unable to interact or even communicate with their environment anymore, especially at the beginning of rehabilitation. Brain-computer interfaces (BCIs) can substitute these temporarily lost communication channels. They also might support rehabilitation by providing an alternative way to control a computer: by thoughts without any muscle activity. This enables the patient to communicate by writing letters on the screen, and stay in social contact with friends or people outside of the rehabilitation facility by participating in games like Second Life© where they may appear as healthy people. Another application is to control items in their room that are connected to the BCI system, like the lights, which can be turned on and off (as can be done in a virtual smart home without leaving the bed). In this paper, the technology of such BCIs and the mentioned applications are described utilizing the P300 approach. A generic BCI interface is presented which allows concurrent control of the different applications and the ability to switch transparently among them. The results of a recent study show that a BCI can be used by patients suffering from cervical spinal cord injury almost as well as by healthy people. This encourages us to think that by enabling the user to socially interact and communicate easily, these applications may assist in rehabilitation and slow down the progress of late syndromes.

Keywords. Brain-computer interface (BCI), P300, visual evoked potentials, speller, Second Life©, virtual smart home

Introduction

Many disorders can affect or even completely damage the usual communication channels a person needs to communicate and interact with their environment. For example, spinal cord injury, stroke and amyotrophic lateral sclerosis (ALS) can result in partial or complete loss of voluntary muscle activities including speech. In such severe cases, a brain-computer interface (BCI) might be the only remaining possibility to communicate [1]. An EEG-based BCI provides a new non-invasive communication channel between the human brain and a computer without using any muscle activity. It measures and analyzes the electrical brain activity during predefined mental tasks and translates them into the corresponding action intended by the user. A BCI can improve quality of life of partially paralyzed patients in rehabilitation by enabling them to control a computer and specially prepared electronic devices and/or stay in contact with friends through social networks and games.

---

[1] Corresponding Author: Dr. Christoph Guger, g.tec Guger Technologies OG, Schiedlberg, Austria 4521; E-mail: guger@gtec.at.

P300 evoked potential based BCIs provide goal-oriented control and are mainly used for spelling devices. Farwell and Donchin were among the first pioneers who used the P300 for communication [2]. Furthermore, this approach can also be used for game control or navigation (e.g., moving a computer mouse) [3,4]. The P300 evoked potential is elicited when an unlikely event occurs randomly between events with high probability. It manifests itself in a positive deflection in the amplitude of the EEG signal around 300 ms after a visual stimulus onset. Different classification techniques have been evaluated for P300 spellers whereby both the Fisher's linear discriminant analysis and the stepwise linear discriminant analysis (LDA) yielded very robust performances [5]. These classification methods need to be trained on each subject in order to adapt to the particular brain activity behavior of a person. Training of such a BCI system can be accomplished within several minutes [6]. Guger et al. demonstrated that more than 70% of a sample population is able to use such a spelling setup with an accuracy of 100% [9].

This paper presents a generic UDP, XML based BCI command interface (according to the recently introduced international BCI interface standard, see www.gtec.at) and its application to implement control interfaces enabling social interactions like spelling, interacting virtually with other participants in Second Life©, operating Twitter© and controlling a virtual smart home. All of these applications are based on the P300 speller principle. Results of a spelling application study done with 100 healthy people will be compared to a recent study also including spinal cord injury patients showing that this type of a BCI would be suited for rehabilitation assistance.

1. Method

For a P300 spelling device, a 6 x 6 matrix of different characters and symbols is commonly presented on a computer screen [7]. In single-character mode, all characters are flashed in a random order, displaying only one character after the other (Figure 1a). In row-column mode, a whole row or column flashes at one time (Figure 1b). The subject has to concentrate on a specific letter he or she wants to write. The flashing of exactly this character or the corresponding row or column is a relative unlikely event which induces a P300 component in the EEG signal, reaching its maximum amplitude around 300 ms after the onset of the flash. For all other characters, rows or columns, no such P300 component is elicited because they are not relevant to the subject at that moment.

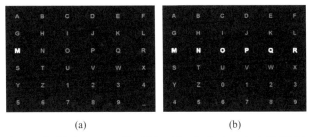

(a)   (b)

Figure 1. Screen layout of a 36-character speller. Either (a) a single character is highlighted at a certain time or (b) a whole row or column is highlighted.

To measure the P300 component acquisition of EEG signals from eight electrode positions mostly over occipital and parietal regions is sufficient (Figure 2) [8]. To train the BCI system, an arbitrary word like LUCAS is announced to the system to be aware of which characters the subject is supposed to concentrate on (targets) and which are not supposed to be concentrated on (non-targets). Each letter, row and column flashes several times (e.g., 100 ms per flash). The subject focuses on each of these letters, one after the other, and continues a mental count whenever the letter of interest flashes. EEG data of a specific time interval around each flash is then sent to an LDA classifier to learn to distinguish the typical EEG signal form of the target characters from the typical signal form of all other non-targets.

After the classifier has been trained this way, the subject can concentrate on any character in the matrix without telling the system. After each row and column has flashed several times, the system sends the EEG data to the trained LDA classifier that is now able to identify the target character by the rule built previously during training. Note that only a few targets are sufficient for training to get a good classifier, rather than training to LDA to all 36 possible characters. The applications described in the following were solely tested with healthy people. All of the following applications are based on the same principle and setup. The applications differ in the content of the matrix, where letters may be replaced by symbols or phrases to control the associated applications. EEG data were recorded with a g.MOBIlab+ bio-signal amplification unit (g.tec medical engineering GmbH, Austria) at 256 Hz sample rate and transferred to the computer wirelessly via Bluetooth®.

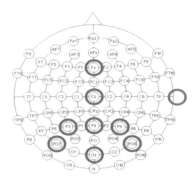

Figure 2. Common electrode setup for P300 spellers according to [8]. Eight EEG electrodes are placed at Fz, Cz, P3, Pz, P4, PO7, Oz and PO8. The ground electrode is mounted on the forehead at Fpz (yellow circle) and the reference electrode is attached to the right ear lobe (blue circle).

A MATLAB/Simulink model controls the interface masks and processes the received data via a specific device driver. A notch filter (50 Hz or 60 Hz) and a band pass filter were applied to the signals in order to eliminate possible artifacts before they were down-sampled to 64 Hz. Data from 100 ms before each flash onset to 700 ms afterwards were filtered and down-sampled again to get 12 feature values (i.e., samples) per channel and flash. These data sets were sent to the LDA to determine if a target character flashed or not. The subjects sat in front of a computer screen and were instructed to relax as much as possible, except for the virtual smart home study where the subjects used the BCI from a standing position. Additionally, the speller application itself, with a modified character matrix, has been tested with patients suffering from spinal cord injury and locked-in syndrome [6].

1.1. Second Life© Control

Second Life© is a free 3-D online virtual world developed by the American company Linden Lab launched on June 23, 2003. After five years, the platform had about 15 million registered users with an average of 60,000 online users at the same time. Only a free client software and account are necessary to participate.

Second Life© aims at socializing with other "residents," which represent persons of the real world. Residents are able to communicate via text and voice chats as well as by gestures. They can perform different actions like taking pictures, attending courses, holding business meetings and so on. With an appropriate interface, handicapped people can participate like any other user. Therefore, we utilized and modified the P300 base system from Figure 1 to provide control for Second Life©.

Three different hierarchical nested control masks were designed. A typical Second Life© scene and the corresponding main control mask of the P300 interface are shown in Figure 3. Letters have been replaced by 31 different commands (classes) to select. Two further control masks for chatting (55 classes) and searching (40 classes) can be accessed through the main control mask. When a certain icon is selected via the P300 interface, Second Life© will be notified to execute the associated action by using keyboard events.

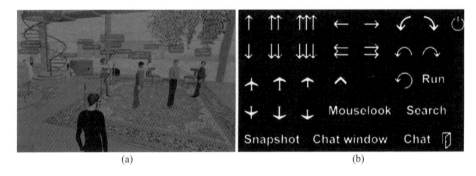

(a)   (b)

Figure 3. Screenshot of a typical Second Life© scene (a) and the corresponding main control mask (b) for the P300 interface. The mask allows to select between commands for walking forward and backward, turning left and right, climbing, teleporting home, showing the map, turning around, activating/deactivating running mode, starting/stopping flying, activating/deactivating mouselook view, entering the search mask, taking a snapshot, starting a chat, etc.

Login	Logout	Line	Search	Friends	Post
Inbox	Send	Follow	Leave	Delete	Enter
A	B	C	D	E	F
G	H	I	J	K	L
M	N	O	P	Q	R
S	T	U	V	W	X
Y	Z	0	1	2	3
4	5	6	7	8	9
,	.	!	?	☺	_

Figure 4. The extended P300 interface control mask for Twitter[©].

1.2. P300 Twitter[©] Interface

Through the social network Twitter Inc.[©], users can exchange messages. These messages can be sent over the Twitter[©] website via smart phones or SMS (Short Message Service). They are displayed on the author's profile page and are limited to 140 characters per message. Interfacing possibilities can be extended through the application-programming interface provided by Twitter[©].

The P300 control mask was extended to add the necessary Twitter[©] control commands in the first two rows. The resulting Twitter[©] control contains a total of 54 possible symbols (Figure 4). The corresponding Unified Modeling Language (UML) state diagram is used to identify the actions and commands required for using the Twitter[©] service (Figure 5).

In the example shown in Table 1, the system was initially trained with 10 target symbols for the BCI user. After the training was finished, another user was asking questions through the web-based Twitter[©] interface and the BCI user answered each question the next day. A total of nine questions were asked, meaning that the BCI user had to use the P300 interface on nine different days. During this period, the BCI user selected between six and 36 characters each day.

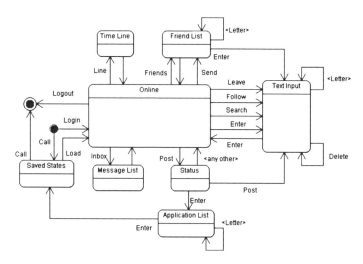

Figure 5. UML diagram of the actions required to use the Twitter[©] service.

1.3. Virtual Smart Home Control

A virtual 3-D representation of a smart home was designed based on the eXTreme Virtual Reality (XVR) environment developed at the University of Pisa [10, 11]. Seven different control masks were developed for the P300 BCI in order to control the virtual smart home environment.

Figure 6 shows two views of the virtual apartment and their corresponding control masks. The pictures in Figure 6a and Figure 6c show a 3-D view of the living room and the corresponding main control mask, which allows the user to access and control some of the devices in the living room, like the TV set, room light and telephone. The picture in Figure 6c shows a bird's-eye view of the virtual apartment. The living room can be found in the top left corner of the bird's-eye view, the top right corner represents the kitchen, the bedroom is in the bottom left corner and in the bottom right corner are the bathroom and entrance door. Using the "Go to" P300 BCI control mask, which is shown in Figure 6d, the users can beam themselves to 21 different locations in the apartment.

With the seven control masks, it is possible for users to switch the light on and off, open and close the doors and windows, control the TV set, use the phone, play music, operate the video camera at the entrance, walk around in the house and move to a specific place in the apartment.

A total of 12 healthy subjects participated in the case study. The system was trained on 42 selected target symbols for each subject. In contrast to the previous applications, the subjects used this BCI from an upright position. The control computer with the screen for the control masks was placed in front of them. A 3-D power wall was installed next to the subjects for projection of the virtual smart home. The subjects were instructed to avoid unnecessary movements and to accomplish some specific tasks like opening the front door, moving to specific places in the apartment or manipulating the light source or room temperature.

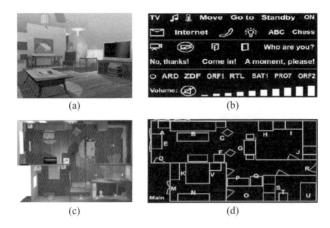

(a)   (b)

(c)   (d)

Figure 6. The living room (a) and the bird's-eye (c) view of the virtual smart home. The smart home environment was developed by Mel Slater and Chris Groenegress [11]. The figures (c) and (d) show the corresponding control masks.

1.4. Generic Control Interface

The interface was designed with the intention of controlling multiple applications and devices simultaneously and providing a common way of sharing BCI control in a consistent manner. The various applications, like Twitter© (section 0), differ in the content of the P300 BCI matrix where letters may be replaced by symbols or phrases to control the associated applications.

In the first state, the possible control states and commands available in order to move on to the next state are identified using UML diagrams, which yield a simple and clear overview of all required elements (Figure 5). Based on the diagrams, the detailed descriptions of the states and actions to be taken (including the transition to the next state), an XML file describing the required masks, the position of the different symbols within the mask and the commands to call are generated for each application. Upon startup, the interface descriptions of the different applications are merged and symbols are added for switching among them. Figure 5 shows the UML diagram for the Twitter© application and Figure 4 shows the P300 mask resulting thereof. Whenever the user selects a control symbol or character, the BCI emits the command or character string associated with the symbol or executes the related action.

2. Results

The interface was implemented for and tested with Twitter©, Second Life© and the virtual smart home application presented above. For the three systems, the control states were identified using UML state diagrams. Based on these, the control mask descriptions were generated and merged. The symbols for switching between the different applications were added. For the Twitter© application, the switching was accomplished by a consecutive selection of "Post" and "Enter" instead. This symbol combination opened the list of applications to select from. With this approach, the control mask, which was designed for the standalone version of the Twitter© applications, could be used without any change (Figure 4). In the following sections, some of the results achieved for each of the applications are discussed.

2.1. P300 Twitter Interface

Table 1 shows the results of the answers from the BCI user (bold sentences) to the nine questions (italic sentences). The improvement of the user's performance from the first session to the last one is interesting. For the first session it took the user 11:09 minutes to spell 13 characters with three mistakes. The user was instructed to correct any mistake yielding an average of 51 seconds selection time for each character. In contrast to this, the last session was accomplished in a time of 6:38 minutes for 27 characters with only one mistake resulting in an average selection time of 15 seconds per character. The number of flashes per character decreased from eight to three flashes as well.

2.2. Virtual Reality Control

Compared to the Twitter© application, three different hierarchically arranged control masks are required for the Second Life© application. The P300 control interface for

Second Life© has been tested in first setups. Preliminary results indicate a very similar performance to the virtual smart home study conducted by Edlinger et al. [10].

In the virtual smart home study, the subjects needed between three and 10 flashes per character (mean 5.2 flashes per character) to achieve an accuracy of 95% in single-character mode [10]. Table 2 lists the accuracy of all subjects for each of the seven control masks among other parameters. Increased amplitudes of the P300 components in the EEG signals yielding better accuracies can be observed on the larger masks compared to the smaller ones. This can be explained by the decreased probability of occurrence for each single character and therefore increased time that is required to flash all symbols. Interestingly, the subjects achieved only 26.39% accuracy for the "Go to" mask, which is quite bad compared to the other control masks. We think this is due to its differing layout. While all the other control masks were arranged in a matrix layout, the "Go to" mask was the only one where the symbols were placed at apparently irregular positions dependent on the appearance of the virtual apartment. More detailed results of the virtual smart home study can be found in [10].

Table 1. Questions and text input with the P300 twitter interface.

Tweets	No. Characters	Duration [mm:ss]	Errors	No. Flashes	Time per character [s]
Friend: Which kind of Brain-Computer Interface do you use?					
BCI: P300 GTEC BCI	13	11:09	3	8	51
Friend: Are you using the g.GAMMAsys?					
BCI: EXACTLY!	7	06:18	1	8	54
Friend: Active or passive electrodes? For explanation: the active system avoids or reduces artifacts and signal noise.					
BCI: ACTIVE ELECTRODES	17	06:10	0	5	22
...					
Friend: How long does it take to code the software for the BCI for TWITTER?					
BCI: 3 WEEKS	7	03:13	1	4	28
Friend: How many characters are you able to write within a minute?					
BCI: 3 TO 4	6	03:15	0	5	33
Friend: Did you get faster in writing during this period?					
BCI: YES, FROM 2 TO 4 CHARACTERS	27	06:38	1	3	15

Table 2. Accuracy, Number of symbols, occurrence probability per symbol, number of flashes per symbol and mask (e.g., 25 x 15 = 375) and selection time per symbol for each mask.

Mask	Accu-racy	No. Sym-bols	Proba-bility	No. Flashes	Time per character
Light	65.28%	25	4%	375	33.75 s
Music	76.11%	50	2%	750	67.50 s
Phone	63.89%	30	3.3%	450	40.50 s
Temper-ature	76.39%	38	2.6%	570	51.30 s
TV	65.74%	40	2.5%	600	54.00 s
Move	75.93%	13	7.7%	195	17.55 s
Go to	26.39%	22	4.5%	330	29.70 s

3. Discussion

Extending the standard P300 speller by icons and symbols enables the user to control more complex scenarios. In [10], it is shown that a proper design of interface masks allows control of demotic devices in a virtual smart home study with comparable reliability to what has been reached for the spelling application. This paper discusses the usage of a BCI interface, to take part in social environments like controlling characters and actions in Second Life© or operating other social interaction applications, like sending or answering Twitter© messages. The generic BCI interface that uses XML-based description files simplifies the definition of the control masks. By merging the control masks of several applications like Twitter©, Second Life© and devices and environments like a virtual smart home, it is possible to use the different systems concurrently. To switch to another application, it is sufficient to select the symbol used to load its control mask. If not, the application will be initialized to receive the control commands from the BCI.

In a recent study, Guger et al. evaluated a P300 speller (6 x 6 character matrix) in row-column mode with 100 healthy subjects (32 female and 68 male at the age of 27.9 ± 10.9) using a similar setup as described in this study [9]. Using a subset of 81 subjects, 88.9% of them were able to use the speller with an accuracy level of 80-100% whereas 72.8% reached an accuracy of 100%. The average accuracy level was 91.1% with a spelling time of 28.8 seconds for a single character. Since this speller is based on the same P300 principle, the results indicate that the previously described applications might perform better using row-column mode instead of single-character mode.

However, most of the existing studies were done with healthy subjects so far. Only some include disabled people. Recently, Ortner et al. evaluated the speller application with 10 disabled subjects (six male and four female at the age of 35.6 ± 11.96) in [6] using a similar setup as described in this study. Eight subjects suffered a cervical spinal cord injury between a neurological level of C2 and C6 and two subjects suffered from locked-in syndrome due to brainstem hemorrhagic stroke. However, six of the cervical spinal cord injured subjects were able to control the speller with accuracy levels between 80% and 100% with a mean of 90%. This result is very similar to the previously described study with the 100 healthy people in [9]. Interestingly, one subject suffering from a lesion at C2 achieved 100% accuracy. Because of a complication due to a tracheotomy, the subject is unable to communicate without help. However, the two patients suffering from locked-in syndrome were not able to gain control of the speller with the predefined settings. Thus, a good visual sight and low muscle artifact contamination seem to be a requirement to achieve good performance. Additionally, tuning of the settings for each individual person may lead to an increase in accuracy.

The results of the study show that patients suffering from more severe diseases can also use the P300 BCI. This encourages us to think that a BCI may be helpful during rehabilitation, especially when people are bound to bed or rehabilitation facilities; it is important to keep them socially engaged. This can be very difficult for paralyzed patients. The applications described here help people to keep in touch with friends and others worldwide through popular social networks and platforms like Twitter© and Second Life©. Another important fact is that patients may appear as healthy people in Second Life©, which may be a benefit regarding psychological aspects to let the disability fade from people's minds. Furthermore, a BCI can also be used for wheelchair control, which many authors identify as their target application. However, there are still some minimum requirements to operate a BCI. In fact, there is a certain percentage of the population (including healthy individuals) that is unable to operate a specific type of BCI at all, which may have various reasons [13].

Acknowledgments
The research leading to these results has received funding from the European Community's, Seventh Framework Programme FP7/2007-2013 under BrainAble project, grant agreement n° 247447. The authors further gratefully acknowledge the funding by the European Commission under contract FP7-ICT-2009-247935 (Brain-Neural Computer Interaction for Evaluation and Testing of Physical Therapies in Stroke Rehabilitation of Gait Disorders) and under contract IST-2006-27731 (PRESENCCIA).

References

[1]   J. R. Wolpaw, N. Birbaumer, D. J. McFarland, G. Pfurtscheller, and T. M. Vaughan, "Brain-computer interfaces for communication and control," Clin. Neurophysiol., vol. 113, no. 6, pp. 767-791, June 2002.
[2]   L. A. Farwell, and E. Donchin, "Talking off the top of your head: toward a mental prosthesis utilizing event-related brain potentials," Electroencephalogr. Clin. Neurophysiol., vol. 70, no. 6, pp. 510-523, December 1988.
[3]   A. Finke, A. Lenhardt, and H. Ritter, "The MindGame: A P300-based brain-computer interface game," Neural Networks, vol. 22, no. 9, pp. 1329-1333, November 2009.
[4]   L. Citi, R. Poli, C. Cinel, and F. Sepulveda, "P300-Based BCI Mouse With Genetically-Optimized Analogue Control," IEEE Trans. Neural Syst. Rehabil. Eng., vol. 16, no. 1, pp. 51-61, February 2008.
[5]   D. J. Krusienski, E. W. Sellers, D. J. McFarland, T. M. Vaughan, and J. R. Wolpaw, "Toward enhanced P300 speller performance," J. Neurosci. Methods, vol. 167, no. 1, pp. 15-21, January 2008.
[6]   R. Ortner, M. Bruckner, R. Prückl, E. Grünbacher, U. Costa, E. Opisso, J. Medina, and C. Guger, "Accuracy of a P300 Speller for People with Motor Impairments," Proceedings of the IEEE Symposium Series on Computational Intelligence 2011, in press.
[7]   E. Donchin, K. M. Spencer, and R. Wijesinghe, "The mental prosthesis: assessing the speed of a P300-based brain-computer interface," IEEE Trans. Rehabil. Eng., vol. 8, no. 2, pp. 174-179, June 2000.
[8]   E. W. Sellers, D. J. Krusienski, D. J. McFarland, T. M. Vaughan, and J. R. Wolpaw, "A P300 event-related potential brain-computer interface (BCI): The effects of matrix size and inter stimulus interval on performance," Biological Psychology, vol. 73, no. 3, pp. 242-252, October 2006.
[9]   C. Guger, S. Daban, E. W. Sellers, C. Holzner, G. Krausz, R. Carabalona, F. Gramatica, and G. Edlinger, "How many people are able to control a P300-based brain-computer interface (BCI)?," Neuroscience Letters, vol. 462, no. 1, pp. 94-98, September 2009.

[10] G. Edlinger, C. Holzner, G. Groenegress, C. Guger, and M. Slater, "Goal-Oriented Control with Brain-Computer Interface," in Proceedings of the 5th International Conference on Foundations of Augmented Cognition. Neuroergonomics and Operational Neuroscience. Berlin, Heidelberg: Springer, 2009, pp. 732-740.

[11] C. Guger, C. Holzner, C. Groenegress, G. Edlinger, and M. Slater, "Control of a smart home with a brain-computer interface," presented at the 4th International Brain-Computer Interface Workshop and Training Course, University of Technology Graz, Graz, Austria, 2008.

[12] F. Nijboer, E. W. Sellers, J. Mellinger, M. A. Jordan, T. Matuz, A. Furdea, S. Halder, U. Mochty, D. J. Krusienski, T. M. Vaughan, J. R. Wolpaw, N. Birbaumer, and A. Kübler, "A P300-based brain-computer interface for people with amyotrophic lateral sclerosis," Clin. Neurophysiol., vol. 119, no. 8, pp. 1909-1916, August 2008.

[13] B. Allison, T. Luth, D. Valbuena, A. Teymourian, I. Volosyak, and A. Graser, "BCI Demographics: How Many (and What Kinds of) People Can Use an SSVEP BCI?," IEEE Trans. Neural Syst. Rehabil. Eng., vol. 18, no. 2, pp. 107-116, April 2010.

Coping with Blast-Related Traumatic Brain Injury in Returning Troops
B.K. Wiederhold (Ed.)
IOS Press, 2011
© *2011 The authors and IOS Press. All rights reserved.*
doi: 10.3233/978-1-60750-797-0-140

Traumatic Brain Injury Battlefield and Intensive Care Rapid and Selective Cerebral Hypothermia Using an Integrated Head-Neck Stabilization and Cooling Helmet System

Huan WANG[a, 1] and William ELKINS[b]
a Department of Neurological Surgery, College of Medicine at University of Illinois, 506 South Mathews Ave, Urbana, IL 61801
b Welkins, LLC, 1430 Blue Oaks Blvd., Suite 250, Roseville CA 95747

Abstract. Traumatic Brain Injury (TBI) has been called the "signature wound" of the Iraq and Afghanistan wars. Helmets help, but don't completely protect against the pressure shifts caused by explosives. Flying objects from explosives have caused other head injuries. More allied soldiers are battling TBI now than in any other war. Better protective equipment and emergency care has saved more lives. Of those surviving a blast, 59% have suffered TBI. TBI is often followed by Posttraumatic Stress Disorder (PTSD). It is well recognized that the application of cooling directly to the head and neck region can potentially have a profound favorable effect on the recovery of the patient. A successful pilot study by Dr. Huan Wang, Dr. William Olivero, and William Elkins was conducted in 2001. Significant reduction in brain temperature in excess of 2°C (3.9°F) was achieved within 15 minutes of the application of the head cooling device. Core temperature was maintained at ≈+2°C over brain temperature. No device related complications were noted. Hypothermia is by far the most potent therapeutic neuro-protectant in laboratory studies. Although systemic (whole-body) hypothermia has demonstrated to provide significant neurological benefits in patients with pre-hospital cardiac arrests, its application in head trauma and stroke patients remains controversial. Systemic hypothermia has potentially severe complications that include arrhythmia, coagulopathy and infection. To minimize such systemic side effects induced by whole-body hypothermia, we have focused on techniques that could selectively cool the brain while maintaining the core body temperature in a safe range. Using National Aeronautics and Space (NASA) spin-off technology, we have developed a specialized integrated head-neck cooling and restraint system that allows optimal contact with the cranium and neck regions. In our pilot study involving severe head trauma and stroke patients, this device demonstrated both rapid and selective brain cooling. To maximize the therapeutic potential of selective cerebral hypothermia, ultra-early initiation of

---

[1] Corresponding Author: Huan Wang, M.D., Assistant Professor of Neurological Surgery, College of Medicine at University of Illinois, 506 South Mathews Ave, Urbana, IL 61801; E-mail: John.Wang@carle.com.

brain cooling in the field is necessary. This project is a prospective, controlled feasibility and safety study of applying a cooling head-neck liner integrated with head-neck stabilization and initiating selective cerebral hypothermia in brain injury patients in the field. This is an extension of a pilot study that we conducted in a clinical setting. The results we obtained from our clinical study demonstrated that we could rapidly lower the intracranial temperature to a hypothermic state while maintaining the body core temperature within a safe range. Our pilot study demonstrated that the cooling head cover was effective in rapidly achieving brain cooling and establishing a favorable brain-to-body temperature gradient. Our overall goal is to significantly improve the outcome of brain injured military personnel by rapidly inducing moderate cerebral (28-32°C) hypothermia but mild systemic (32-35°C) hypothermia to maximize the neuro-protective potentials yet minimize the systemic hypothermia induced complications.

Keywords. hypothermia, cooling helmet, head trauma, military

Introduction

Brain injury is one of the foremost causes of morbidity and mortality. The relative lack of effective treatments greatly compromises the well being of patients inflicted with brain injuries each year. To date, hypothermia is by far the most potent neuro-protectant in animal studies [1-8]. Hypothermic full circulatory arrest continues as standard practice during surgeries for complex brain aneurysms, aortic aneurysms, and in correction of congenital heart disease in infants [9, 10]. However, although the neuro-protective effects of hypothermia instituted in both the pre-injury and peri-injury periods are well established, most potential clinical applications of hypothermia would limit its use in the post-injury (resuscitative) period.

Numerous animal studies have demonstrated that a 1-2°C temperature change in the brain can result in significantly different neurological and histological outcomes [1-8, 11, 12]. From these data, it is now established that hyperthermia intensifies the brain injury while hypothermia protects the brain. It has been shown that hyperthermia is an independent predictor of adverse neurologic sequelae and increased resource utilization after brain injury [13]. Hypothermia therapy may therefore accomplish its clinical efficacy via two routes: 1) prophylaxis against hyperthermia; 2) therapeutic hypothermia.

The head and neck cools rapidly when exposed to cold water and has little vasoconstriction as a response to cold (14-17). Standard mathematical and engineering analysis of heat exchange suggests that cooling the neck alone with ice can accomplish a 2°C temperature reduction of the carotid blood prior to its entry into the brain and surface cooling of head and neck could lead to an average brain tissue temperature at least several degrees lower than the body core temperature [18]. In animal models of cardiac arrest, packing the head with ice obtained 2°C reductions in cerebral temperature and produced significant improvement in neurologic recovery from global ischemia [19]. During full circulatory arrest, brain temperature continues to rise slowly from residual metabolic heat generation. The simple and widely used adjunct of packing the head in ice during this arrest period has been clinically proven to decrease post-operative neurological impairment [10, 20].

Resuscitative (post-injury) hypothermia as a potential treatment in brain injury patients remains controversial [21, 22]. However, most clinical studies have examined only whole body hypothermia which has numerous methodological drawbacks. Whole body hypothermia has pronounced physiological side effects such as decreased cardiac output, increased vascular resistance, ventricular fibrillation, increase of myocardial ischemia, impaired coagulation, and impaired immune function [21, 23-27]. The increased risk of systemic complications when using whole body hypothermia may outweigh the neuroprotective benefits of such therapy [21)]. Whole body hypothermia may easily miss the treatment window because it requires ICU monitoring and is not practical in the prehospital settings, where hypothermic protection of the brain can be maximized [28-30]. Therefore, ultra-early delivery of selective cooling of the brain in the field may be a more successful way of treating brain injury patients and needs to be studied.

A new head-and-neck cooling head cover, developed using a NASA spin-off spacesuit technology, may have the potential for use in the pre-hospital setting, and the potential of cooling the brain more than the rest of the body (Figure 1). This technology originated in a NASA program that produced a channeled cooling suit for astronauts. While now used mainly in industrial and military settings that require heavy protective clothing, such as nuclear power plants and steel mills, this technology has started to find numerous applications in sports injuries and in patients with diseases such as hypohydrotic ectodermal dysplasia (HED; born without sweat glands), multiple sclerosis, cystic fibrosis, and severe burns. The same technology was also used in the Desert Storm. An antifreeze solution, cooled by a portable, battery-powered unit with an insertable ice cartridge, is pumped and circulates through tubes to the garments that are snugly fitted against the skin surface using air counter-pressure. We have recently completed an IRB-approved randomized study of using this cooling head cover in brain injury patients and demonstrated significant preferential lowering of the brain temperature over the body temperature. In 2003, the study results were presented in the 53rd Annual Meeting of the Congress of Neurological Surgeons and the 28th International Stroke Conference. In 2004, the study results were published in the Journal of Neurosurgery (J Neurosurg 100:272-277, 2004). No device-related complications were noted.

The proposed pilot study is a prospective, non-randomized study involving 80 brain injury patients. The newly designed head-and-neck cooling head cover has a built-in ASPEN Collar for cervical spine protection. The EMS personnel or the life-flight crew will initiate selective cerebral hypothermia in the field by placing the cooling head cover on the study patients. The cooling will continue in the intensive care unit in severe brain injury patients with intracranial temperature and pressure monitoring. Although the primary end point is feasibility and safety of initial selective brain cooling in the field using this cooling head cover, outcome data will also be collected and analyzed in preparation for multi-center outcome studies.

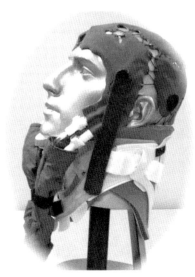

Figure 1. Photograph of the Head-Neck Stabilization and Cooling Assembly. The cooling helmet has an outer pneumatic liner pressurized to allow close contact with the cranium and neck. The device also is adjustable to fit a significant range of head sizes.

Illustrative Case

A 17-year-old female was presented with severe head injury (GCS= 7). Head CT demonstrated traumatic subarachnoid hemorrhage, a small subdural hematoma, and diffuse petechial intraparenchymal hemorrhages consistent with shear injury. Initial ICP was in the mid 30's. The cooling helmet was applied after admission to the hospital. The patient was also intubated, paralyzed and sedated. Neurotrend (Codman & Shurtleff, Inc., Raynham, MA), intra-cranial pressure MicroSensor (Codman & Shurtleff, Inc., Raynham, MA), and pulmonary artery catheter (Abbott Laboratories, North Chicago, IL) were placed to monitor brain intraparenchymal temperature, ICP, cardiac output, and core temperature in addition to bladder temperature and other routine continuous ICU vital sign monitoring.

Brain temperature was slightly higher than core temperature at baseline. Within 15 minutes after the application of the cooling helmet, brain temperature dropped by approximately 20°C while core temperature did not drop below 37°C until 4-5 hours later (Figure 2). The cooling helmet maintained brain temperature about 1.5-2.5°C below core temperature throughout the 48-hour cooling period. When core temperature dropped to 32°C and brain temperature dropped to 29.4°C, active body warming was initiated to minimize the risk of cardiac arrhythmia. Core temperature, as illustrated by the graph (Figure 2), was thereafter maintained at 33-35°C with external warming blankets. After the cooling helmet was removed at hour 48, brain temperature approached core temperature within 1-2 hours and then together both rose gradually to 37°C over a 30-hour period. No deleterious effects, such as arrhythmia, infection, or clinically significant coagulopathy, etc., were observed. At 6-month follow-up visit, patient had gone back to school and resumed cheerleading activities with minor right-sided tremors.

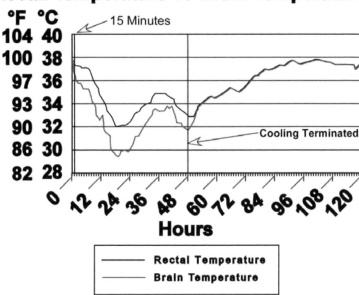

Figure 2. Graph showing that, within 15 minutes after application of the cooling helmet, the brain temperature dropped by approximately 2°C, whereas the core temperature did not drop below 37°C until four to five hours later.

References

[1.]   Barone F, Feuerstein GZ, White RF: Brain cooling during transient focal ischemia provides complete neuroprotection. Neurosci Biobehav Rev 21:31-44, 1996

[2.]   Busto R, Ginsberg MD: The influence of altered brain temperature in cerebral ischemia, in Ginsberg MD, Bogousslavsky J (eds): Cerebrovascular Disease: Pathophysiology, Diagnosis, and management. Malden, MA: Blackwell Science, 1998, pp 287-307

[3.]   Dietrich WD, Busto R, globus MY-T, et al: Brain damage and temperature: cellular and molecular mechanisms. In: Siesjo BK, Wieloch T (eds): Cellular and Molecular Mechanisms of Ischemic Brain Damage. Philadelphia, Pa: Lippincott-Raven, 1996, pp 177-197. Advances in Neurology series.

[4.]   Ginsberg MD, Sternau LL, Blobus MYT, et al: Therapeutic modulation of brain temperature: relevance to ischemic brain injury. Cerebrovasc Brain Metab Rev 4:189-225, 1992

[5.]   Ginsberg MD: The concept of the therapeutic window: a synthesis of critical issues. In: Moskowitz MA, Caplan LR (eds): Cerebrovascular Diseases: Nineteenth Princeton Stroke Conference. Boston, Mass: Butterworth-Heinemann, 1995, pp 331-351

[6.]   Maher J, Hachinski V: Hypothermia as a potential treatment for cerebral ischemia. Cerebrovasc Brain Metab Rev. 5:277-300, 1993

[7.]   Maier C, Sun G, Kunis D: Delayed induction and long-term effects of mild hypothermia in a focal model of transient cerebral ischemia: neurologic outcome and infarct size. Neurosurgery 94: 90-96, 2001

[8.]   Markgraf C, Clifton G, Moody M: Treatment window for hypothermia in brain injury. Neurosurgery 95: 979-983, 2001

[9.]   Spetzler R, Hadley M, Rigamonti D, Carter L, Raudemz P, Shedd S, Wilkinsson E: Aneurysms of the basilar artery treated with circulatory arrest, hypothermia, and barbiturate cerebral protection. J Neurosurg 68:868-879, 1988.

[10.] Randall B, Arisan E, Jock N, Khanh H, Tatu J, Nin C: Use of hypothermic circulatory arrest for cerebral protection during aortic surgery. J Card Surg 1997; 12:312-321.

[11.] Wass CG, Lanier WL, Hofer RE, et al: Temperature changes of ≤ 1 °C alter functional neurologic outcome and histopathology in a canine model of complete cerebral ischemia. Anesthesiology 1995; 83: 325-335.

[12.] Busto R, Dietrich W, Globus M, Valdes I, Scheinberg P, Ginsberg M: Small differences in intraischemic brain temperature critically determine the extent of ischemic neuronal injury. J Cereb Blood Flow Metab 7:729-738, 1987.

[13.] JoAnne E, Jill G, Mark A, Donald H: Early hyperthermia after traumatic brain injury in children: Risk factors, influence on length of stay, and effect on short-term neurologic status. Crit Care Med 2000; 28:2608-2615.

[14.] Kissen AT, Hall JF, Klemm FK: Physiological responses to cooling the head and neck versus the trunk and leg areas in severe hyperthermic exposure. Aerospace Med 42:882-888, 1971

[15.] Nunneley DA, Troutman SJ, Webb P: Head cooling in work and heat stress. Aerospace Med 42:64-68, 1971

[16.] Shvartz E: Effect of a cooling hood on physiological responses to work in a hot environment. J Appl Physiol 29:36-39, 1970

[17.] Williams BA, Shitzer A: Modular liquid cooled head cover liner for thermal comfort. Aerospace Med 45:1030-1036, 1974

[18.] Zhu L, Diao C: Theoretical simulation of temperature distribution in the brain during mild hypothermia treatment for brain injury. Med Biol Engl Comput 39: 681-687, 2001

[19.] Scott T, Clifton W, James M: Noninvasive cerebral cooling in a swine model of cardiac arrest. Acad. Emerg. Med. 1998; 5:25-30.

[20.] Robert B, David Z, Harm V, Richard C: Topical ice slurry prevents brain rewarming during deep hypothermic circulatory arrest in newborn sheep. J Card. Vas. Anes. 1997; 11(5):591-4.

[21.] Clifton GL, Miller ER, Choi SC, et al: Lack of effect of induction of hypothermia after acute brain injury. N Engl J Med 344:556-563, 2001

[22.] Marion DW, Penrod LE, Kelsey, et al: Treatment of traumatic brain injury with moderate hypothermia. N Engl J Med 336:540-546, 1997

[23.] Frank SM, Fleisher LA, Breslow MJ, et al: Perioperative maintenance of normothermia reduces the incidence of morbid cardiac events: A randomized clinical trial. JAMA 277:1127-1134, 1997

[24.] Clifton GL, Allen S, Berry J, et al: Systemic hypothermia in treatment of brain injury. J Neurotrauma 9:S487-495, 1992

[25.] Kruz A, Sessler DI, Lenhardt RA: Study of wound infections and temperature group: perioperative normothermic to reduce the incidence of surgical-wound infection and shorten hospitalization. New Engl J Med 334:1209-1215, 1996

[26.] Kuhnen G, Bauer R, Walter B: Controlled brain hypothermia by extracorporeal carotid blood cooling at normothermic trunk temperatures in pigs. J Neuroscience Methods 89:167-174, 1999

[27.] Schmied H, Kurz A, Sessler DI, et al: Mild intraoperative hypothermia increases blood loss and allogeneic transfusion requirements during total hip arthroplasty. Lancet 347:289-292, 1996

[28.] Kuboyama K, Safar P, Radovsky A, et al: Delay in cooling negates the beneficial effect of mild resuscitative cerebral hypothermia after cardiac arrest in dogs: A prospective, randomized, controlled study. Crit Care Med 1993; 21:1348-1358.

[29.] Maier C, Sun G, Kunis D: Delayed induction and long-term effects of mild hypothermia in a focal model of transient cerebral ischemia: neurologic outcome and infarct size. Neurosurgery 2001; 94: 90-96.

[30.] Markgraf C, Clifton G, Moody M: Treatment window for hypothermia in brain injury. Neurosurgery 2001; 95: 979-983.

Coping with Blast-Related Traumatic Brain Injury in Returning Troops
B.K. Wiederhold (Ed.)
IOS Press, 2011
© 2011 The authors and IOS Press. All rights reserved.
doi: 10.3233/978-1-60750-797-0-146

Biofeedback/Neurofeedback Treatment of Psychiatric Disturbances Following Traumatic Brain Injury: Case Reports

Dragica KOZARIC-KOVACIC[a,1], Andrea JAMBROSIC SAKOMAN[a]
and Igor MARINIC[a]

[a] *University Hospital Dubrava, Department of Psychiatry, Referral Centre for Stress Related Disorders of the Ministry of Health and Social Welfare of the Republic of Croatia, Regional Center for Psychotrauma, Zagreb, Croatia*

Abstract. Traumatic Brain Injury (TBI) is often comorbid with psychiatric disturbances that impede patients' recovery and everyday functioning. We present two case studies of patients who exhibited psychiatric disorders after TBI. Both patients were included in psychiatric treatment for approximately one year without improvement in anxiety, depressive symptoms, and quality of life in everyday functioning, before we decided to apply biofeedback/neurofeedback (BFB/NFB) treatment as add-on therapy. Protocols of BFB/NFB treatment are described in the paper. BFB/NFB treatment showed clinical improvement in anxiety, depressive symptoms, and overall functioning, which was confirmed by psychophysiological measures and clinical scales, as well as by patients' subjective reports.

Keywords. Traumatic Brain Injury, depressive disorder, anxious disorders, biofeedback/neurofeedback treatment, case reports

Introduction

Traumatic Brain Injury (TBI) is an acquired brain injury which occurs when a sudden trauma causes temporary or permanent damage to the brain and can result in mild, moderate or severe symptoms. TBI among the civilian population is most commonly the result of traffic accidents, sport injuries, and falls, while blast trauma is an important issue in war affected areas.

Recent studies showed that several factors could contribute to etiology and symptoms of TBI. These include physical injury, followed by various potentially citotoxic events on a cellular level that could lead to injury or death of neurons, changes in neurotransmitter levels, and intracranial or systemic complications [1-5].

TBI can manifest itself through somatic and neuropsychiatric symptoms, and they may differ regarding the localization and extent of the injury, medical and psychiatric comorbidities that may exist, and psychosocial factors [6].

---

[1] Corresponding Author. Prof. Dragica Kozarić-Kovačić, MD, PhD, University Hospital Dubrava, Department of Psychiatry, Referral Centre for the Stress-related Disorders of the Ministry of Health and Social Welfare, Regional Centre for Psychotrauma, Avenija Gojka Suska 6, 10 000 Zagreb, Croatia, Phone no.: +385-1-290-26-18, Fax.: +385-1-290-3700; E-mail: dkozaric_kovacic@yahoo.com.

Neuropsychiatric disturbances consist of behavioral, emotional, and cognitive symptoms [1, 7, 8].

Behavioral symptoms, such as impulsivity, amotivation, agitation, and aggression can occur after TBI, as well as personality changes [9-12].

The most commonly observed psychiatric illnesses among patients suffering from TBI are mood disorders. Studies show that the prevalence of major depression following moderate to severe TBI varies from 25-40%, as opposed to 17% in the general population [1, 13, 14]. Depression rates one year after TBI are about 14% [15]. It should be taken into account that sometimes it is not clear weather depression is a result of TBI and its effect on the brain, or it is a result of changes in overall functioning, cognitive, social, psychological or economic [6, 16].

Extensive research into depression has pointed to differences in activation between the left and the right prefrontal cortex [17]. Studies also identified frontal asymmetry with more left frontal alpha activity in individuals biologically predisposed to depression [18]. Some authors have expressed the belief that this frontal asymmetry may represent a state marker of depression [19-21], as well as reflecting a biological or trait marker of a vulnerability to depression [22, 23].

Henriques and Davidson showed an association of the left hemisphere with approach behavior and motivation, while the right hemisphere was connected to withdrawal behavior [23]. Studies were conducted with an intent to establish a link between location of the brain area that was injured and psychiatric and cognitive symptoms manifested by the patients, in order to provide more adequate treatment.

Some of the studies that examined electroencephalogram (EEG) in patients after closed head injury showed generalized slowing of the EEG, most predominately at the site of injury. Frequencies in the 4-7 Hz range were often higher at the site of injury [24].

It should also be noted that changes in EEG differ with time after TBI, do not always correspond to clinical findings, and should not be used to objectify brain injury [25].

Anxiety disorders also occur in a significant proportion of patients with TBI and frequently coexist with depressive disorder. Prevalence of anxiety disorders – generalized anxiety disorder, posttraumatic stress disorder (PTSD), and panic disorder – after mild TBI is estimated to be 24%, compared to 7% in the general population [6, 26]. Two or more psychiatric disorders have been reported in 40% of TBI victims [27]. The consequences of high prevalence of psychiatric comorbidity are reduced functioning, as well as a poorer rehabilitation outcome.

Impairments in cognitive functioning, such as difficulties in information processing, problem solving, memory deficits, impairment in attention, and executive functioning can be detected in sufferers of TBI, depending on trauma severity [9]. Some authors are also pointing out the issue of the effect of mood disorders on cognitive functioning in patients with TBI [16]. One of the studies researching that problem showed that depressive patients with TBI were performing poorer in the tasks of working memory, processing speed, verbal memory, and executive functions than non-depressed patients with TBI [28].

With regards to somatic symptoms, headache is one of the most common, with an estimated frequency from 25-90% in patients with TBI [6, 29-31]. Another common somatic complaint in TBI patients is fatigue, which is considered to be linked with depression and anxiety, sleep disorders, and decreased cognitive functioning [6, 32-34].

Frequent somatic symptoms also include dizziness or nausea, sleep disturbances and seizures [6, 35, 36].

Psychophysiological studies of traumatized victims in the acute and chronic phase of trauma have shown changes in psychophysiological parameters [37, 38].

Preliminary research on biofeedback (BFB)/neurofeedback (NFB) is encouraging for treatment of different symptoms stemming from TBI such as anxiety, depression, cognitive difficulties (memory, concentration, attention), impulsiveness, and sleep disorders, but more rigorous research is needed to corroborate such reports [39, 40].

The aim of this paper is to show our experiences with BFB/NFB treatment through case studies of two patients who developed psychiatric disorders and cognitive impairment after TBI.

1. Methods and Participants

1.1. Participants

We present two case studies of individuals who developed psychiatric disorders, as well as cognitive deficits, after TBI. Both patients were treated through inpatient and outpatient treatment programs that included pharmacotherapy, individual and group psychotherapy, anxiety management, and psycho-education. Since their symptoms of anxiety and depression were resistant to treatment approximately one year into treatment, we decided to apply add-on BFB/NFB.

1.2. Pre-treatment Evaluation

Before entering the BFB/NFB program, patients were assessed by the psychiatrist who performed clinical evaluation and applied the Mini International Neuropsychiatric Interview, Croatian version (MINI) [41], Hamilton Depression Scale (HAMD) [42], Hamilton Anxiety Scale (HAMA) [43], and Clinician-Administered PTSD Scale (CAPS) [44]. Neuropsychological assessment was done by the psychologist using a battery of neuropsychological tests. Full cap EEG was conducted using Neurofax, BFB/NFB was done using BioGraph Infinity software, and also basic psychophysiological assessment was done prior to the decision on the BFB treatment.

Basic psychophysiological assessment was performed to gain insight into physiological response to different stressors for each of the participants. Seven steps evaluation protocol was done. Each step lasted two minutes, beginning with baseline recording, color words, mental math test followed, and finally, imagining a stress producing situation. Two minutes of recovery period followed each of the steps. After basic physiological assessment both patients underwent BFB training based upon parameters drawn in the assessment.

1.3. Biofeedback/neurofeedback Settings

Skin conductance (SC) was measured by placing a silver/silver chloride sensor on the palm surface of the distal part of the index and ring finger of the non-dominant hand. Heart rate (HR) and blood volume pulse (BVP) were measured by placing a sensor (plethysmograph) on the thumb of the non-dominant hand. Respiration was measured by placing the band across the abdomen while degree of stretching is monitored [45]. Respiratory sinus arrhythmia (RSA), which pertains to the synchrony between pulse rate and respiration, was also monitored. Electromyography was measured by placing a ground electrode in between two active electrodes on the muscle of choice.

EEG in NFB session was recorded with one scalp electrode placed at the skull at the vertex (Cz) against an electrode clip placed on the right and left ear lobe, one used as the reference and the other as a ground. Each lead was checked separately. Impedance was acceptable when each electrode impedance was below 5 kohms.

After preparation was done, five minutes of baseline EEG was recorded with eyes opened and eyes closed condition. During the baseline EEG assessment, the participant received no auditory stimulation, and in a couple of sessions was taught to recognize EEG patterns for different band widths, as well as to recognize artifacts. An EEG analysis was done after removing the artifacts by the trainer. Frequency analysis was performed using a Fast Fourier Transform (FFT).

The frequency bands used were: theta, 4.0-7.0 Hz; alpha, 8.0-12.0 Hz; sensory-motor rhythm (SMR), 13.0-15.0 Hz, and beta, 15.0-18.0 Hz.

Before treatment both of the patients signed consent for treatment.

2. Case 1

2.1. Medical History

Male patient aged 48 years, without developmental difficulties, tertiary educated, married, father of two children, well adapted and functioning, running family business. His medical history showed no serious physical illnesses or psychiatric disorders.

After a fall from approximately five meters in September 2009, he was hospitalized at the Department of neurosurgery. Multislice computed tomography (MSCT) of the brain was performed which showed lesions in the left temporobasal region and the left mesial hypocampal region corresponding to intracerebral haematoma. He was discharged from the hospital after twelve days with a diagnosis of cerebral contusion of medial frontotemporal region, cerebral concussion, intracerebral haematoma of left temporal region, multi-fragment fracture of sphenoid bone, and posttraumatic ophthalmoplegia of the left eye. He was then referred to a rehabilitation facility.

EEG conducted in November 2009 showed general slowing, predominantly in the left frontotemporal region. Neuropsychological testing conducted in January 2010 showed indicators of organic cerebral dysfunction, reflected in the specific deficits of organization, integration, planning, speed, memory, and new learning, as well as personality changes, emotional lability, and adaptation.

He was referred to a psychiatrist by the neurosurgeon in January 2010. During the first psychiatric examination the patient presented a depressive mood, affective lability, anxiety, memory and concentration difficulties, concern for the future, pessimistic thoughts about his condition and deterioration in professional and family roles, difficulties in adaptation to current condition and reduced abilities. He was diagnosed with an organic mood disorder (International Classification of Diseases 10) and followed as an outpatient. He also complained of severe headaches that followed the TBI.

Since June 2010 he was hospitalized three times because of worsening of his symptoms, and at each hospitalization presented with worsening of anxiety, depressed mood, behavioral changes, memory, and concentration difficulties. He had persisting problems with adaptation to current psychiatric condition, changes in professional and family roles, and reduction in level of functioning. Family was also reluctant to accept his condition.

2.2. Biofeedback/neurofeedback Protocol

After approximately one year of initial treatment, we decided to include BFB/NFB training in order to address anxiety and depressive symptoms which did not improve adequately with prior treatment, as well as memory and concentration difficulties which did not show expected speed of recovery. Prior to entering BFB/NFB program he was receiving pharmacotherapy that consisted of escitalopram 20 mg/day and oxazepam as needed, up to 30 mg/day.

Before entering the program, an assessment was done, as described above. At the time that the patient was included in the BFB/NFB treatment his dominant psychiatric symptoms were anxiety and depression. He achieved 31 points on HAMA scale and 37 points on HAMD scale. Memory impairment was objectified by neuropsychological testing.

Stress evaluation protocol showed that during the stressful event recall his heart rate rose to 106/beats per minute (bpm) from an average of 75/bpm in all other tasks, and respiration became irregular and rapid and rose to 17 breaths per minute as opposed to 11 breaths per minute in the other stress tasks. SC was stable, from 1 to 2 μSiemens, throughout the entire assessment.

Gradually, patient mastered the diaphragmatic breathing of seven breaths per minute and produced good RSA. That was combined with frontalis EMG which he managed to bring down, also using the relaxation techniques that he was acquainted with before starting the training. Patient found audio and visual feedback from the monitor very useful in achieving this goal. He was trained in increasing SC in order to be alert, while relaxed, which was also needed for the NFB that followed.

After that, NFB treatment was planned at left frontal (F3) and right frontal (F4) sites, but as baseline assessment of EEG done at Cz, F3 and F4 exhibited excessive eye blink artifacts, training was started at Cz.

Training protocol was based on work of Tansey and Byers [40, 46-48]. Following preparation, a five-minute baseline EEG was recorded for an eyes opened and eyes closed condition. High theta was shown, as well as a low SMR. First 15 NFB training sessions were aimed at enhancing SMR, and simultaneously suppressing the theta frequency in the eyes opened condition. The mean amplitude of SMR activity (13-15 Hz) and theta activity (4-7 Hz) that was gathered during baseline was used as the threshold during NFB training. Diaphragmatic breathing and relaxation training preceded each NFB session.

In the each of the NFB sessions feedback a tone was given to the patient if SMR amplitude equaled or exceeded the threshold setting, and if theta band was kept below level that was set. Auditory feedback signal was denied if the theta band exceeded pre-set level, even if SMR threshold was exceeded. Both of the bands (SMR and theta) settings were adjusted during the session in order to keep the tone about 70-80% of the time. The first aim was to increase mean amplitude of SMR activity (13-15 Hz), while the second aim was to extend the time that patient could hold the SMR activity above the threshold. The training was conducted with eyes open watching a bar graph on the monitor, and the patient was given the instruction to enhance the SMR frequency and suppress the theta frequency. Each of the sessions lasted for 30 minutes, and was conducted twice a week. Patient was given the instructions to find the mental strategy that would keep SMR frequency above the threshold and theta frequency below. He was also instructed to try to reduce limb movement in order to reduce artifacts.

2.3. Results

After 15 NFB sessions, patient managed to raise the mean amplitude of SMR activity and suppress theta frequency while being relaxed. Patient reported that he learned to empty his mind, yet stay focused. He further reported that he was able to connect better with his family, which helped to somewhat alleviate his depressive symptoms. No improvements were noted regarding his memory deficits.

Future plan is to proceed with NFB training at the F3 for the next 20 sessions.

HAMD and HAMA scores after 15 NFB sessions were lower than at the beginning of the training, 20 and 16 points, respectively.

3. Case 2

3.1. Medical History

Female patient aged 50, without developmental difficulties, grew up in a dysfunctional family with a physically and verbally aggressive father. Parents divorced when she was 14, she remained living with her mother, until mother's death 11 years ago, and currently is living with her brother. She had completed elementary and high school. She has worked as a shop assistant since 1980, and she was well functioning at her workplace. Since 2007 she was treated for hypertension and heart problems.

Patient was a victim of armed robbery at the workplace three times. First time, in 2000, she did not seek psychiatric help. Second time, in 2006, she was hit in the head with a blunt object during the robbery, was evaluated in the emergency room, and diagnosed with a concussion. After the incident she began having memory and concentration difficulties, and sought psychiatric help for the first time.

She was treated through an outpatient clinic and daily hospital program from 2006, with the diagnosis of adjustment disorder followed by mixed anxiety and depression. During the treatment, the patient achieved a prolonged stable condition and was functioning adequately, both in the family role and the workplace. Due to the improvement of her condition, in May 2009, she stopped taking antidepressant treatment that she had been on for two years. Some minor memory and concentration difficulties persisted.

Patient returned for a psychiatric evaluation during December 2009 after she was again exposed to armed robbery at the workplace. She was displaying symptoms of acute stress reaction with dominant symptoms of fear, anxiety, sleep disturbances, intrusive thoughts concerning the traumatic event, and loss of appetite. Memory and concentration difficulties had intensified, and she was having symptoms of increased vegetative activity such as tremor of the hands, sleep reduction, concentration difficulties, sweating, and palpitations. During the outpatient treatment there was no reduction in the intensity of the symptoms, and she was reporting significantly compromised functioning, with no reduction in the intensity of vegetative symptoms. Memory and concentration difficulties were accentuated due to worsening of the psychiatric condition. She presented herself with symptoms of mixed anxiety and depression and PTSD with mild TBI symptoms. Because of her condition the patient was hospitalized twice.

3.2. Biofeedback Protocol

Due to treatment resistance we decided to include NFB training as add-on therapy. Symptoms of anxiety were not subsiding. Prior to starting BFB/NFB treatment the patient was receiving psychopharmacotherapy in the form of duloxetine 60 mg/d, mirtazapine 15 mg/d, and alprazolam 1 mg/d.

As described above, psychiatric assessment, psychiatric scales, neurophysiological assessment, and basic psychophysiological assessment were performed. Activation of autonomic nerve system was registered clinically, objectified by psychophysiological assessment, HAMD (score: 29), and HAMA (score: 37).

Stress assessment showed that during the math task HR rate rose to 188/bpm, averaging about 102/bpm, and skin conductance averaged at 5 µSiemens, while baseline recordings showed that average HR was 81/bpm, and SC was 3 µSiemens. She refused to recall any stressful event, because she was overwhelmed with extreme increased arousal during remembering, as she had later explained. BFB treatment was aimed at teaching her diaphragmatic and regular breathing at about eight breaths per minute, while monitoring for RSA and blood volume pulse, and maintaining SC in a middle range. She was also taught to drop her trapezius EMG. At the beginning of the training she felt that she could partially influence only her breathing in order to calm herself, but with no lasting success.

3.3. Results

After 16 training sessions that were done once a week and lasted 40 minutes, she managed to breathe regularly at eight breaths per minute. She could think of a stressful event, as well as complete a math task and remain calm, which could also be observed in measured variables as well as by her subjective report. The prescribed dose of benzodiazepines was reduced as a result of such progress.

Patient said that being able to gain some mastery of her anxiety symptoms, which she found paralyzing before, was the most important achievement of this training. That was objectified by lowering HAMD score to 19, and HAMA score to 23.

Future plan for the patient is to proceed to NFB training.

4. Conclusions

Patients showed clinical improvement of targeted symptoms (anxiety and depression), improvement in HAMA, and HAMD scores. Both patients have learned to better control their autonomic system response, which resulted in better coping with anxiety producing stressors. This improved their quality of life and overall functioning. They found the ability to have better control of their symptoms, which impeded their functioning, to be very important.

BFB and NFB treatment for psychiatric disorders following TBI in persons resistant to the standard treatment is promising.

References

[1]   J.M. Silver, T.W. McAllister and D.B. Arciniegas, Depression and cognitive complaints following mild traumatic brain injury, *Am J Psychiatry*, **166** (2009), 653-661.
[2]   J.T. Povlishock and D.I. Katz, Update of neuropathology and neurological recovery after traumatic brain injury, *J Head Trauma Rehabil*, **20** (2005), 76-94.
[3]   J.M. Meythaler, J.D. Peduzzi, E. Eleftheriou and T.A. Novack, Current concepts: diffuse axonal injury-associated traumatic brain injury, *Arch Phys Med Rehabil*, **82** (2001), 1461-1471.
[4]   D.B. Arciniegas and J.M. Silver, Pharmacotherapy of posttraumatic cognitive impairments, *Behav Neurol*, **17** (2006), 25-42.
[5]   T.W. McAllister, L.A. Flashman, B.C. McDonald and A.J. Saykin, Mechanisms of working memory dysfunction after mild and moderate TBI: evidence from functional MRI and neurogenetics, *J Neurotrauma*, **23** (2006), 1450-1467.
[6]   S. Riggio and M. Wong, Neurobehavioral sequelae of traumatic brain injury, *Mt Sinai J Med*, **76** (2009), 163-172.
[7]   W.A. Gordon, M. Brown, M. Sliwinski, M.R. Hibbard, N. Patti, M.J. Weiss, R. Kalinsky and M. Sheerer, The enigma of "hidden" traumatic brain injury, *J Head Trauma Rehabil*, **13** (1998), 39-56.
[8]   M.R. Hibbard, S. Uysal, M. Sliwinski and W.A. Gordon, Undiagnosed health issues in individuals with traumatic brain injury living in the community, *J Head Trauma Rehabil*, **13** (1998), 47-57.
[9]   S. Vaishnavi, V. Rao and J.R. Fann, Neuropsychiatric problems after traumatic brain injury: unraveling the silent epidemic, *Psychosomatics*, **50** (2009), 198-205.
[10] E. Kim, E.C. Lauterbach, A. Reeve, D.B. Arciniegas, K.L. Coburn, M.F. Mendez, T.A. Rummans and E.C. Coffey, Neuropsychiatric complications of traumatic brain injury: a critical review of the literature (a report by the ANPA Committee on Research), *J Neuropsychiatry Clin Neurosci*, **19** (2007), 106-127.
[11] E. Kim, Agitation, aggression, and disinhibition syndromes after traumatic brain injury, *NeuroRehabilitation*, **17** (2002), 297-310.
[12] M.R. Hibbard, J. Bogdany, S. Uysal, K. Kepler, J.M. Silver, W.A. Gordon and L. Haddad, Axis II psychopathology in individuals with traumatic brain injury, *Brain Inj*, **14** (2000), 45-61.
[13] J.M. Rogers and C.A. Read, Psychiatric comorbidity following traumatic brain injury, *Brain Inj*, **21** (2007), 1321-1333.
[14] R. van Reekum, T. Cohen and J. Wong, Can traumatic brain injury cause psychiatric disorders?, *J Neuropsychiatry Clin Neurosci*, **12** (2000), 316-327.
[15] S. Deb, I. Lyons, C. Koutzoukis, I. Ali and G. McCarthy, Rate of psychiatric illness 1 year after traumatic brain injury, *Am J Psychiatry*, **156** (1999), 374-378.
[16] K.E. Thornton and D.P. Carmody, Quantitative Electroencephalography in the Assessment and Rehabilitation of Traumatic Brain Injury, in: *Handbook of Integrative Clinical Psychology, Psychiatry and Behavioral Medicine*, R.A. Carlstedt, ed, Springer Pub., New York, 2009, pp. 463-508.
[17] R.J. Davidson, Anterior electrophysiological asymmetries, emotion, and depression: conceptual and methodological conundrums, *Psychophysiology*, **35** (1998), 607-614.
[18] D.C. Hammond and E. Baehr, Neurofeedback for the treatment of depression: current status of theoretical issues and clinical research, in: *Introduction to quantitative EEG and neurofeedback: advanced theory and applications*, T. Budzynski, ed, Elsevier, Amsterdam; Boston, 2009.
[19] E. Baehr, J.P. Rosenfeld and R. Baehr, The clinical use of an alpha asymmetry neurofeedback protocol in the treatment of depression: Two case studies, *J Neurother*, **2** (1997), 10-23.
[20] J.P. Rosenfeld, E. Baehr, R. Baehr, I.H. Gotlib and C. Ranganath, Preliminary evidence that daily changes in frontal alpha asymmetry correlate with changes in affect in therapy sessions, *Int J Psychophysiol*, **23** (1996), 137-141.
[21] J.H. Askew, The diagnosis of depression using psychometric instruments and quantitative measures of electroencephalographic arousal. Unpublished doctoral dissertation, University of Tennessee, 2001.
[22] J.B. Henriques and R.J. Davidson, Regional brain electrical asymmetries discriminate between previously depressed and healthy control subjects, *J Abnorm Psychol*, **99** (1990), 22-31.
[23] J.B. Henriques and R.J. Davidson, Left frontal hypoactivation in depression, *J Abnorm Psychol*, **100** (1991), 535-545.
[24] M.E. Ayers, Electro-encephalic neurofeedback and closed head injury of 250 individuals, in: *National Head Injury Foundation Annual Conference*, 1987.

[25] M.R. Nuwer, D.A. Hovda, L.M. Schrader and P.M. Vespa, Routine and quantitative EEG in mild traumatic brain injury, *Clin Neurophysiol*, **116** (2005), 2001-2025.

[26] G. Mooney and J. Speed, The association between mild traumatic brain injury and psychiatric conditions, *Brain Inj*, **15** (2001), 865-877.

[27] M.R. Hibbard, S. Uysal, K. Kepler, J. Bogdany and J. Silver, Axis I psychopathology in individuals with traumatic brain injury, *J Head Trauma Rehabil*, **13** (1998), 24-39.

[28] M.J. Rapoport, S. McCullagh, P. Shammi and A. Feinstein, Cognitive impairment associated with major depression following mild and moderate traumatic brain injury, *J Neuropsychiatry Clin Neurosci*, **17** (2005), 61-65.

[29] J.M. Uomoto and P.C. Esselman, Traumatic brain injury and chronic pain: differential types and rates by head injury severity, *Arch Phys Med Rehabil*, **74** (1993), 61-64.

[30] L. Baandrup and R. Jensen, Chronic post-traumatic headache-a clinical analysis in relation to the International Headache Classification 2nd Edition, *Cephalalgia*, **25** (2005), 132-138.

[31] C. Paniak, S. Reynolds, K. Phillips, G. Toller-Lobe, A. Melnyk and J. Nagy, Patient complaints within 1 month of mild traumatic brain injury: a controlled study, *Arch Clin Neuropsychol*, **17** (2002), 319-334.

[32] J.B. Cantor, T. Ashman, W. Gordon, A. Ginsberg, C. Engmann, M. Egan, L. Spielman, M. Dijkers and S. Flanagan, Fatigue after traumatic brain injury and its impact on participation and quality of life, *J Head Trauma Rehabil*, **23** (2008), 41-51.

[33] M.C. Ouellet, S. Beaulieu-Bonneau and C.M. Morin, Insomnia in patients with traumatic brain injury: frequency, characteristics, and risk factors, *J Head Trauma Rehabil*, **21** (2006), 199-212.

[34] T.A. Ashman, J.B. Cantor, W.A. Gordon, L. Spielman, M. Egan, A. Ginsberg, C. Engmann, M. Dijkers and S. Flanagan, Objective measurement of fatigue following traumatic brain injury, *J Head Trauma Rehabil*, **23** (2008), 33-40.

[35] L. Chamelian and A. Feinstein, Outcome after mild to moderate traumatic brain injury: the role of dizziness, *Arch Phys Med Rehabil*, **85** (2004), 1662-1666.

[36] V. Rao and P. Rollings, Sleep Disturbances Following Traumatic Brain Injury, *Curr Treat Options Neurol*, **4** (2002), 77-87.

[37] D. Kozarić-Kovačić, A. Jambrošić-Sakoman and T. Jovanovic, Psychophysiological indicators of acute stress disorder and posttraumatic stress disorder: Predictive value of peritraumatic dissociation, *JCR*, **3** (2010), 154-156.

[38] D. Kozaric-Kovacic, A. Jambrosic Sakoman, T. Jovanovic and G. Milas, Psychophysiological indicators of acute stress disorder, *Stud Health Technol Inform*, **154** (2010), 185-189.

[39] M. Ayers, A controlled study of EEG neurofeedback training and clinical psychotherapy for right hemispheric closed head injury, *Biofeedback Self Regul*, **18** (1993), 3.

[40] A.P. Byers, Neurofeedback Therapy for a Mild Head Injury, *J Neurother*, **1** (1995), 22-37.

[41] Y. Lecrubier, E. Weiller, T. Hergueta, P. Amorim, L.I. Bonora, J.P. Lépine, D. Sheehan, J. Janavs, R. Baker, K.H. Sheehan, E. Knapp and M. Sheehan, *Mini international neuropsychiatric Interview (MINI). Croatian version 5.0.0 /DSM-IV/ current.*, August 1998.

[42] M. Hamilton, A rating scale for depression, *J Neurol Neurosurg Psychiatry*, **23** (1960), 56-62.

[43] M. Hamilton, The assessment of anxiety states by rating, *Br J Med Psychol*, **32** (1959), 50-55.

[44] D.D. Blake, F.W. Weathers, L.M. Nagy, D. Kaloupek, G. Klauminzer, D.S. Charney, T.M. Keane and T.C. Buckley, *Clinician-Administered PTSD Scale (CAPS) Instruction Manual.*, Boston, MA: National Center for PTSD., 2000.

[45] M. Thompson and L. Thompson, *The neurofeedback book: an introduction to basic concepts in applied psychophysiology*, Association for Applied Psychophysiology and Biofeedback, Wheat Ridge, CO, 2003.

[46] M.A. Tansey, EEG sensorimotor rhythm biofeedback training: some effects on the neurologic precursors of learning disabilities, *Int J Psychophysiol*, **1** (1984), 163-177.

[47] M.A. Tansey, The response of a case of petit mal epilepsy to EEG sensorimotor rhythm biofeedback training, *Int J Psychophysiol*, **3** (1985), 81-84.

[48] M.A. Tansey, Brainwave signatures-an index reflective of the brain's functional neuroanatomy: further findings on the effect of EEG sensorimotor rhythm biofeedback training on the neurologic precursors of learning disabilities, *Int J Psychophysiol*, **3** (1985), 85-99.

© 2011 The authors and IOS Press. All rights reserved.
doi: 10.3233/978-1-60750-797-0-155

Acute and Long-term Sequelae of Blast Exposure in Dutch Soldiers Deployed in Afghanistan; Preliminary Results

Eric VERMETTEN [a,b,c,1], Pieter F. ELAND [a,d], Wim WERTHEIM [e], Yolande SMITH[e] and Cisca F.H.H. LINN [b,c,f]

[a] Military Mental Health Research, Utrecht, The Netherlands
[b] Rudolf Magnus Institute of Neurosciences, Utrecht, The Netherlands
[c] University Medical Center Utrecht, The Netherlands
[d] Vincent van Gogh Institute for Psychiatry, Venray, The Netherlands
[e] Military Rehabilitation Center Doorn, The Netherlands
[f] Central Military Hospital, Utrecht, The Netherlands

Abstract. Introduction: Troops deployed to Iraq and Afghanistan are at high risk for exposure to combat events. The occurrence of Posttraumatic Stress Disorder (PTSD) and Traumatic Brain Injuries (TBI) or concussion related to these events is of interest. In the last two decades much interest has been given to the prevalence of PTSD in returning soldiers. The Dutch deployment in Uruzgan was also characterized by the frequent occurrence of blasts caused by improvised explosive devices (IEDs). A timely and proper assessment of the impact of an IED blast is necessary for the health and sustainability of military personnel during missions. OBJECTIVE: We designed and implemented a protocol for the assessment of comorbid PTSD or depression and long term follow-up of soldiers who were exposed to blast of IED. **Method:** From November 2009 to August 2010 all Dutch soldiers who were exposed (during deployment in Afghanistan) to a blast from IED or grenades within 25 meters were assessed with the Military Acute Concussion Evaluation (MACE, McCrea, 2001)). This was performed within 24 hours (T1) in theatre, by a specially trained nurse or doctor. Three to six months after their return (T2) home this group of non-injured soldiers (n=106) was invited to be reassessed by a series of self-report and clinical instruments. After the test a clinical interview was performed with a clinical neuropsychologist to assess PTSD or depression. Concurrent treatment in hospital or in the outpatient department was not influenced and if necessary, the patient was referred to the psychiatrist for PTSD, rehabilitation center or other specialist for medical problems. RESULTS: In the acute phase, MACE was helpful to structure the assessment. Immediate in-theatre assessment will prevent retrospective bias when asked about event-related aspects later. Preliminary results of all MACE assessment on T1 (n=98), as well as the detailed follow-up assessment (T2) in the first cohort of 56 Dutch soldiers show few cases of PTSD (n=2), and no cases of mTBI on clinical assessment. Fatigue and subjective concentration problems were found in respectively, 12 and 21%. Impact of the event was reported as mild in most cases. **Conclusions:** These first results show mild effects on subjective symptom reporting after blast exposure, except for fatigue and subjective concentration. Extensive neuropsychological assessment indicated a reduced ability to store new information and an impairment of the long-term memory in a significant group. A

---

[1] Corresponding Author: Eric Vermetten, Military Mental Health Research, Utrecht, The Netherlands; E-mail: hgjm.vermetten@mindef.nl.

limitation for the interpretation of these data is the absence of a control group, yet, the performance is remarkable and will need to be followed up. Careful recording of effects of blast exposure through targeted screening and structured assessment is essential to evaluate symptom onset, and long-term effects.

Keywords: mild Traumatic Brain Injury, blast, Posttraumatic Stress Disorder, neuropsychology, combat, military, Military Acute Concussion Evaluation

Disclaimer: The views expressed in this document are those of the authors and do not necessarily reflect views of the agencies or institutions with which the authors are affiliated, including the Dutch Department of Defense. This work is not an official document, guidance, or policy of the Dutch government, and no official endorsement should be inferred.

1. Introduction

Troops deployed to Iraq and Afghanistan are at high risk for exposure to combat events. Dutch participation in NATO Operation Enduring Freedom Deployment in Afghanistan was marked by frequent blasts caused by Improvised Explosive Devices (IEDs). The occurrence of mild Traumatic Brain Injury (mTBI) or concussion and Posttraumatic Stress Disorder (PTSD) related to these events is of interest. The last two decades the prevalence of PTSD is investigated in returning soldiers. In addition, there is also increasing awareness of the pathogenesis, neurobiology and treatment of this disorder [1]. Recently, in particular since the "Global War on Terror," "Operation Iraqi Freedom" and "Operation Enduring Freedom," the focus is on the prevalence of traumatic brain injuries (TBIs), due to exposure to blasts e.g. by IEDs. The reported incidence rates of TBI vary greatly among NATO countries, ranging from 3.7-59%, so that TBI is called the "signature" injury of conflicts, next to PTSD, amputations and burns [2, 3]. Reviewing the current data shows that the widely divergent incidence figures are based on differences in definitions screening and reporting methods. Yet, the longer-term impact of combat-related concussion/mTBI and comorbid PTSD on troops' health and well being, as well as operational fitness, is largely unknown.

In the last decade many armed forces have invested in research studies in the area of PTSD, which are contributing to knowledge about pathogenesis, neurobiology and treatment of this disorder, in particular, in a military setting. The symptoms of this disorder such as intrusions, avoidance and hypervigilance, are well characterized and fit in a biological framework. For the Dutch population prevalence data on PTSD are well known, while data are not known for concussion or mTBI. The prevalence of both PTSD and mTBI for some other international partners is known [4, 5]. Yet, prevalence figures vary in cohorts of wounded soldiers from Iraq between 2004-2005 to 15.8% meeting criteria for TBI (13.4% mild, 2.4% moderate-severe TBI), and other head injury 35.0%, while 49.2% had no head/brain injury. In this literature, the importance of good differential diagnosis between PTSD and mTBI is described through focusing on the use of validated instruments. One in three patients with mTBI could also possibly have comorbid PTSD symptoms.

Despite increased academic interest there are still important gaps in knowledge about the epidemiology, diagnosis, pathogenesis, and the relationship of mTBI with comorbid PTSD and depression. Furthermore, knowledge is still lacking concerning optimal treatment. The Dutch deployment in Uruzgan was also characterized by the frequent occurrence of blasts caused by IEDs. A timely and proper assessment of the impact of an IED blast is necessary for the health and sustainability of military personnel during missions.

IED explosions are characterized by a physical component (pressure wave) and psychological component ("appraisal" of vital threat involving a stress response: derealization, dissociation, tremor, anxiety, panic). The physical component is predictable and calculable in a sense; the psychological component is not predictable, highly variable and differs from person to person. The physical effects may be expressed in brain trauma, the psychological effects in acute stress symptoms, and these may contribute to posttraumatic stress symptoms, fatigue or depression.

TBI after blast exposure is a complex clinical syndrome, and is caused by the combination of all blast effects, that is, from primary to quaternary blast mechanisms. It is called a "Grand Challenge" in TBI research [6]. The blast effects may lead to a scale from pathophysiologic changes: hemorrhages (subarachnoid, intraparenchymal, microbleeds), vasospasm, and increased intracranial pressure from edema (vasogenic and cytotoxic) inflammation, metabolic phenomena, such as excitotoxicity and abnormalities in cellular and membrane abnormalities [7, 8]. Remarkably, blast injury is usually manifested in the form of poly-trauma, meaning injury involving multiple organs or organ systems involved. In addition, pulmonary, gastrointestinal and cerebral haemorraghies are described. There is a large variance in the injuries sustained due to such exposures, classified in severity and staging in primary, secondary, tertiary and quaternary (requires some explanation, related to exposures), and guided by the Glasgow Coma Scale; duration of unconsciousness and posttraumatic amnesia in mild, moderate and severe, TBI is about breakdown phenomena [9]. Thus, blast injuries may – as blows to the head – cause damage with potential severe neurological effects.

Definition blast injury: injury that occurs due to the detonation of explosives, including vehicle-borne and person-borne explosives, rocket-propelled grenades and improvised explosives

Primary (overpressure)   blast: lung; eardrum rupture, middle ear damage and injury, abdominal bleeding and perforation; eye tear, non-impact, blast-induced mTBI

Secondary (projectiles): Ballistic penetration (fragmentation) or blunt trauma; eye penetration

Tertiary (relocation of victims, blast wind): Fractures and traumatic amputations, closed and open brain injury, blunt injuries, crush

Quaternary (all other injuries): Burns, damage or effect of inhaled toxic gases, and disease or injury caused by chemical, biological, radiological contaminants (e.g. "dirty bombs")

Figure 1. Definition and classification of blast reactions [10].

Criteria	mild	moderate	severe
CGS	13-15	9-12	3-8
LOC	0-30 min	> 30 min – 24 hours	> 24 hours
PTA	0-24 hours	> 24 hours – 7 days	> 7 days

Figure 2. Classification of brain injury on basis of severity (McCrea et al., 2008). GCS – Glasgow Coma Scale; LOC – loss of consciousness; PTA – posttraumatic amnesia.

Exposed individuals often show loss of memory for events before and after the explosion, confusion, headache, but more importantly for military personnel: reduced sense of reality, and impaired executive functions. There is a risk for sudden unexpected cerebral edema or persistent traumatic focal cerebral vasospasm despite careful monitoring. The degree of loss of consciousness immediately after exposure to a blast is an indicator of the severity of the TBE. In cases where this loss of consciousness occurs for less than 15 minutes without focal neurological injury, this constitutes a mild traumatic brain injury (mTBI).

Although the first signs of blast-induced neurotrauma usually appear immediately, it can sometimes take months or years after the initial trauma before the symptoms are manifested. These are vague symptoms like extreme fatigue, attention and concentration problems, memory problems, irritability, insomnia, tinnitus, and mood swings. The wide variety of symptoms includes weight loss, hormonal problems, chronic fatigue, headaches and memory problems, speech and balance problems. These changes are often debilitating and slowly but surely start to interfere with daily activities. Because these complaints by victims are underestimated, time is lost for secondary prevention and/or timely rehabilitation. However, it is unclear what component of the blast carries more of an impact on health and operational fitness in the long term: physical, emotional or neuropsychological aspects [11]. Our objective was to design and implement a protocol for the assessment of mTBI, comorbid PTSD or depression, and long term follow-up of soldiers that were exposed to an IED blast.

2. Method

From November 2009 to August 2010 all Dutch soldiers deployed in Afghanistan that were exposed to a blast from an IED or grenades (within 25 meters) were assessed with the Military Acute Concussion Evaluation (MACE, [12]). This was intended as a tool for identifying TBI (in this article we have used this term as a synonym for concussion) and post-traumatic cognitive impairment, and was performed within 24 hours (T1) in theatre by a specially trained nurse or doctor. This resulted in a group of seriously injured and immediately repatriated soldiers and a group of non-to mild injured soldiers.

Three to six months after their return (T2) home this group of non-to mild injured soldiers (n=106) was invited to be reassessed by a series of self-report and clinical instruments: the four dimensional symptom questionnaire (4DSQ, [13], the Chalder fatigue scale [14] and the impact of events scale (IES, [15]. In addition, the following neuropsychological assessments were performed: 15 Word Test (immediate recall), Stroop Color Word Test I, II and III [16, 17], 15 Word Test (with delayed recall and recognition) [18], Symbol Substitution (WAIS III) and Digit Span (WAIS III) [19, 20]. After the test a clinical interview was performed with a clinical neuropsychologist to assess for PTSD or depression.

For the above research objective, we implemented TBI assessment in two phases:
1. *Phase one: during deployment*: Assessment at the Role 1/2. This was performed during deployment: all soldiers who were exposed to a blast within 25 meters were assessed with the MACE by the local military doctor or nurse within 24-48 hours post

blast, and data were entered into the Defense Medical Information System. Clinical care was performed as usual.

2. *Phase two: 3-6 months after return from deployment*: This assessment was made at the Military Rehabilitation Center in Doorn. A return screening protocol was prepared in cooperation with the disciplines of neurology, psychiatry, and rehabilitation medicine. If symptoms were reported the participant was referred to the specific discipline or medical specialty.

3. *Phase three: 12 months after return from deployment*: Assessment will be performed at the same location as assessment two. A similar assessment package will be used to assess the individual soldier.

3. Instruments

The following instruments were used in a standard manner according to the instructions of the various manuals:

• *Military Acute Concussion Evaluation (MACE, [12].* This instrument consists of two parts. The first part consists of medical history questions concerning the description of the incident causing the injury, whether or not the individual was wearing a helmet and/or belt, the existence of retrograde and posttraumatic amnesia and loss of consciousness. This also includes questions about the presence of possible early symptoms of concussion or TBI, such as drowsiness/confusion, headache, dizziness, balance disturbances, nausea/vomiting, difficulty concentrating, irritability, visual difficulties, tinnitus, hearing loss and anxiety/fear. The second part of the MACE tool consists of neuropsychological test questions and a brief examination of some neurological functions. The test site is based on the SAC (Standardized Assessment of Concussion) (McCrea, 2001) that has been validated on concussions resulting from sports injuries.

• *Four Dimensional Symptom Questionnaire (4DSQ, [13].* The primary goal of this questionnaire is for general practitioners to differentiate between stress-related syndromes (such as stress, burnout) and psychiatric disorders (such as depression and anxiety disorders). The measurement scores four dimensions of psychopathology: distress, depression, anxiety and somatization. The depression scale and the anxiety scale consist of 12 and six items, respectively. The distress and anxiety scale items, both 16. The items are rated on a five-point scale.

• *Chalder Fatigue Scale (CFS, [14].* The CFS is a validated questionnaire that measures both mental and physical fatigue, using six and eight items, respectively. The items are scored on a two-point scale. Fatigue is defined as a score of at least four on the total CFS.

• *Impact of Events Scale (IES, 15,16].* The IES/SVL identifies the impact of an event. The measurement scores two central dimensions in the psychological reactions to an event. On the one hand, it helps to relive the event. On the other hand, it helps to avoid unpleasant feelings or memories of the event. Answers are scored on a four-point scale. The focus is on feelings and thoughts during the past seven days. The items are filled out with respect to a specific event, in this case the IED/blast incident. The IES can be used to support the diagnosis of PTSD.

• *15 Word Test [19].* The subject receives 15 unrelated words presented verbally five times in a row, in which, after each series, the subject is asked to reproduce as many words as possible. After 20-30 minutes the subject is asked to reproduce as many words as possible from those 15 words. Afterwards, the subject will complete a recognition task to indicate whether the word was in the original list or not. The test measures: verbal short and long term memory, learning and recognition [6]. The standard data sets of Van der Elst et al. [20] are used.

• *Digits [21].* The subject is asked to verbally reproduce a series of numbers in a specific forward order, after the specific order is verbally presented. In the Digit Span Backwards, the subject is asked to reproduce the numbers in the reverse order of the order verbally presented. Forward Digits is a task to measure attention span [22]. The standard data of the WAIS III are applied, in which age and educational level are taken into account [21].

• *Stroop Color Word Test I, II and III [17, 18].* The subject receives three cards in succession with one hundred items each, printed over ten columns. On the first card, the subject is asked to read the names of different colors, printed in black, as quickly as possible. The second card shows colored boxes and the subject is asked to name the colors as fast as possible. On the third there are names of colors written in color. The subject is asked to name the color of the ink, in which the color word is printed (and not to read the word). The speed of information processing is measured (Stroop I and II) and the ability to select and attention, while inhibiting an impulse (Stroop III score given the Stroop II). The standard data from Schmand, Houx and The King (2003) are used.

• *Symbol Substitution (part of the WAIS III) [21].* This test consists of a string of numbers (one through nine) with associated symbols. The participant is instructed to use this key and to place symbols in a string of numbers within two minutes. The speed of information processing is measured [22].

4. Statistical Analysis

The descriptive statistic was calculated for all variables from the MACE. The missing values for each specific part of the questionnaires were not replaced by another value and are not included in the statistical analysis. The correlation between the results of the various neuropsychological tests was assessed with the Pearson (Product-Moment) correlation coefficient. Preliminary analyses were performed to prevent violation of the assumptions for normality, linearity and homoscedasticity. An independent t-test was performed in order to make a comparison between the MACE-scores of soldiers with different scores on the neuropsychological subtasks. Finally, a Chi-square test was performed in order to assess significant differences between groups with different demographic variables such as age, wearing a helmet, mounted or unmounted patrol or not wearing a seat belt. Statistical analyses were performed using IBM SPSS 18 for Windows.

5. Results

During the period from 1 August, 2006 to 1August, 2010 the Netherlands Armed Forces acted to lead the nation's activity in the province of Uruzgan. Approximately 350 IED-blast hits were reported by NLD/AUS in Uruzgan in this period. In the period from January 2007 to August 2010, 24 Dutch soldiers were killed in action; over 140 soldiers were wounded in action. The exact grand total of servicemen exposed to blasts from an IED (non-injured) is unknown.

5.1. Phase One, In Theatre; MACE Assessment

The study population (n = 98) consisted of 96 men and two women. It is important to note that this is not the total population exposed to an IED. The soldiers that survived the explosion but were injured were not part of this assessment since they were immediately repatriated. This number is estimated to be equal to the number of this sample. The mean age of the current non-inured sample was 25.7 years old (SD = 4.9, range: 20-46). In our sample, in 90 cases injury was caused by an IED and in nine cases, by the explosion of a grenade. In 72.4% of the military sample (n = 71) a helmet was worn at the time of the blast. Of 44 mounted soldiers (44.4%) and 54 unmounted soldiers (n = 55), 1.8% (n = 9) were wearing a safety belt at the time of the blast.

Two soldiers experienced loss of consciousness for a few minutes. In one soldier this was accompanied by a retrograde (five minute) and a posttraumatic amnesia (10 minutes). The frequency of individual symptoms of mTBI is reported in Table 1. In general, the frequency of reported symptoms is consistent with what has been reported in the literature. The three most commonly reported symptoms include anxiety (41.8%), headache (33.7%) and pain in the locomotor system (26.5%). The three lowest scoring symptoms include dizziness (3.1%), blurred vision (3.1%) and concentration problems (6.1%). However, soldiers showed no abnormalities during the neurological screen. In three soldiers there were neurological abnormalities. One soldier had eye tracking problems, mild word finding problems, and vestibular problems; two others had problems with eye tracking and word findings. All others had no abnormalities.

The neurological test questions were completed by 92 soldiers (93.9%), in which an average score on the MACE was found to be 27.6 (SD = 2.25, range 18 to 30). Broken down into different parts, we found the following scores: orientation 4.8 (SD = 0.45, range 3-5), immediate memory 14.5 (SD = 0.93, range 11 to 15), concentration 4.1 (SD = 0.97, range 2 to 5), and delayed memory 4.1 (SD = 1.03, range 1 to 5).

Of the 98 soldiers 56 have been reassessed to-date at follow-up after 3-6 months. This group consisted of 54 men and two women. The average age of these soldiers was 25.4 years old (SD = 4.8, range = 20-46). Of this group of 56 soldiers, 44 (79%) completed training at the lower level education. Twelve soldiers (21%) had a higher level education at the high school level to university education (Table 2).

All soldiers reported to the doctor and the clinical neuropsychologist that they did not have any complaints in their daily life, and that they had no problems in exercising their current jobs.

Sample	96 male, 2 female
Mean age	25.7 (SD=4.9; range20-46)
In all cases blast-explosion	90 by IED, 9 by handgranate
Helmet during blast	71 (72.4 %)
Mounted	44 cases
Unmounted	54 cases
	(in unmounted cases 1.8 %
	(n=9) was wearing safety belt)
LOC	n=2 (2.0%)
Reported symptoms	
Fear	n= 41 (41.8%)
Headache	n= 33 (33.7%)
Tinnitus	n=15 (15.3%)
Nausea	n= 15 (15.3%)
Somnolent	n=12 (12.2%)
At ease	n= 8 (8.2%)
Dizziness	n= 6 (6.1%)
Vertigo	n= 3 (3.1%)
Blurred vision	n= 3 (3.1%)
*Other**	n= 26 (26.5%)
*Abnormal neurological screen***	n= 3 (3.1%)
Score neurological test	
Orientation (max score 5)	4.8 (SD=0.5; range= 3-5)
Immediate Recall (max score 15)	14.5 (SD=0.9; range 11-15)
Concentration (max score 5)	4.1 (SD=1.0; range 2-5)
Delayed recall (max score 5)	4.1 (SD=1.0; range 1-5)
Total (max score 30)	27.6 (SD=2.3; range 18-30)

* Reported symptoms: pain in musculoskeletal system, chest pain, schrapnel injuries
** Found abnormalities: eye tracking, mild word finding problems and vertigo.

Table 1. Results Phase one, MACE, in theatre.

5.2. Phase Two; 3-6 month Follow-up

General symptoms, 4DSQ - The mean scores on the four dimensions of 4DSQ are shown in Table 2. For distress, two soldiers had a moderately elevated score (> 10), in which one soldier was associated with moderately elevated scores on depression. One soldier had a significantly increased score (> 20) on distress, accompanied by a moderately high score on somatization. On the depression dimension one soldier had a moderately elevated score (> 2). A highly elevated score (> 5) was not found. On the anxiety dimension no elevations (> 8) were found. On the somatization dimension seven soldiers showed a moderately increased score (> 10). A highly elevated score (> 20) was not found here.

Fatigue, CFS - On the CFS we saw an average score of 1.3 (SD = 1.71, range = 0-6). In total, seven soldiers (12.6%) scored above the cut-off score of four, which is considered an indication for the existence of severe fatigue. Twelve soldiers (21.4%) indicated concentration problems on the CFS subjective. Some soldiers had doubts about the quality of their memory, but none of them reported subjective memory complaints.

Impact, IED - The impact of the IED/blast incident was assessed with the IES. The mean scores on the dimension on reliving are shown in Table 2. The mean total subjective stress score was 3.3 (SD 7.15, range 0-41). The degree of subjective stress for 87.5% (n = 49) of the soldiers was subclinical (score: 0-8), for (n = 6) 10.7% mild and for (n = 1) 1.8% moderate. None of the soldiers scored for severe (score 44 +) on the IES.

Neuropsychological Assessment - The number of soldiers with a score of weak to very low average on the various neuropsychological subtasks is shown in Table 2. In total, eight soldiers (14.3%) had a score below average on the Stroop Test Card I, Stroop Card II and on the Symbol Substitution Test (part of the WAIS III), indicative of delayed information processing. On the Stroop Test Card III, corrected for their individual speed of information processing given the score on Card II, 17 soldiers (30.4%) had a reduced score (very poor to low average), indicative of increased distractibility. On Digit Span (part of the WAIS III) four (4.7%) soldiers had a corrected, reduced score (very low to low average), indicative of reduced working memory capacity. On the overall score of the 15 Word list 25 soldiers (44.6.9%) had a reduced score below the fourth decile (very low to low average), and on the delayed recall of the 15 Word test15 soldiers showed relative to age, education and gender a reduced performance score below the fourth decile. Both tests are indicative of a reduced ability to store new information and an impairment in long-term memory. Of the soldiers (n = 21) with a below average score, indicative of concentration problems (Digit and Stroop Color Word Test III Data Card II), only three soldiers reported subjective concentration complaints on the CFS.

The relationship between neuropsychological subtasks was examined with the Pearson (Product Moment) correlation-coefficient to consider normality, linearity and homoscedasticity. These were the only two strong positive correlations. Namely, between the percentile score on the Stroop II card and the raw score on the symbol substitution, r = .55, n = 56, p = <.0005 and between the percentile score on Stroop Card II and the corrected score on the Symbol Substitution r = .50, n = 56, p = <.0005. The three tests measure the mental speed of information processing in explaining the fact that high scores on the Stroop Card II are associated with high scores (raw and corrected) on symbol substitution. A total of 39 soldiers scored a score below the low average on at least one of the neuropsychological subtasks.

An independent t-test was performed to make a comparison between the total scores of the MACE of soldiers with and without at least one score below the low average on one of the neuropsychological subtasks. There was a significant difference in the scores for the soldiers with a good score on the neuropsychological subtasks (M = 28.80, SD = 1.48) and the soldiers with a poor score on neuropsychological subtasks (M = 26.54, SD = 2.58, t (47) = 2.65, p = .01, two-tailed). The magnitude of the differences between the average (mean difference = 2.26, 95% CI: 0.54 to 3.98) was large (eta squared = 0.13).

Those not wearing a helmet were significantly associated with two or more neurological sub-tasks with a score below the low average, $\chi2$ (1, n = 49) = 7.4, p = .01, phi = -. 43. This significance was not found between those not wearing a helmet and one or more neurological sub-tasks with a score below the low average, $\chi2$ (1, n = 49) = 2.6, p = .11, phi = -. 28. For other variables, such as unmounted patrol or wearing a seat belt, no significant group differences were found.

Sample	54 male, 2 female
Mean age	25.4 (SD=4.8; range=20-46)
Education	
lower	n=44 (79%)
higher	n=12 (21%)
4DKL	
distress	3.1 (SD=4.6; range= 0-21)
Depression	0.3 (SD=0.7; range=0-3)
anxiety	0.7 (SD=1.3; range= 0-6)
Somatization	2.9 (SD=4.5; range=0-19)
CFS	1.3 (SD=1.7; range=0-6)
SVL/IES	
intrusions	2.1 (SD=3.6; range=0-14)
shock	1.3 (SD=4.2; range=0-27)
total	3.3 (SD=7.2; range=0-41)
Below is a report of the number of subjects that scored < 40e percentile; score Symbol Substitution and Numbers < 8; score Word list < 4 decile	
Stroop	
Stroop Test Card I	20 (35.7%)
Stroop Test Card II	17 (30.4%)
Stoop Test Card III#	17 (30.4%)
Symbol Substitution	8 (14.3%)
Numbers	4 (4.7%)
15 Wordtest	
Total correct	25 (44.6%)
Delayed recall	15 (26.8%)
Somatic symptoms**	
Psychological complaints***	

corrected for individual speed of information processing, relative to score on Card II
** predominant chronic back complaints e.g. not earlier diagnosed compression fracture L5
*** both soldiers were referred because of PTSD symptoms to Military Mental Health Service

Table 2. Results Phase two, 3-6 months post deployment screen.

A Chi-square test of independence (with Yates Continuity Correction) showed that two soldiers reported chronic back pain after the blast/IED incident. Both were referred for X-ray screening. In one soldier a compression fracture (L5) was found. Both soldiers were referred for follow-up assessment to the rehabilitation center. In total, two soldiers were referred to military mental health professionals because of posttraumatic stress disorder symptoms, despite the fact that both soldiers' scores were subclinical on the degree of subjective stress.

5.3. Phase Three: 12 Months Post-deployment

No data on phase three are available at this moment.

6. Discussion

This study is, to the best of our knowledge, the first study on the acute and long-term sequelae of exposure to a blast/IED incident, using the MACE-instrument in the immediate period after blast exposure and extensive neuropsychological test research at the long-term phase.

These data are the first preliminary data from an ongoing study that started in November 2009 when all Dutch soldiers exposed to single blast/IED were screened on a mandatory basis and followed up for health assessment. To-date, February 2011, we are at approximately 50% of blast exposed soldiers; 56 soldiers have been reassessed at 3-6 months. The MACE is a good, useful assessment, most importantly perhaps for Part 1, which contains careful history assessment, as well as assessment of consciousness and first symptoms. However, the MACE lacks specificity and the scale is not validated. Yet, its use in theatre may prevent retrospective bias when patients present symptoms later.

At follow-up (FU) after 3-6 months most soldiers volunteered to report that they were very satisfied with the assessment. It was remarkable that almost all of the soldiers that were reassessed at FU had no complaints. At this moment of assessment, we could not find evidence of discrete mTBI (yet) by self-reported symptoms. Yet, a significant portion of the studied population had a very weak performance on the neuropsychological battery that was used, in particular information processing, and memory performance. This finding could be explained by several factors. First, the fact that they all were exposed to a blast, and the effect we measured, was attributable to this. Several studies hypothesize a direct effect of blast on neurocircuitry involved in these processes [23, 24]. Secondly, it could be a secondary phenomenon. The soldiers could have scored low on these parameters predeployment. The Dutch military does not routinely screen using a neuropsychological performance assessment, or does this as a standard screen prior to deployment. Other military services, e.g. the United States Army, use the ANAM in a militarized version to assess neuropsychological performance prior to deployment [25]. Thirdly, demand characteristics could also contribute to the results. It could well be that participants were nervous, which contributed to a demand characteristic in which their performance was compromised. For these factors to be answered we need to report at this stage that we are lacking a premorbid screen, and have no control group in our database yet. This is a limiting factor for the interpretation of our results. Also, we may have to further look into factors like education that could contribute to an explanation of the reported results.

We conclude that careful reporting (e.g. in an electronic data reporting system) during a sustained blast exposure and targeted screening are essential to evaluate immediate impact, and evaluate long-term effects. Of key importance is the implementation of a "Blast Tracking Database" as well as a "Wounded in Action" database (e.g. how many blasts, how many soldiers have been exposed, injured) in following up on the health and operational fitness of those that are injured (according to one of the recommendations in the literature). This information may be difficult to obtain, and availability is compromised at a time when this can be considered classified information. Also, entering blast dosimeters or helmet detectors could be used to correlate with the impact on health parameters.

In PTSD it is known that there is an autonomic dysregulation (manifesting in disorders of cognitive and emotional disinhibition, sleep and arousal) that drives the symptoms in the disorder. The neurobiological correlates are known, and the central and peripheral dysregulation has been well studied [see e.g. 26]. This is also very well known in moderate and severe TBIs, but not yet sufficiently studied in the mild forms of TBI. There are candidate biomarkers, proteomics, for TBI (the UCH-L1 protein, MAP-2, and tau), that may be extended to contribute to explain symptoms in mild forms of TBI. Yet, there presently no known diagnostic or prognostic value for mTBI [27]. In addition, it is possible that a distinction needs to be made between single and repetitive military blast exposures. Recently it was found that only soldiers with repetitive blast repetitive exposures showed a cerebrocerebellar hypometabolism similar to the clinical data of patients with cerebellar lesions [28].

In summary, careful reporting of effects of blast exposure through targeted screening is essential to evaluate symptom onset, and long-term effects. Implementations of the MACE as a screening instrument for TBI, as well as posttraumatic cognitive symptoms, can provide an opportunity for structured assessment of the effects of blast on the health and operational fitness of the individual soldier. Importantly, they should also contribute with guidelines to line commanders addressing when to call for return to duty after soldiers are exposed to an IED-related blast. Yet, we feel that there are still gaps in knowledge that prevent us from a complete and definite answer to the long-time impact of blast exposure on deployed soldiers. The outstanding research efforts (predominantly initiated by the United States) that have been initiated over the last five years are expected to resolve at least some of these issues.

Acknowledgements:
The authors thank Jessie Smulders, MSc and line commanders for assistance with recruitment of participants.

References

[1]   Menon, D. K., Schwab, K., Wright, D. W., & Maas, A. I. (2010). Position statement: Definition of traumatic brain injury. Archives of Physical Medicine and Rehabilitation, 91(11), 1637-1640.
[2]   Elder, G. A., & Cristian, A. (2009). Blast-related mild traumatic brain injury: Mechanisms of injury and impact on clinical care. Mount Sinai Journal of Medicine, 76(2), 111-118. doi:10.1002/msj.20098
[3]   Moore, D. F., & Jaffee, M. S. (2010). Military traumatic brain injury and blast. NeuroRehabilitation, 26(3), 179-181.
[4]   MacGregor, A. J.; Shaffer, R. A.; Dougherty, A. L.; Galarneau, M. R.; Raman, R.; Baker, D. G.; Lindsay, S. P.; Golomb, B. A., and Corson, K. S. Prevalence and psychological correlates of traumatic brain injury in operation iraqi freedom. J Head Trauma Rehabil. 2010 Jan-2010 Feb 28; 25(1):1-8.
[5]   Carlson, K. F.; Nelson, D.; Orazem, R. J.; Nugent, S.; Cifu, D. X., and Sayer, N. A. Psychiatric diagnoses among Iraq and Afghanistan war veterans screened for deployment-related traumatic brain injury. J Trauma Stress. 2010 Feb; 23(1):17-24.
[6]   Risling, M. Blast Induced Brain Injuries - A Grand Challenge in TBI Research. Front Neurol. 2010; 1:1.
[7]   Saljo, A.; Mayorga, M.; Bolouri, H.; Svensson, B., and Hamberger, A. Mechanisms and pathophysiology of the low-level blast brain injury in animal models. Neuroimage. 2011 Jan; 54 Suppl 1:S83-8.
[8]   Courtney, A. C., & Courtney, M. W. (2009). A thoracic mechanism of mild traumatic brain injury due to blast pressure waves. Medical Hypotheses, 72(1), 76-83. doi:10.1016/j.mehy.2008.08.015
[9]   Tellier, A.; Marshall, S. C.; Wilson, K. G.; Smith, A.; Perugini, M., and Stiell, I. G. The heterogeneity of mild traumatic brain injury: Where do we stand? Brain Inj. 2009 Oct; 23(11):879-87.
[10] Kocsis, J. D. and Tessler, A. Pathology of blast-related brain injury. J Rehabil Res Dev. 2009; 46(6):667-72.

[11] Vanderploeg, R. D.; Belanger, H. G., and Curtiss, G. Mild traumatic brain injury and posttraumatic stress disorder and their associations with health symptoms. Arch Phys Med Rehabil. 2009 Jul; 90(7):1084-93.

[12] McCrea, M. (2001). Standardized mental status assessment of sports concussion. Clinical Journal of Sport Medicine, 11(3), 176-181.

[13] Terluin, B., van Marwijk, H. W. J., Adèr, H. J., de Vet, H. C. W., Penninx, B. W. J. H., Hermens, M. L. M., Stalman, W. A. B. (2006). The four-dimensional symptom questionnaire (4DSQ): A validation study of a multidimensional self-report questionnaire to assess distress, depression, anxiety and somatization. BMC Psychiatry, 6

[14] Chalder, T., Berelowitz, G., Pawlikowska, T., Watts, L., Wessely, S., Wright, D., & Wallace, E. P. (1993). Development of a fatigue scale. Journal of Psychosomatic Research, 37(2), 147-153.

[15] Horowitz, M., Wilner, N., & Alvarez, W. (1979). Impact of event scale: A measure of subjective stress. Psychosomatic Medicine, 41(3), 209-218.

[16] Van Der Ploeg, E., Mooren, T. T. M., Van Der Velden, P. G., Kleber, R. J., & Brom, D. (2004). Construct validation of the dutch version of the impact of event scale. Psychological Assessment, 16(1), 16-26. doi:10.1037/1040-3590.16.1.16

[17] Stroop, J. R. (1935). Studies of interference in serial verbal reactions. Journal of Experimental Psychology, 18, 421-457.

[18] Hammes, J. (1973). De stroop kleur-woord test: Handleiding [the stroop color-word test: Manual]. Amsterdam: Swets & Zeitlinger.

[19] Saan, R. J., & Deelman, B. G. (1998). Nieuwe 15-woorden test A en B. In A. Bouma, J. Mulder & J. Lindeboom (Eds.), Handboek neuropsychologische diagnostiek (). Lisse: Swets & Zeitlinger.

[20] Van der Elst, W., van Boxtel, M. P., van Breukelen, G. J., & Jolles, J. (2005). Rey's verbal learning test: Normative data for 1855 healthy participants aged 24-81 years and the influence of age, sex, education, and mode of presentation. Journal of the International Neuropsychological Society: JINS, 11(3), 290-302.

[21] Wechsler, D. (2004). WAIS III. afname en scorehandleiding. Nederlandstalige bewerking. (4e druk ed.). Lisse: Swets & Zeitlinger.

[22] Eling, P., De Haan, E. H. F., Hijman, R., & Schmand, B. (2003). Cognitieve neuropsychiatrie. Amsterdam: Boom.

[23] Koliatsos, V. E.; Cernak, I.; Xu, L.; Song, Y.; Savonenko, A.; Crain, B. J.; Eberhart, C. G.; Frangakis, C. E.; Melnikova, T.; Kim, H., and Lee, D. A mouse model of blast injury to brain: initial pathological, neuropathological, and behavioral characterization. J Neuropathol Exp Neurol. 2011 May; 70(5):399-416.

[24] Kwon, S. K.; Kovesdi, E.; Gyorgy, A. B.; Wingo, D.; Kamnaksh, A.; Walker, J.; Long, J. B., and Agoston, D. V. Stress and traumatic brain injury: a behavioral, proteomics, and histological study. Front Neurol. 2011; 2:12.

[25] Reeves, D. L.; Winter, K. P.; Bleiberg, J., and Kane, R. L. ANAM genogram: historical perspectives, description, and current endeavors. Arch Clin Neuropsychol. 2007 Feb; 22 Suppl 1:S15-37.

[26] Vermetten, E. and Bremner, J. D. Circuits and systems in stress. II. Applications to neurobiology and treatment in posttraumatic stress disorder. Depress Anxiety. 2002; 16(1):14-38.

[27] Dash, P. K.; Zhao, J.; Hergenroeder, G., and Moore, A. N. Biomarkers for the diagnosis, prognosis, and evaluation of treatment efficacy for traumatic brain injury. Neurotherapeutics. 2010 Jan; 7(1):100-14.

[28] Peskind, E. R.; Petrie, E. C.; Cross, D. J.; Pagulayan, K.; McCraw, K.; Hoff, D.; Hart, K.; Yu, C. E.; Raskind, M. A.; Cook, D. G., and Minoshima, S. Cerebrocerebellar hypometabolism associated with repetitive blast exposure mild traumatic brain injury in 12 Iraq war Veterans with persistent post-concussive symptoms. Neuroimage. 2011 Jan; 54 Suppl 1:S76-82.

Section IV

Quality of Life

© 2011 The authors and IOS Press. All rights reserved.
doi: 10.3233/978-1-60750-797-0-171

12-month Outcome of Mild Traumatic Brain Injury and Polytrauma in U.S. Military Service Members

Rael T. LANGE[a, b, c, 1], Tracey A. BRICKELL[a], Grant L. IVERSON[a, c],
Glenn PARKINSON[a, b], Aditya BHAGWAT[a, b, d] and Louis M. FRENCH[a, b, e]
[a]*Defense and Veterans Brain Injury Center*
[b]*Walter Reed Army Medical Center*
[c]*University of British Columbia*
[d]*United States Public Health Service*
[e]*Uniformed Services University of the Heath Sciences*

Abstract. This study examined 12-month outcome following polytrauma and mild Traumatic Brain Injury (MTBI) in injured service members who were evaluated at the Walter Reed Army Medical Center following injuries sustained in combat theater during Operations Iraqi Freedom or Enduring Freedom (OIF/OEF). Patients (N=48) completed the Neurobehavioral Symptom Inventory within 2 months of injury (M=15.9 days, SD=13.6) and a telephone interview at 12 months post injury (M=13.1, SD=0.8). More than half of the sample met DSM-IV criteria for Postconcussional Disorder within 2 months (54.2%) and 12 months post injury (55.6%). Over time, 20.8% showed an improvement of symptoms, 16.7% worsened, and 33.3% had persistent symptoms. At 12 months, most were on active duty (79.2%), reported that they were satisfied with life (81.3%), and indicated that their health status was either "excellent," "very good," or "good" (66.7%). However, a substantial percentage reported that they continued to take medications (81.3%), experienced bodily pain (72.9%), needed help with daily activities (29.2%), and were currently in treatment with a mental health professional (39.6%). A small percentage reported that they had recently had suicidal or homicidal thoughts (10.4%). Extended follow-up is recommended for service members who sustain an MTBI in the context of polytrauma.

Keywords: postconcussion symptoms, mild Traumatic Brain Injury, military service members

Author notes: Portions of these data were presented at the NATO Wounds of War III conference in Vienna, Austria, February 2011. The views expressed in this article are those of the authors and do not reflect the official policy of the Department of Defense or U.S. Government.

---

[1] Corresponding Author: Rael T. Lange, Defense and Veterans Brain Injury Center, Walter Reed Army Medical Center, Building #1, Room B207, 6900 Georgia Ave NW, Washington, DC, 20307. Phone: 240-997-5284; Email: rlange@dvbic.org.

Introduction

Improvised explosive devices, the weapons of choice for insurgent enemies in Operation Iraqi Freedom (OIF) and Operation Enduring Freedom (OEF), are the leading cause of death and injury in service members [1-3]. More than 79% of all injuries sustained in the Iraq/Afghanistan conflicts are reportedly due to explosive devices [1]. With advances in protective body armor, helmet design, battlefield medical procedures, and rapid medical evacuation, more service members are surviving injuries and amputations that were otherwise fatal in past conflicts. Consequently, a larger number of service members are returning home and learning to come to terms with multiple severe concurrent blast-related impairments or polytrauma injuries [4-6].

Service members injured by blasts often experience multiple injuries and residual problems rather than isolated injuries [6]. Common polytrauma injuries include traumatic brain injury, amputation/s, open wounds, musculoskeletal or orthopedic injuries, disfigurement, spinal cord injury, chronic pain, auditory and visual impairment, and mental health problems [4, 7]. These injuries can occur concurrently in two or more body parts or systems and often result in cognitive, physical, psychological, or psychosocial impairments [8].

Traumatic brain injury (TBI) is common in returning service members and frequently cited as the signature injury of the conflicts in Iraq/Afghanistan [2, 6, 9-15]. A study of service members injured in OIF/OEF who were medically evacuated to Walter Reed Army Medical Center (WRAMC) found that 28% of those injured in combat had sustained a TBI (WRAMC Work Unit # 05-71029) [16]. Mild TBI has been reported as the most common TBI with post-deployment screening estimates ranging between 11.2% and 22.8% [6, 7, 17, 18]. Recently, the Department of Defense (DoD) reported that there were 195,547 brain injuries coded by the DoD Health Care System in the first 10 years of the Iraq/Afghanistan conflicts; 76.8% of these were classified as mild (n=150,222). These data, however, likely underestimate the true prevalence of the mildest forms of brain injury in this population because some military personal likely never seek medical treatment [19].

Mild TBI is generally not associated with long-term neuropsychological impairment. Recovery to baseline is usually reported within a few months following injury, with only a small percentage (3-5%) reporting persistent postconcussion symptoms [12]. The majority of service members who sustain a mild TBI on the battlefield will have time-limited symptoms. In the short-term recovery phase, the service member might experience a temporary impairment in performance including slowed reaction time, headache, dizziness, inattention, impaired judgment, modest physical limitations relating to vision and balance, or other postconcussion symptoms [20]. These symptoms may have implications for the service member's cognitive and behavioral fitness for duty. Returning to the battlefield before service members are combat-ready could have consequences for their personal welfare (e.g., exposure to further blasts and brain injury before the brain has had time to heal) and also the safety of the service member's unit. It is important to appreciate, however, that postconcussion symptoms are not specific to mild TBI and are often reported in the absence of a brain injury [20, 21]. Symptoms of mild TBI (concussion) overlap with symptoms of acute stress and heightened anxiety (e.g., confusion, inattention, disorientation, being dazed, or having brief amnesia) that are commonly experienced during episodes of high combat exposure, even in the absence of a TBI [22, 23].

Of concern, an increasing number of service members returning from OIF/OEF with a history of mild TBI are experiencing symptoms beyond normal recovery and in excess of expectations [24, 25]. High rates of depression, PTSD, and substance abuse have been reported by researchers, especially in those service members exposed to, or wounded in, combat [26-29]. Even in the absence of brain injury, polytrauma patients endorse high rates of psychological and neurobehavioral symptoms, including memory problems, significant mood symptoms, and amotivation [30].

Given the high rates of TBI and other bodily injuries, there is considerable concern about harmful long-term effects of TBI on OIF/OEF service members and veterans. TBI and associated polytrauma in returning service members may complicate treatment and rehabilitation outcomes, and reintegration to civilian and family life. At this stage, the long-term effects are relatively unknown making it challenging to plan for health care and social service requirements. These concerns prompted the U.S. Congress to include a requirement in the National Defense Authorization Act for a 15-year longitudinal study of service members who sustained a TBI in theater, in an effort to address the long-term needs of injured service members and veterans.

Evidence regarding long-term outcomes of TBI, particularly mild TBI, is limited and is largely focused on civilian populations. In service members, some information is available regarding longer-term outcomes in those who have sustained a TBI during peacetime and previous conflicts [31-36]. However, similar longitudinal data pertaining to service members injured during the Iraq/Afghanistan conflicts are limited. Although many of the issues related to recovery from TBI in a civilian setting or past military conflicts may be applicable today, there are potentially unique issues associated with mild TBI in OIE/OEF military populations that limit the generalizability of previous literature in predicting long-term outcomes. The purpose of this study is to examine 12-month outcome following mild TBI in service members injured in OEF/OIF.

1. Method

1.1 Participants

Participants were 48 patients who sustained an uncomplicated mild TBI (n=36) or complicated mild TBI (n=12) who were evaluated at the Walter Reed Army Medical Center (WRAMC), Washington, DC following injuries sustained in the combat theater during OIE/OEF. Patients were selected from a larger sample of 571 U.S. military service members who were evaluated at WRAMC between December 2005 and May 2008 following a suspected or confirmed TBI sustained during OEF/OIF, and who had agreed to the use of their clinical data for research purposes. The majority (75%) of the sample sustained a mild TBI due to a blast-related injury (25% non-blast related injury—falls, motor vehicle accident, etc). All participants had sustained multiple bodily injuries that ranged from minor (10.4%), moderate (35.4%), serious (25.0%), severe (27.1%), to critical (2.1%; based on a modified Injury Severity Score from the Abbreviated Injury Scale—see "Measures and Procedures" section below). Patients typically were medically evacuated for limb loss or systemic injuries, rather than mild TBI per se.

Table 1. Demographic and injury severity characteristics.

	Uncomplicated Mild TBI		Complicated Mild TBI		Total		
	M	SD	M	SD	M	SD	p
Age	26.3	5.7	27.1	7.4	26.5	6.1	.705
Days post-injury: T1	15.3	12.4	17.8	17.2	15.9	13.6	.575
Months post-injury: T2	13.1	0.8	13.0	0.9	13.1	0.8	.610
ISS$_{mod}$	9.9	6.4	13.1	7.8	10.7	6.9	.171
	F	%	f	%			
Gender							
Male	35	97.2	12	100	47	97.9	--
Female	1	2.8	0	0	1	2.1	
Loss of Consciousness							
None	9	25.0	2	16.7	11	22.9	--
< 1 min	19	52.8	5	41.7	24	50.0	
1-15 minutes	5	13.9	2	16.7	7	14.6	
Unknown	3	8.3	3	25.0	6	12.5	
Post-Traumatic Amnesia							
<1 min	14	38.9	5	41.7	19	39.6	--
1-15 minutes	9	25.0	0	0	9	18.8	
16-59 minutes	5	13.9	2	16.7	7	14.6	
1-24 hours	4	11.1	1	8.3	5	10.4	
1-7 days	4	11.1	4	33.3	8	16.7	
Mechanism of Injury							
Non-Blast	7	19.4	5	41.7	12	25.0	--
Blast	29	80.6	7	58.3	36	75.0	
Bodily Injuries							
Minor (ISS$_{mod}$ 1-3)	3	8.3	2	16.7	5	10.4	--
Moderate (ISS$_{mod}$ 4-8)	16	44.4	1	8.3	17	35.4	
Serious (ISS$_{mod}$ 9-15)	9	25.0	3	25.0	12	25.0	
Severe (ISS$_{mod}$ 16-24)	7	19.4	6	50.0	13	27.1	
Critical (ISS$_{mod}$ 25-75)	1	2.8	0	0.0	1	2.1	
Where Wounded							
OIF	34	94.4	12	100	46	95.8	--
OEF	2	5.6	0	0	2	4.2	
Deployment Number							
First	24	66.7	9	75.0	33	68.8	--
Second	5	13.9	2	16.7	7	14.6	
Third	7	19.4	1	8.3	8	16.7	

Note: N=48 (36 uncomplicated MTBI, 12 complicated MTBI); Abbreviations: T1 = Time 1 and T2 = Time 2. ISS$_{mod}$ = a modified version of the Injury Severity Score from the Abbreviated Injury Scale that includes extracranial injuries only. The ISS$_{mod}$ bodily injury severity groups are based on categories proposed by Stevenson et al (2001)[37]: Minor (ISS 1-3), Moderate (ISS 4-8), Serious (ISS 9-15), Severe (ISS 16-24), and Critical (ISS 25-75). OIF = Operation Iraqi Freedom and OEF = Operation Enduring Freedom.

Patients were included in the selected sample if they (a) had sustained a closed TBI (n=544, 95.3% of total sample), (b) had sufficient information available that could be used to confidently classify them as having sustained an uncomplicated or complicated mild TBI (n=390, 68.3% of total sample), (c) were wounded during OEF/OIF (n=503, 88.1% of total sample), (d) had been deployed three or fewer occasions (n=435, 76.2% of total sample), (e) had an Abbreviated Injury Scale [38] score completed by a clinical staff member (n=504, 88.3% of total sample), (f) had completed the Neurobehavioral

Symptom Inventory [39] within two months post injury (n=333, 58.3% of total sample), and (g) had completed a follow-up interview within 12-14 months post-injury (n=91, 15.9% of total sample). Demographic and injury characteristics for the total sample, including the two mild TBI subgroups, are presented in Table 1.

Patients were classified into uncomplicated mild TBI and complicated mild TBI groups based on duration of loss of consciousness (LOC), duration of post-traumatic amnesia (PTA), and reported intracranial abnormalities on computed tomography (CT) or magnetic resonance imaging (MRI) scans undertaken within the first few days and/or weeks post injury. Uncomplicated mild TBI was defined as PTA<24 hours, LOC<15 minutes, and the absence of intracranial abnormality on CT or MRI scan. Complicated mild MTBI was defined as PTA<24 hours, LOC<15 minutes, and the presence of intracranial abnormality on CT or MRI scan. It was our preference to apply diagnostic criteria for mild TBI based on the American Congress of Rehabilitation Medicine [40], World Health Organization [41], or Department of Defense [42] guidelines. However, there were two limitations of the available data that prevented use of these criteria. First, Glasgow Coma Scale (GCS) scores were not available. GCS scores are often not available shortly after combat-related injuries and could not be used here. Second, the available information regarding LOC was limited to categorical data that did not allow us to differentiate between those patients with LOC greater or less than 30 minutes (i.e., LOC categories: <15 minutes and 16-60 minutes). As such, a criterion of LOC<15 minutes was applied. Note, however, that in some circumstances the minority of patients (n=8) were classified as sustaining a mild TBI when their PTA fell in the moderate range, and their LOC fell in the mild range. For these cases, duration of LOC was used as the primary criterion for final classification because estimates of PTA might have been confounded by routinely administered sedative medication at the time of injury. Unfortunately, information relating to this variable was not available.

1.2 Measures and Procedure

Participants completed the Neurobehavioral Symptom Inventory (NBSI) within 2 months following injury (M=15.9 days, SD=13.6, range=3 to 60; 87.5% evaluated within first 30 days) and a telephone interview at approximately 12 months post injury (M=13.1, SD=0.8, range=12-14 months; 12 months=27.1%, 13 months=35.4%, 14 months=37.5%). The Abbreviated Injury Scale (AIS) was completed by a physician's assistant within the first 3-9 months post injury.

The NBSI [39] is a 22-item measure designed to evaluate self-reported postconcussion symptoms (e.g., headache, balance problems, nausea, fatigue, sensitivity to noise, irritability, sadness, nervousness, difficulty concentrating, difficulty remembering, visual problems). The NBSI requires the test taker to rate the presence/severity of each item on a 5-point scale as follows: 0=none, 1=mild, 2=moderate, 3=severe, and 4=very severe. A total score is obtained by summing the ratings for the 22 items. For the purposes of this study, items on the NBSI were classified as "present" when endorsed as mild or greater.

The brief telephone interview is an unpublished, 10-15 minute, semi-structured questionnaire developed specifically for this study. The interview was designed to provide a "snap-shot" of key outcome variables commonly examined following TBI. These variables include: (a) marital and living situation (e.g., marital status, change in marital status, who living with), (b) health status (e.g., bodily pain, seizures, medications, medication effectiveness), (c) access to services (e.g., help with daily activities, receiving mental health treatment), (d) alcohol use (e.g., consumption, family complaints), (e) satisfaction with life, (f) suicidal and homicidal thoughts, (g) medical board proceedings, and (h) postconcussion symptoms (e.g., headache, dizziness, balance, memory, fatigue, attention, irritability, depression, concentration, sleep, anxiety, ringing in ears, mood lability, limb weakness, intrusive thoughts, sensitivity to noise). For the 16 postconcussion symptoms, each symptom was read aloud to the participant and he/she was required to confirm the presence or absence of the symptom. Severity ratings were not obtained.

The AIS [38] is an anatomically-based, consensus-derived, global severity scoring system that classifies injuries to the body categorized into six main regions [i.e., (i) head or neck, (ii) face, (iii) chest, (iv) abdominal or pelvic contents, (v) extremities or pelvic girdle, and (vi) external]. Injuries are rated on a 6-point ordinal scale that classifies injury severity as minor (1), moderate (2), serious (3), severe (4), critical (5), or maximal (6). The AIS is traditionally interpreted using the Injury Severity Score (ISS). The ISS is calculated by summing the squares of the highest AIS severity codes in each of the three most severely injured body regions (range = 1-75). For the purposes of this study, a modified ISS score was calculated (ISS_{mod}) designed to include only bodily injuries. All AIS codes that related to intracranial injuries were not included in the calculation of ISS_{mod}. The ISS_{mod} was calculated in the same manner as the ISS score described above. ISS_{mod} scores were classified into five categories as recommended by Stevenson and colleagues [37]: Minor (ISS 1-3), Moderate (ISS 4-8), Serious (ISS 9-15), Severe (ISS 16-24), and Critical (ISS 25-75).

2. Results

2.1 Demographic and Injury Characteristics

Descriptive statistics of demographic and injury characteristics for the total group, and mild TBI subgroups, are presented in Table 1. There were no significant main effects for age (p=.705), days tested post injury at Time 1 (p=.575), months tested post injury at follow-up (p=.610), or bodily injury severity score (ISS_{mod}, p=.171). For the remaining variables, formal statistical comparisons (i.e., chi-square analyses) were not possible due to the large number of groups and small sample sizes. Neither chi-square statistics (due to small sample sizes in many cells) nor Fisher exact tests (maximum of 2 groups x 2 categories allowed) could be appropriately interpreted. Nonetheless, an informal comparison of these variables revealed few appreciable differences between groups, with the exception of (a) mechanism of injury (Blast: 80.6% uncomplicated mild TBI, 58.3% complicated mild TBI) and (b) ISS_{mod} severity categories (ISS_{mod} Serious or higher: 45.3% uncomplicated mild TBI, 75.0% complicated mild TBI).

2.2 Post-concussion Symptoms

The prevalence of endorsed symptoms was examined by considering all 22 individual NBSI symptoms simultaneously at Time 1, and all 16 individual PCS symptoms simultaneously at 12-month follow-up. The cumulative percentages of the number of participants who endorsed symptoms as "mild or greater" (i.e., present) in each group at Time 1 are presented in Table 2. The cumulative percentages of the number of participants who endorsed symptoms as 'present' in each group at follow-up are presented in Table 3. Postconcussion symptom reporting was common within the first two months post-injury (Time 1) and at 12 months post-injury (follow-up).

Table 2. Number of individual NBSI items endorsed (present) by group: Time 1.

Number of symptoms	Total Cum %	Uncomplicated Mild TBI Cum %	Complicated Mild TBI Cum %	% Difference Comp/Uncomp
20 symptoms	2.1	2.8	--	2.8
19 or more	12.5	13.9	8.3	5.6
18 or more	14.6	16.7	8.3	8.4
17 or more	20.8	25.0	8.3	16.7
16 or more	22.9	27.8	8.3	19.5
15 or more	25.0	30.6	8.3	22.3
14 or more	31.3	36.1	16.7	19.4
13 or more	35.4	36.1	33.3	2.8
12 or more	37.5	36.1	41.7	-5.6
11 or more	45.8	47.2	41.7	5.5
10 or more	52.1	47.2	66.7	-19.5
9 or more	56.3	50.0	75.0	-25
8 or more	62.5	58.3	75.0	-16.7
7 or more	64.6	61.1	75.0	-13.9
6 or more	66.7	63.9	75.0	-11.1
5 or more	70.8	69.4	75.0	-5.6
4 or more	81.3	83.3	75.0	8.3
3 or more	89.6	91.7	83.3	8.4
2 or more	89.6	91.7	83.3	8.4
1 or more	93.8	94.4	91.7	2.7
0 symptoms	100	100.0	100	0

Note: N=48 (36 uncomplicated MTBI, 12 complicated MTBI). Abbreviations: NBSI = Neurobehavioral Symptom Inventory. 22 symptoms maximum.

Table 3. Number of PCD symptoms endorsed as present by group at 12-month follow-up.

Number of Symptoms	Total (%)	Uncomplicated Mild TBI (%)	Complicated Mild TBI (%)	% Difference Complicated/Uncomplicated
15 symptoms	6.3	5.6	8.3	-2.7
14 or more	16.7	13.9	25.0	-11.1
13 or more	22.9	22.2	25.0	-2.8
12 or more	31.3	30.6	33.3	-2.7
11 or more	35.4	36.1	33.3	2.8
10 or more	43.8	47.2	33.3	13.9
9 or more	50.0	52.8	41.7	11.1
8 or more	56.3	58.3	50.0	8.3
7 or more	62.5	63.9	58.3	5.6
6 or more	66.7	66.7	66.7	0
5 or more	72.9	69.4	83.3	-13.9
4 or more	77.1	75.0	83.3	-8.3
3 or more	83.3	83.3	83.3	0
2 or more	89.6	86.1	100	-13.9
1 or more	97.9	97.2	100	-2.8
0 symptoms	100	100.0	100	0

Note: N=48 (36 uncomplicated MTBI, 12 complicated MTBI). 16 symptoms maximum.
PCD = Post-concussive Disorder

For example, at Time 1 (using the 22-item NBSI), eight or more symptoms were reported by 62.5% of the sample (58.3% Uncomplicated MTBI, 75.0% Complicated MTBI; p>.05). At 12-month follow-up (using a 16-item symptom checklist), eight or more symptoms were reported by 56.3% of the sample (58.3% Uncomplicated MTBI, 50.0% Complicated MTBI; p>.05). Chi-square analyses revealed no significant differences   (all p>.05) in the proportion of patients in the uncomplicated and complicated mild TBI groups who endorsed symptoms at any number of low score criteria (likely due to small sample sizes). Nonetheless, it is interesting to note that within the first two months post injury, a larger proportion of patients in the uncomplicated mild TBI group endorsed 14 or more (19.4% difference), 15 or more (22.3% difference), and 16 or more symptoms (19.5% difference), compared to the complicated mild TBI group (e.g., 15 or more symptoms: 30.6% uncomplicated mild TBI, 8.3% complicated mild TBI). In comparison, these differences were not apparent between groups at the 12-month follow-up (difference = 0-13.9%).

Table 4. Prevalence and comparison of sample meeting DSM-IV criteria for Postconcussional Disorder at Time 1 and 12 month follow-up.

	No Change: No PCS (Absent-Absent)	Worsened (Absent-Present)	Improved (Present-Absent)	No change: Persistent PCS (Present-Present)	Total
Prevalence					
Time 1 (NBSI) mild or greater					
Uncomplicated Mild TBI	--	--	--	--	50.0
Complicated Mild TBI	--	--	--	--	66.7
All Mild TBIs	--	--	--	--	54.2
Follow-up (phone interview items)					
Uncomplicated Mild TBI	--	--	--	--	55.6
Complicated Mild TBI	--	--	--	--	33.3
All Mild TBIs	--	--	--	--	50.0
Comparison of T1 to T2					
TBI Severity					
Uncomplicated Mild TBI	30.6	19.4	13.9	36.1	--
Complicated Mild TBI	25.0	8.3	41.7	25.0	--
All Mild TBIs	29.2	16.7	20.8	33.3	--
Bodily Injury Severity					
Mild (n=5)	20.0	20.0	0	60.0	--
Moderate (n=17)	17.6	5.9	23.5	52.9	--
Serious (n=12)	41.7	25.0	16.7	16.7	--
Severe/Critical (n=14)	35.7	21.4	28.6	14.3	--

Note: N=48 (36 uncomplicated MTBI, 12 complicated MTBI). Abbreviations: NBSI = neurobehavioral Symptom Inventory; PCD = DSM-IV research criteria for Postconcussional Disorder; MTBI = mild traumatic brain injury.

Table 5. Percentage* of sample with symptoms individual improved (IMP), worse (WO), or no change (NC) from Time 1 to 12 month follow-up.

	Uncomplicated Mild TBI				Complicated Mild TBI				All Mild TBI			
	NC Nil	WO	IMP	NC PCD	NC Nil	WO	IMP	NC PCD	NC Nil	WO	IMP	NC PCD
Headache	19.4	25.0	11.1	44.4	8.3	33.3	8.3	50.0	16.7	27.1	10.4	45.8
Dizziness	38.9	11.1	27.8	22.2	41.7	25.0	8.3	25.0	39.6	14.6	22.9	22.9
Balance	47.2	16.7	19.4	16.7	50.0	25.0	8.3	16.7	47.9	18.8	16.7	16.7
Memory	19.4	25.0	13.9	41.7	16.7	25.0	8.3	50.0	18.8	25.0	12.5	43.8
Fatigue	33.3	25.0	13.9	27.8	25.0	8.3	16.7	50.0	31.3	20.8	14.6	33.3
Attention	22.2	16.7	16.7	44.4	0	16.7	50.0	33.3	16.7	16.7	25.0	41.7
Irritability	11.1	30.6	11.1	47.2	25.0	8.3	8.3	58.3	14.6	25.0	10.4	50.0
Depression	38.9	13.9	33.3	13.9	58.3	16.7	16.7	8.3	43.8	14.6	29.2	12.5
Concentration	22.2	16.7	16.7	44.4	8.3	8.3	41.7	41.7	18.8	14.6	22.9	43.8
Sleep	13.9	13.9	25.0	47.2	25.0	33.3	8.3	33.3	16.7	18.8	20.8	43.8
Anxiety	36.1	19.4	30.6	13.9	33.3	25.0	25.0	16.7	35.4	20.8	29.2	14.6

Note: N=48 (36 uncomplicated MTBI, 12 complicated MTBI). Abbreviations: (a) NC Nil = No Change/No PCD (no PCD at Time 1 or Follow-up); (b) WO = Worsening symptoms (Time 1 = PCD Absent; Follow-up = PCD Present); (c) IMP = Improvement of symptoms (Time 1 = PCD Present; Follow-up = PCD Absent); (d) NC PCD = No Change/Persistent PCD symptoms (Time 1 = PCD Present; Follow-up = PCD Present). PCD = Postconcussional Disorder.
*Each cell refers to the percentage of people in each group (i.e., Uncomplicated MTBI, Complicated MTBI, and All Mild TBI) whose symptom worsened, improved, or remained stable.

The percentage of each group that met DSM-IV research criteria for Postconcussional Disorder (PCD) was calculated based on symptom reporting. A person was classified as meeting DSM-IV criteria for PCD if they (a) endorsed three or more of the Category C symptoms, and (b) endorsed subjective complaints of attention or memory (Category D criteria requires *objective* evidence of cognitive impairment in attention or memory. For the purposes of this study, *subjective* reports of these cognitive complaints were used as a proxy because all the subjects did not undergo neuropsychological testing). Note that only those symptoms that directly overlapped between Time 1 and follow-up were used here to enable direct comparison between both time points (i.e., headache, dizziness, balance, memory, fatigue, attention, irritability, depression, concentration, sleep, and anxiety). Only the first six of the eight Category C symptom criteria for Post-concussive Disorder can be addressed by these items.

The percentages of the sample meeting DSM-IV criteria for PCD at Time 1 and follow-up are presented in Table 4. Within the first 2 months following injury, 54.2% of the sample met DSM-IV symptom research criteria for PCD (50.0% uncomplicated mild TBI, 66.7% complicated mild TBI; p>.05). At 12-month follow-up, 55.6% met criteria for PCD (55.6% uncomplicated mild TBI, 33.3% complicated mild TBI; p>.05). There were no between-group differences in the proportion of patients who met DSM-IV criteria for PCD at Time 1 or follow-up (p>.05). However, it is noted that more than half (55.6%) of the uncomplicated mild TBI group met PCD criteria at follow-up compared to a third (33.3%) of the complicated mild TBI group (22.3% difference). A within groups comparison revealed a significant decrease in the proportion of patients meeting PCD criteria at follow-up, compared to Time 1, in the complicated mild TBI group (p<.05; 33.4% difference), but not in the uncomplicated mild TBI group (p>.05; 5.6% difference).

A comparison of PCD status, and endorsement of individual symptoms, from Time 1 to follow-up (see Tables 4 and 5) was undertaken by calculating the number of people whose symptoms improved, worsened, or remained stable over time. Overall, in the entire sample, (a) 29.2% did not meet PCD criteria at Time 1 or follow-up (no change-no PCD), (b) 20.8% showed an improvement of symptoms (from PCD present to PCD absent), (c) 16.7% showed an increase in symptoms (from PCD absent to PCD present), and (d) 33.3% had persistent ongoing symptoms from Time 1 to follow-up (no change-persistent PCD). However, there were some important differences between groups. A larger proportion of the complicated mild TBI group (41.7%) showed an improvement in PCD status from Time 1 to follow-up (p<.05), compared to the uncomplicated MTBI group (13.9%). Overall, individual symptoms that improved most frequently included depression (29.2%), anxiety (29.2%), and attention (25.0%). Individual symptoms that worsened most frequently were headaches (27.1%), irritability (25.0%), and memory (25.0%).

2.3 Bodily Injury and Symptom Reporting

The relation between bodily injury severity (ISS_{mod}) and postconcussion symptom reporting was examined using Pearson product-moment correlation analyses. Within the first 2 months post injury, there was a significant negative association between ISS_{mod} and the number of NBSI symptoms endorsed ($r = -.377$, $p=.009$) and the number of DMS-IV criteria met ($r = -.433$, $p=.002$). As bodily injury severity increased, there was a decrease in self-reported postconcussion symptoms. At 12 months post injury, however, there was no association between ISS_{mod} and the number of PCS symptoms endorsed ($r = -.177$, $p=.234$).

2.4 Other Outcome Variables

Other outcome variables at 12-month follow-up are presented in Table 6. The majority of the patients were on active duty (79.2%), most reported that they were satisfied with life (81.3%), and most indicated that their health status was either 'excellent', 'very good', or 'good' (66.7%). However, substantial percentages of the sample reported that they continue to take medications (81.3%), were experiencing bodily pain (72.9%), and needed help with daily activities (29.2%). A small percentage of the sample reported that they had recently had suicidal or homicidal thoughts (10.4%). More than one-third (39.6%) reported to be currently in treatment for mental health issues.

3. Discussion

To date, there are very limited longitudinal data on outcome for service members who sustained a mild TBI in a combat environment in Iraq and Afghanistan. The purpose of this study was to examine 12-month outcome following mild TBI and polytrauma in service members injured in OEF/OIF. Overall, these results show that at 2 months post injury and 12 months post injury, more than half of the service members in this sample reported symptoms consistent with DMS-IV criteria for Postconcussional Disorder (54.2% at 2 months, 55.6% at 12 months). However, it is important to note that the people who met PCD criteria at 2 months post injury were not necessarily the same people who met criteria at 12-month follow-up. In other words, not all of those reporting symptoms in the first two months of injury continued to report these symptoms at one year. Specifically, one-third (33.3%) of the sample reported post-concussive symptoms at both points in time (2 and 12 months post injury).

Table 6. Outcome variables at 12-month follow-up.

		Uncomplicated MTBI	Complicated MTBI	Total
Active Duty Status	Active Duty	77.8	83.3	79.2
	Retired/Reserve/Other	22.2	16.7	20.8
Medical Board Pending?	Yes	30.6	50.0	35.4
Help with daily activities?	Yes	27.8	33.3	29.2
Marital Status	Married	63.9	50.0	60.4
	Single	25.0	41.7	29.2
	Divorced	11.1	8.3	10.4
Change in Marital Status	Yes	11.1	8.3	10.4
Health Status	Excellent/Good/V.Good	69.5	58.3	66.7
	Fair/Poor	30.5	41.7	32.3
Bodily Pain?	Yes	77.8	58.3	72.9
Presence of Seizures?	Yes	2.8	16.7	6.3
Taking medications?	Yes	80.6	83.3	81.3
Medication helping symptoms?	Yes	66.7	75.0	68.8
Alcohol consumption	None	33.3	33.3	33.3
	1-2 times/week	27.8	16.7	25.0
	1-2 days/month	38.9	50.0	41.7
Family complained of drinking?	Yes	5.6	8.3	6.3
Satisfied with Life	Yes	83.3	75.0	81.3
Considered Suicide/Homicide?	Yes	11.1	8.3	10.4
Seeing a counsellor or Psychiatrist?	Yes	44.4	83.3	39.6

Note: N=48 (36 uncomplicated MTBI, 12 complicated MTBI)

Approximately one-fifth of the sample (20.8%) who reported symptoms at two months post injury reported that they had *improved* at 12 months. Conversely, approximately one-fifth of the sample (16.7%) reported a *decline* over time; that is, they met criteria for PCD at one year but not at two months post injury. A substantial minority of the sample (29.2%) did not report experiencing significant postconcussion symptoms at either two months post injury or at 12 months post injury. Overall, a substantial portion of the sample (more than 50%) reported significant symptoms 12 months post injury.

With more than 50% of the service members in our sample meeting criteria for Postconcussional Disorder at 12 months following injury, our findings confirm previous concerns of a higher than normal number of service members returning from OIF/OEF with persistent postconcussion symptoms beyond expected recovery times (i.e., 1-3 months) [24, 25]. When considering long-term outcome from mild TBI, it is important to appreciate that there are many non-TBI factors that can cause or maintain self-reported symptoms (e.g., co-morbidities, social-psychological factors, or legal factors) [4, 9, 12, 25, 43]. Post-concussive symptoms are not unique to TBI and the symptom profile often overlaps with a number of pre-existing or comorbid conditions. Post-concussive symptoms have been reported among clinical groups with PTSD, depression, orthopedic injuries, chronic pain, psychiatric diagnoses, sleep problems, or medication side-effects, and even samples of healthy adults [44]. Among returning service members, mental health comorbidity (in particular PTSD and depression) is frequently reported in combination with mild TBI [7, 18, 24, 45]. Recovery from mild TBI in a military setting is complex and often confounded by exposure to emotionally traumatic events and co-morbid physical injuries. Mental health problems can manifest at varying time points and tend to intensify with time [46-51]. Research indicates that PTSD and depression might be a better explanation than mild TBI to account for persistent post-concussive symptoms in some people [24, 45, 52, 53]. In this study, a large percentage of the sample was reporting medication use (81.3%) and ongoing pain (72.9%). In addition, more than one-third of the sample was receiving treatment for mental health issues (39.6%). Given that there are several studies indicating that postconcussion-like symptoms are common in patients with mental health problems and chronic pain, the presence of these comorbidities in the present sample likely accounts for some of the symptom reporting.

It is interesting to note that in the first two months post injury, there was an inverse relationship between severity of bodily injury and self-reported symptoms. That is, greater bodily injuries were associated with lesser postconcussion-like symptom reporting. Similar findings have also been found by researchers examining symptom reporting in OIF/OEF service members [54, 55]. Kennedy and colleagues [54] found that PTSD and postconcussion symptom ratings within the first three months post injury were highest in those OIF service members who sustained a mild TBI and no other physical injury, compared to those who sustained a mild TBI and associated physical injuries. These authors concluded that having an observable physical injury with systematic rehabilitation and measurable improvements might provide a protective factor against emotional and somatic symptoms. In a replication and expansion of this study, French and colleagues [55] examined PTSD and postconcussion symptom reporting in 137 service members who experienced multiple bodily injuries and an uncomplicated mild TBI (73.7% tested within 3 months). They were stratified by four bodily injury severity groups (defined by a modified ISS score that excluded intracranial injury codes; i.e., minor, moderate, serious, severe/critical). There was a significant negative linear association between bodily injury severity and symptom reporting. As bodily injury severity increased, there was a decrease in self-reported symptoms. French and colleagues hypothesized a number of reasons to account for these findings (see [55] for a further discussion).

In the present study, however, the inverse relationship between severity of bodily injury and self-reported symptoms found within the first few months of injury was not evident at 12 months post injury. As posited by French et al., the reporting of fewer symptoms in the severely injured group may mean that as physical wounds heal, symptom reporting in this group may increase to "normal" levels as they become less focused on their physical recovery. Based on this rationale, we might expect to see a larger portion of those patients with more severe injuries report PCD symptoms at 12 months post injury, but not at Time 1 (i.e., Time 1 = PCD absent, 12 months post injury = PCD Present). In partial support of this hypothesis, 25.0% and 21.4% of patients with bodily injuries in the 'Serious' and 'Severe/Critical' ISS_{mod} classification range had this pattern of symptom reporting. In contrast, only 5.9% of patients with bodily injuries in the 'Moderate' range had this pattern of symptom reporting. Inconsistent with this hypothesis, however, 20% of patients with bodily injuries in the 'Mild' classification range also had this pattern of symptom reporting. However, the sample size of the Mild group was very small [n=5] and is unlikely to be representative of this group.

Of further interest to this study was the comparison of uncomplicated and complicated mild TBI groups. Overall, there was a tendency for the uncomplicated mild TBI group to report a greater number of PCD symptoms at Time 1 (e.g., 15 or more symptoms = 30.6%) when compared to the complicated mild TBI group (8.3%), but not at 12-month follow-up. However, when considering DSM-IV criteria for PCD, there were no differences in the proportion of patients who met DSM-IV criteria at Time 1, but there was a lower proportion of the complicated mild TBI group that met criteria at 12 months post injury. The complicated mild TBI group also had a greater proportion of the sample that improved diagnostically from Time 1 to follow-up. Conventionally, patients who sustain a complicated mild TBI are more likely to have worse acute symptoms and a slower recovery trajectory [56]. These results are inconsistent with civilian studies. It is important to point out, however, that more than 75% of the complicated mild TBI group had bodily injuries in the 'Serious' or 'Severe/Critical' range, compared to only 45.3% of the uncomplicated mild TBI group. As seen in this study and reported elsewhere [54, 55], bodily injury severity can influence symptom reporting. Though, in this case, we would expect to see lower reporting of symptoms in the complicated mild TBI group (i.e., the more severely injured group); which was not the case here. Although we made an attempt to compare these two groups, the sample size of the complicated mild TBI group was very small and any formal statistical comparisons, or informal comparisons, should be considered speculative at best. The small sample size of the complicated mild TBI group is considered to be a substantive limitation of this study, but has been included for descriptive purposes.

A primary focus of this study was postconcussion symptom reporting. However, this study provides other important information regarding outcome from mild TBI in service members who sustain multiple bodily injuries. These data further show that there is a substantial minority of people at 12 months post injury who are reporting significant distress. Specifically, 39.6% are currently in treatment for a mental health problem, 37.5% report having a worse quality of life than before their injury, 32.3% report their health to be only fair or poor, 29.2% need help with their daily activities, 18.7% are not satisfied with their current life, and 10.4% have had recent thoughts of suicide or homicide. In addition to these patients, a large portion of the sample continues to experience bodily pain (72.9%) and take medications (81.3%).

In conclusion, in this sample of 48 service members who sustained a mild TBI and polytrauma in the OIF/OEF combat theater, more than 50% met Category C research criteria for DSM-IV Postconcussional Disorder at 12 months post injury. The prevalence of this diagnosis is much greater than expected based on the natural history of recovery from mild TBI [56]. Depending on how the condition is diagnosed, a large percentage of healthy adults [57], patients with chronic pain [58], and patients with depression [59] will endorse symptoms consistent with Postconcussional Disorder. Of course, a mild TBI is not necessary (and often not sufficient) to produce the constellation of symptoms and problems that comprise the postconcussion syndrome at 12 months post injury. In addition, recovery from mTBI in a military setting is complex and often confounded by dual exposure to blast and traumatic stressors that make it difficult to disentangle other potential causes for postconcussion-like symptoms, such as mental health comorbidity, chronic pain, or medication use. These and other contributing factors need to be considered when evaluating the etiology of symptom reporting in this population. Nonetheless, the etiology of these symptoms should not be a critical factor in determining a treatment plan. Self-reported symptoms in service members who have sustained a mild TBI in the context of polytruama, regardless of etiology, require treatment. Extended follow-up is recommended.

References

[1]   Owens, B.D., et al., *Combat wounds in operation Iraqi Freedom and operation Enduring Freedom.* J Trauma, 2008. **64**(2): p. 295-9.
[2]   Snell, F.I. and M.J. Halter, *A signature wound of war: mild traumatic brain injury.* J Psychosoc Nurs Ment Health Serv, 2010. **48**(2): p. 22-8.
[3]   Wallace, D., *Improvised explosive devices and traumatic brain injury: the military experience in Iraq and Afghanistan.* Australas Psychiatry, 2009. **17**(3): p. 218-24.
[4]   Brenner, L.A., R.D. Vanderploeg, and H. Terrio, *Assessment and diagnosis of mild traumatic brain injury, posttraumatic stress disorder, and other polytrauma conditions: burden of adversity hypothesis.* Rehabilitation Psychology, 2009. **54**(3): p. 239-46.
[5]   Jaffee, M.S. and K.S. Meyer, *A brief overview of traumatic brain injury (TBI) and post-traumatic stress disorder (PTSD) within the Department of Defense.* Clin Neuropsychol, 2009. **23**(8): p. 1291-8.
[6]   Lew, H.L., et al., *Prevalence of chronic pain, posttraumatic stress disorder, and persistent postconcussive symptoms in OIF/OEF veterans: polytrauma clinical triad.* J Rehabil Res Dev, 2009. **46**(6): p. 697-702.
[7]   Belanger, H.G., J.M. Uomoto, and R.D. Vanderploeg, *The Veterans Health Administration's (VHA's) System of Care for mild traumatic brain injury: costs, benefits, and controversies.* J Head Trauma Rehabil, 2009. **24**(1): p. 4-13.
[8]   (IOM), I.o.M., ed. *Returning Home from Iraq and Afghanistan: Preliminary Assessment of Readjustment Needs of Veterans, Service Members, and Their Families.* 2010, The National Academies Press.
[9]   Benzinger, T.L., et al., *Blast-related brain injury: imaging for clinical and research applications: report of the 2008 st. Louis workshop.* Journal of Neurotrauma, 2009. **26**(12): p. 2127-44.
[10] Rosenfeld, J.V. and N.L. Ford, *Bomb blast, mild traumatic brain injury and psychiatric morbidity: a review.* Injury, 2010. **41**(5): p. 437-43.
[11] Elder, G.A. and A. Cristian, *Blast-related mild traumatic brain injury: mechanisms of injury and impact on clinical care.* Mt Sinai J Med, 2009. **76**(2): p. 111-8.
[12] Howe, L.L., *Giving context to post-deployment post-concussive-like symptoms: blast-related potential mild traumatic brain injury and comorbidities.* Clinical Neuropsychology, 2009. **23**(8): p. 1315-37.
[13] Uomoto, J.M. and R.M. Williams, *Post-acute polytrauma rehabilitation and integrated care of returning veterans: toward a holistic approach.* Rehabilitation Psychology, 2009. **54**(3): p. 259-69.
[14] MacGregor, A.J., et al., *Prevalence and psychological correlates of traumatic brain injury in operation iraqi freedom.* Journal of Head Trauma Rehabilitation, 2010. **25**(1): p. 1-8.
[15] Dausch, B.M. and S. Saliman, *Use of family focused therapy in rehabilitation for veterans with traumatic brain injury.* Rehabil Psychol, 2009. **54**(3): p. 279-87.
[16] Warden, D., *Military TBI during the Iraq and Afghanistan wars.* Journal of Head Trauma Rehabilitation, 2006. **21**(5): p. 398-402.
[17] Iverson, G.L., *Clinical and methodological challenges with assessing mild traumatic brain injury in the military.* Journal of Head Trauma Rehabilitation, 2010. **25**(5): p. 313-9.
[18] Kennedy, J.E., et al., *Posttraumatic stress symptoms in OIF/OEF service members with blast-related and non-blast-related mild TBI.* NeuroRehabilitation, 2010. **26**(3): p. 223-31.

[19] *TBI Numbers.* 2010 [cited 2010 December 29th 2010]; Available from: http://www.dvbic.org/images/pdfs/TBI-Numbers/2009-2010Q3-updated-as-of/2000-2010Q3-Updated-as-of-15-NOV-2010.aspx.

[20] Fear, N.T., et al., *Symptoms of post-concussional syndrome are non-specifically related to mild traumatic brain injury in UK Armed Forces personnel on return from deployment in Iraq: an analysis of self-reported data.* Psychological Medicine, 2009. **39**(8): p. 1379-87.

[21] Meares, S., et al., *Mild traumatic brain injury does not predict acute postconcussion syndrome.* Journal of Neurology, Neurosurgery and Psychiatry, 2008. **79**(3): p. 300-6.

[22] Iverson, G.L., et al., *Challenges associated with post-deployment screening for mild traumatic brain injury in military personnel.* Clinical Neuropsychology, 2009. **23**(8): p. 1299-314.

[23] Reeves, R.R., *Diagnosis and management of posttraumatic stress disorder in returning veterans.* J Am Osteopath Assoc, 2007. **107**(5): p. 181-9.

[24] Schneiderman, A.I., E.R. Braver, and H.K. Kang, *Understanding sequelae of injury mechanisms and mild traumatic brain injury incurred during the conflicts in Iraq and Afghanistan: persistent postconcussive symptoms and posttraumatic stress disorder.* Am J Epidemiol, 2008. **167**(12): p. 1446-52.

[25] Iverson, G.L., N.D. Zasler, and R.T. Lange, *Post-Concussive Disorder*, in *Brain Injury Medicine*, N.D. Zasler, D.I. Katz, and R.D. Zafonte, Editors. 2007, Demos Medical Publishing: New York. p. 373-405.

[26] Baker, D.G., et al., *Trauma Exposure, Branch of Service, and Physical Injury in Relation to Mental Health Among U.S. Veterans Returning From Iraq and Afghanistan.* Military Medicine, 2009. **174**(8): p. 773-778.

[27] Koren, D., et al., *Increased PTSD risk with combat-related injury: a matched comparison study of injured and uninjured soldiers experiencing the same combat events.* American Journal of Psychiatry, 2005. **162**(2): p. 276-82.

[28] Ferrier-Auerbach, A.G., et al., *Predictors of emotional distress reported by soldiers in the combat zone.* Journal of Psychiatric Research, 2009. **44**(7): p. 470-476.

[29] Grieger, T.A., et al., *Posttraumatic stress disorder and depression in battle-injured soldiers.* American Journal of Psychiatry, 2006. **163**(10): p. 1777-83; quiz 1860.

[30] Frenisy, M.C., et al., *Brain injured patients versus multiple trauma patients: some neurobehavioral and psychopathological aspects.* Journal of Trauma, 2006. **60**(5): p. 1018-26.

[31] Ommaya, A.K., et al., *Outcome after traumatic brain injury in the U.S. military medical system.* Journal of Trauma, 1996. **41**(6): p. 972-5.

[32] Grafman, J., et al., *Intellectual function following penetrating head injury in Vietnam veterans.* Brain, 1988. **111 (Pt 1)**: p. 169-84.

[33] Koenigs, M., et al., *Focal brain damage protects against post-traumatic stress disorder in combat veterans.* Nature Neuroscience, 2008. **11**(2): p. 232-7.

[34] Raymont, V., et al., *Demographic, structural and genetic predictors of late cognitive decline after penetrating head injury.* Brain, 2008. **131**(Pt 2): p. 543-58.

[35] Schwab, K., et al., *Residual impairments and work status 15 years after penetrating head injury: report from the Vietnam Head Injury Study.* Neurology, 1993. **43**(1): p. 95-103.

[36] Salazar, A.M., K. Schwab, and J.H. Grafman, *Penetrating injuries in the Vietnam war. Traumatic unconsciousness, epilepsy, and psychosocial outcome.* Neurosurgery Clinics of North America, 1995. **6**(4): p. 715-26.

[37] Stevenson, M., et al., *An overview of the injury severity score and the new injury severity score.* Injury Prevention, 2001. **7**: p. 10-13.

[38] *Rating the severity of tissue damage. I. The abbreviated scale.* JAMA, 1971. **215**(2): p. 277-80.

[39] Cicerone, K.D. and K. Kalmar, *Persistent postconcussion syndrome: The structure of subjective complaints after mild traumatic brain injury.* J Head Trauma Rehabil, 1995. **10**(3): p. 1-17.

[40] Mild Traumatic Brain Injury Committee, American Congress of Rehabilitation Medicine, and Head Injury Interdisciplinary Special Interest Group, *Definition of mild traumatic brain injury.* Journal of Head Trauma Rehabilitation, 1993. **8**(3): p. 86-87.

[41] Carroll, L.J., et al., *Methodological issues and research recommendations for mild traumatic brain injury: the WHO Collaborating Centre Task Force on Mild Traumatic Brain Injury.* Journal of Rehabilitation Medicine, 2004(43 Suppl): p. 113-25.

[42] Managment of Concussion/nTBI Working Group, *VA/DoD Clinical Practice Guidline for Managment of Concussion/Mild Traumatic Brain Injury.* 2009, Department of Veterans Affairs/Department of Defense.

[43] Stein, M.B. and T.W. McAllister, *Exploring the convergence of posttraumatic stress disorder and mild traumatic brain injury.* American Journal of Psychiatry, 2009. **166**(7): p. 768-76.

[44] Iverson, G.L. and R.T. Lange, *Post-Concussion Syndrome*, in *The little Black Book of Neuropsychology: A syndrome-Based Approach*, M.R. Schoenberg and J.G. Scott, Editors. *In Press*, Springer Science+Business Media, LLC.

[45] Hoge, C.W., et al., *Mild traumatic brain injury in U.S. Soldiers returning from Iraq.* New England Journal of Medicine, 2008. **358**(5): p. 453-63.

[46] Batten, S.V. and S.J. Pollack, *Integrative outpatient treatment for returning service members.* Journal of Clinical Psychology, 2008. **64**(8): p. 928-39.

[47] Belanger, H.G., et al., *Cognitive sequelae of blast-related versus other mechanisms of brain trauma.* Journal of the International Neuropsychological Society, 2009. **15**(1): p. 1-8.

[48] Hoge, C.W., et al., *Combat duty in Iraq and Afghanistan, mental health problems, and barriers to care.* New England Journal of Medicine, 2004. **351**(1): p. 13-22.

[49] Marx, B.P., et al., *Association of time since deployment, combat intensity, and posttraumatic stress symptoms with neuropsychological outcomes following Iraq war deployment.* Archives of General Psychiatry, 2009. **66**(9): p. 996-1004.

[50] Milliken, C.S., J.L. Auchterlonie, and C.W. Hoge, *Longitudinal assessment of mental health problems among active and reserve component soldiers returning from the Iraq war.* Journal of the American Medical Association, 2007. **298**(18): p. 2141-8.

[51] Seal, K.H., et al., *Getting beyond "Don't ask; don't tell": an evaluation of US Veterans Administration postdeployment mental health screening of veterans returning from Iraq and Afghanistan.* American Journal of Public Health, 2008. **98**(4): p. 714-20.

[52] Fear, N.T., et al., *Symptoms of post-concussional syndrome are non-specifically related to mild traumatic brain injury in UK Armed Forces personnel on return from deployment in Iraq: an analysis of self-reported data.* Psychol Med, 2009. **39**(8): p. 1379-87.

[53] Pietrzak, R.H., et al., *Subsyndromal posttraumatic stress disorder is associated with health and psychosocial difficulties in veterans of Operations Enduring Freedom and Iraqi Freedom.* Depress Anxiety, 2009. **26**(8): p. 739-44.

[54] Kennedy, J.E., et al., *Symptoms in military service members after blast mTBI with and without associated injuries.* NeuroRehabilitation, 2010. **26**(3): p. 191-7.

[55] French, L.M., et al., *Influence of Bodily Injuries on Symptom Reporting following Uncomplicated Mild Traumatic Brain Injury in U.S. Military Service Members.* Journal of Head Trauma Rehabilitation, under review.

[56] Iverson, G.L., et al., *Mild TBI,* in *Brain Injury Medicine,* N.D. Zasler, D.I. Katz, and R.D. Zafonte, Editors. 2007, Demos Medical Publishing: New York. p. 333-371.

[57] Iverson, G.L. and R.T. Lange, *Examination of "postconcussion-like" symptoms in a healthy sample.* Applied Neuropsychology, 2003. **10**(3): p. 137-44.

[58] Smith-Seemiller, L., et al., *Presence of post-concussion syndrome symptoms in patients with chronic pain vs mild traumatic brain injury.* Brain Injury, 2003. **17**(3): p. 199-206.

[59] Iverson, G.L., *Misdiagnosis of the persistent postconcussion syndrome in patients with depression.* Archives of Clinical Neuropsychology, 2006. **21**(4): p. 303-10.

© 2011 The authors and IOS Press. All rights reserved.
doi: 10.3233/978-1-60750-797-0-187

Loneliness and Emptiness - Reorientation Syndrome after Traumatic Brain Injury Mechanism: Access and Solutions to This Underestimated Problem After Traumatic Brain Injury

Nikolaus STEINHOFF[a, b, 1]
[a]Federal Hospital Lower Austria LK Hochegg
[b]Austrian Association for Brain Injury

Abstract. A brain undergoing Traumatic Brain Injury (TBI) suffers damage to almost all areas, and the pattern of lesions reflects the forces on the skull at the moment of the trauma; different symptoms result after every single trauma. The common problem for those afflicted by TBI is how to overcome the sudden change in emotions and how to accept their new situation with memories in the body still corresponding to the time before the accident. Members of the Austrian Association of TBI suffering from TBI were questioned concerning their situation after TBI. The change in life affects personal capacities, family and work relationships, ability to work, and financial/social situation and results in a change in relationships with key people in their life. The burden of change is more important if the person was previously a strong, body-oriented person who had to define himself through a hierarchic system, e.g. military organisation. The TBI patient may feel a resulting emptiness in their life, inside and out, and has to reorient himself with a reduced brain capacity. Most people, the injured and families alike, feel a sense of loneliness after TBI. Caregivers and case managers are not skilled enough to deal with emptiness, reorientation, the mourning process and the issue of responsibilities resulting from medical, therapeutic and social consequences after TBI. Reorientation Syndrome is a considerable condition after each TBI that has to be respected to understand how to help TBI patients and their families successfully reintegrate into a functional life after TBI.

Keywords. Traumatic Brain Injury, reorientation syndrome, re-adaptation

Introduction

At the moment Traumatic Brain Injury (TBI) occurs, the brain suffers damage to most of its areas in one second. Consequently, the pattern of lesions reflects the forces on the skull at the moment of the injury, which results in different symptoms after every single trauma; in the population suffering from TBI, every degree and combination of

---

[1] Corresponding Author: Nikolaus Steinhoff, Federal Hospital Lower Austria LK Hochegg, Austria; E-mail: Nikolaus.Steinhoff@hochegg.lknoe.at.

handicap can be found. A common problem for TBI sufferers and their families, as well as for case managers, is to overcome the sudden change in emotions and address how to adapt to the new situation with memories in the body corresponding to the time before the accident. In addition, the attack against normal life, incurred at the moment of the physical trauma, leaves a psychological trauma that might extremely influence recovery if it is not taken into account. TBI results in a profound and very individual change in life. This includes change in personal capacities (mobility, communication, psychology, emotions), change in family and work situation (position, treatment), change of key persons, and change in the financial and social situation (legal, personal status). Despite the wide range of patterns of lesions, TBI cases are quite similar and the question comes up very often of what the changes are and the similarities between those injured and their situation after the trauma. This, and the single steps of adaptation to the new life after the trauma, was the goal of our investigation, following the need to better understand the single steps of reintegration and to ensure the consequence of a high level of rehabilitation after TBI. This article describes the long term and still on-going investigation and presents the vertices of the Re-adaptation Syndrome after TBI.

1. Method

The approach to the research utilized a questionnaire given to TBI injured members of the Austrian Association of TBI, as well as relatives, caregivers and medical and therapeutic professionals, and also members of the European Association of TBI, and concerned persons in other European countries. The first hypothesis concerning the situation after TBI was that there is a resulting feeling emptiness and loneliness, as well as other reasons influencing the emotional situation after TBI, including the fact of long-term rehabilitation, and the correlation to the degree and to the relation to families, caregivers and the attending professionals – also within the National Health Organisations or insurance companies.

The questionnaire consisted of the following points: 1) What is the new situation after TBI, 2) Is there Emptiness and/or Loneliness, 3) Definition, 4) Reasons and 5) Solutions.

2. Results

2.1. Reorientation

The new situation after TBI becomes a strain mostly at key moments, when the injured and the family realize the physical and neuropsychological changes, the change of interaction with the relatives and others, and when the change in emotions and the reality of how previous life was conducted is realized. The burden of change is more important if the person was previously a strong, body-oriented person and had to define himself through a hierarchic system, e.g. military organization.

Those suffering from TBI may experience the feeling of emptiness, inside and out, and have to re-orient themselves with a reduced brain capacity. Emptiness, compared to the situation before and similar to depression, is felt when suddenly, nothing around an individual is satisfying. Equivalent to the adaptation to a normal new situation in life, life after TBI has to be refilled with new contents. Correlating to the individual situation before and after TBI, there is an undulating and varying degree of emptiness.

Reorientation is a condition with different negative and positive influencing factors: 1) UNDERSTANDING the new situation (injured, family and professionals), 2) SOCIETY – change of interests, mobility, communication, 3) TIME – there is a lot of time (thinking, substance abuse), lack of occupation, 4) CONFIDENCE – "it's not working like before", loss of confidence in own emotions and reaction of others, loss of confidence in daily living, 5) ACTIVITY – being frightened, loss of initiative and impulsion, retreat as self protecting reaction, 6) SPIRIT and EMOTION with self-pity, dark ideas and rumination, 7) EXISTENCE – lack of solution and keys to solve problems of new life, 8) HELP – concerning legal, organizational and management solutions. Loneliness is a frequent result of many of these factors. Emptiness leads to loneliness. Loneliness might lead to emptiness, but doesn't have to, and BOTH are part of the Reorientation Syndrome.

Influencing factors can also be the premorbid personal situation, the results of the brain lesion resulting from TBI, family, legal and social situations, resulting quality of life or harassment and secondary syndromes such as burn-out or depression.

This applies to the injured as well as the relatives. Also, relatives describe harassment and burn-out, as well as loneliness and emptiness. They have the same influencing factors, changing life after TBI.

Consequences in life are retreat and isolation, lack of sense of life, depression, Posttraumatic Stress Disorder, aggression and bitterness, substance abuse (alcohol, medication, drugs), loneliness (families separated, others) and suicide.

The old memories persist in the body. There is a need to find new solutions and match these with positive emotions, and to integrate new information and fill the feeling of emptiness with new content.

Adaptation to new situations is normal in daily life. But through central nervous lesions, the capacity of re-adaptation to the new situation after trauma is reduced. The Reorientation Syndrome is unique for each individual through the individual type of lesions and its consequences, the premorbid personality and the very special family and social situation after TBI.

2.2. Two Phases of Reorientation

Phase of Retreat: There is a need to retreat to define solutions for a new situation. It often appears very suddenly, and might be triggered by the problems that are becoming more and more obvious, and lead to fear as well as affect the behavior of surrounding persons.

Phase of Adaptation: Recalibration of "internal norms" leads to new emotional orientation and reduces fear. The acceptance of letting go of pre-trauma body memories and accepting existing situations of internal and external emptiness leads to acquiring new emotions, as well as starting to develop personal responsibilities to result in a reduction of suffering. This process corresponds to a mourning process. Here, finding the keys for new defined problems and defining new contents leads to re-adaptation to the situation after TBI.

Injured patients and their families describe very good support in the immediate time after TBI. However, during long-term care and during the Re-adaptation Syndrome phase, the understanding of the situation by carers, doctors, therapists and case-managers is not enough to support TBI-related persons in a satisfying way.

Approach to support: Through case management the Reorientation Syndrome symptoms can be reduced by paying attention to and addressing the feeling of emptiness. Reducing feelings of emptiness in the phases of re-adaptation corresponds to teamwork and prevention after TBI.

3. Conclusion

In conclusion, one can say that most persons, injured and families alike, feel some sort of emptiness after TBI. Caregivers and case managers are not skilled enough to deal with emptiness, reorientation, the mourning process and the issue of responsibilities resulting from medical, therapeutic and social consequences after TBI.

The general attitude toward those suffering from TBI and their families is still a problem to be solved. The adaptation to the new situation is hindered through handicaps after central nervous lesions such as depression or PTSD. Isolation influences the feelings of emptiness and loneliness and these emotions sometimes mutually interact.

The two phases of the Reorientation Syndrome, Retreat and Adaptation, should be realized early in the rehabilitation process. To get emotionally reoriented takes time and the risk of burn-out for injured/families as well as harassment, exists at all levels. The trainers are to be trained and the cooperation between injured, family, trainers, doctors and NHO respected.

The Reorientation Syndrome becomes individual through the individual type of lesions, the premorbid personality and the very special family and social situation after TBI. It applies to the injured and the families; both have to become reoriented after TBI.

The Reorientation Syndrome is a considerable condition after each TBI that has to be respected in order to understand how to help those injured by TBI and their families. The Reorientation Syndrome also applies to other traumatic situations that strongly affect emotions and lead to a new situation in life.

References

[1] R. Brunner, F. Resch, Dissoziative und somatoforme Störungen. Herpertz-Dahlmann B et al., *Entwicklungspsychiatrie, Biopsychologische Grundlagen und die Entwicklung psychischer Störungen.* Schattauer, Stuttgart, New York (2003)

[2] A.M. Owen et al., Detecting Awareness in the Vegetative State. *Science* 8 September 2006: Vol. 313. no. 5792, p. 1402

[3] R. Korinthenberg, J. Schreck , J. Weser , G. Lehmkuhl, Post-traumatic syndrome after minor head injury cannot be predicted by neurological investigations. *Brain Dev.* 2004 Mar;26(2):113-7.

[4] R.T. Katz, J. DeLuca, Sequelae of minor traumatic brain injury, *Am Fam Physician.* 1992 Nov;46(5):1491-8.

[5] N.D. Zasler, D.I. Katz, R.D. Zafonte, *Brain injury medicine: principles and practice,* Demos, NY, 2007

[6]   H. Paşaoglu, E. Inci Karaküçük, A. Kurtşoy, A. Paşaoğlu, Endogenous neuropeptides in patients with acute traumatic head injury, I: cerebrospinal fluid beta-endorphin levels are increased within 24 hours following the trauma, *Neuropeptides*. 1996 Feb;30(1):47-51.

[7]   G.E. Jaskiw, J.F. Kenny, Limbic cortical injury sustained during adulthood leads to schizophrenia-like syndrome, *Schizophr Res*. 2002 Dec 1;58(2-3):205-12.

Coping with Blast-Related Traumatic Brain Injury in Returning Troops
B.K. Wiederhold (Ed.)
IOS Press, 2011
© 2011 The authors and IOS Press. All rights reserved.

Subject Index

Author Index